Novel Research in Sexuality and Mental Health

Novel Research in Sexuality and Mental Health

Editor

Angel L. Montejo

MDPI • Basel • Beijing • Wuhan • Barcelona • Belgrade • Manchester • Tokyo • Cluj • Tianjin

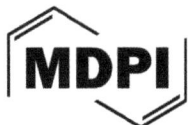

Editor
Angel L. Montejo
International Academy of Sexual Medicine (AISM)
Spain

Editorial Office
MDPI
St. Alban-Anlage 66
4052 Basel, Switzerland

This is a reprint of articles from the Special Issue published online in the open access journal *Journal of Clinical Medicine* (ISSN 2077-0383) (available at: https://www.mdpi.com/journal/jcm/special_issues/research_sexuality_mentalhealth).

For citation purposes, cite each article independently as indicated on the article page online and as indicated below:

LastName, A.A.; LastName, B.B.; LastName, C.C. Article Title. *Journal Name* **Year**, *Article Number*, Page Range.

ISBN 978-3-03943-356-8 (Hbk)
ISBN 978-3-03943-357-5 (PDF)

© 2020 by the authors. Articles in this book are Open Access and distributed under the Creative Commons Attribution (CC BY) license, which allows users to download, copy and build upon published articles, as long as the author and publisher are properly credited, which ensures maximum dissemination and a wider impact of our publications.

The book as a whole is distributed by MDPI under the terms and conditions of the Creative Commons license CC BY-NC-ND.

Contents

About the Editor vii

Angel L. Montejo
Sexuality and Mental Health: The Need for Mutual Development and Research
Reprinted from: *J. Clin. Med.* **2019**, *8*, 1794, doi:10.3390/jcm8111794 1

Armin Soave, Sebastian Laurich, Roland Dahlem, Malte W. Vetterlein, Oliver Engel, Timo Nieder, Peer Briken, Michael Rink, Margit Fisch and Philip Reiss
Negative Self-Perception and Self-Attitude of Sexuality Is a Risk Factor for Patient Dissatisfaction Following Penile Surgery with Small Intestinal Submucosa Grafting for the Treatment of Severe Peyronie's Disease
Reprinted from: *J. Clin. Med.* **2019**, *8*, 1121, doi:10.3390/jcm8081121 5

Charlotte Gibbels, Christopher Sinke, Jonas Kneer, Till Amelung, Sebastian Mohnke, Klaus Michael Beier, Henrik Walter, Kolja Schiltz, Hannah Gerwinn, Alexander Pohl, Jorge Ponseti, Carina Foedisch, Inka Ristow, Martin Walter, Christian Kaergel, Claudia Massau, Boris Schiffer and Tillmann H.C. Kruger
Two Sides of One Coin: A Comparison of Clinical and Neurobiological Characteristics of Convicted and Non-Convicted Pedophilic Child Sexual Offenders
Reprinted from: *J. Clin. Med.* **2019**, *8*, 947, doi:10.3390/jcm8070947 15

Angel L. Montejo, Joemir Becker, Gloria Bueno, Raquel Fernández-Ovejero, María T. Gallego, Nerea González, Adrián Juanes, Laura Montejo, Antonio Pérez-Urdániz, Nieves Prieto and José L. Villegas
Frequency of Sexual Dysfunction in Patients Treated with Desvenlafaxine: A Prospective Naturalistic Study
Reprinted from: *J. Clin. Med.* **2019**, *8*, 719, doi:10.3390/jcm8050719 29

Arne Dekker, Frederike Wenzlaff, Anne Daubmann, Hans O. Pinnschmidt and Peer Briken
(Don't) Look at Me! How the Assumed Consensual or Non-Consensual Distribution Affects Perception and Evaluation of Sexting Images
Reprinted from: *J. Clin. Med.* **2019**, *8*, 706, doi:10.3390/jcm8050706 47

Rodrigo J. Carcedo, Daniel Perlman, Noelia Fernández-Rouco, Fernando Pérez and Diego Hervalejo
Sexual Satisfaction and Mental Health in Prison Inmates
Reprinted from: *J. Clin. Med.* **2019**, *8*, 705, doi:10.3390/jcm8050705 59

Carlos Cuenca-Barrales, Ricardo Ruiz-Villaverde and Alejandro Molina-Leyva
Sexual Distress in Patients with Hidradenitis Suppurativa: A Cross-Sectional Study
Reprinted from: *J. Clin. Med.* **2019**, *8*, 532, doi:10.3390/jcm8040532 77

Marina Letica-Crepulja, Aleksandra Stevanović, Marina Protuđer, Božidar Popović, Darija Salopek-Žiha and Snježana Vondraček
Predictors of Sexual Dysfunction in Veterans with Post-Traumatic Stress Disorder
Reprinted from: *J. Clin. Med.* **2019**, *8*, 432, doi:10.3390/jcm8040432 89

Daniel Turner, Peer Briken and Daniel Schöttle
Sexual Dysfunctions and Their Association with the Dual Control Model of Sexual Response in Men and Women with High-Functioning Autism
Reprinted from: *J. Clin. Med.* **2019**, *8*, 425, doi:10.3390/jcm8040425 107

Noelia Fernández-Rouco, Rodrigo J. Carcedo, Félix López and M. Begoña Orgaz
Mental Health and Proximal Stressors in Transgender Men and Women
Reprinted from: *J. Clin. Med.* **2019**, *8*, 413, doi:10.3390/jcm8030413 . . . . **119**

Meda Veronica Pop and Alina Simona Rusu
Couple Relationship and Parent-Child Relationship Quality: Factors Relevant to Parent-Child Communication on Sexuality in Romania
Reprinted from: *J. Clin. Med.* **2019**, *8*, 386, doi:10.3390/jcm8030386 . . . . **135**

Carlos Llanes, Ana I. Álvarez, M. Teresa Pastor, M. Ángeles Garzón, Nerea González-García and Ángel L. Montejo
Sexual Dysfunction and Quality of Life in Chronic Heroin-Dependent Individuals on Methadone Maintenance Treatment
Reprinted from: *J. Clin. Med.* **2019**, *8*, 321, doi:10.3390/jcm8030321 . . . . **149**

Jannis Engel, Maria Veit, Christopher Sinke, Ivo Heitland, Jonas Kneer, Thomas Hillemacher, Uwe Hartmann and Tillmann H.C. Kruger
Same Same but Different: A Clinical Characterization of Men with Hypersexual Disorder in the Sex@Brain Study
Reprinted from: *J. Clin. Med.* **2019**, *8*, 157, doi:10.3390/jcm8020157 . . . . **161**

Yanira Santana, Angel L. Montejo, Javier Martín, Ginés LLorca, Gloria Bueno and Juan Luis Blázquez
Understanding the Mechanism of Antidepressant-Related Sexual Dysfunction: Inhibition of Tyrosine Hydroxylase in Dopaminergic Neurons after Treatment with Paroxetine but Not with Agomelatine in Male Rats
Reprinted from: *J. Clin. Med.* **2019**, *8*, 133, doi:10.3390/jcm8020133 . . . . **179**

Aleksandra Diana Dwulit and Piotr Rzymski
The Potential Associations of Pornography Use with Sexual Dysfunctions: An Integrative Literature Review of Observational Studies
Reprinted from: *J. Clin. Med.* **2019**, *8*, 914, doi:10.3390/jcm8070914 . . . . **197**

Nerea M. Casado-Espada, Rubén de Alarcón, Javier I. de la Iglesia-Larrad, Berta Bote-Bonaechea and Ángel L. Montejo
Hormonal Contraceptives, Female Sexual Dysfunction, and Managing Strategies: A Review
Reprinted from: *J. Clin. Med.* **2019**, *8*, 908, doi:10.3390/jcm8060908 . . . . **213**

Safiye Tozdan, Peer Briken and Arne Dekker
Uncovering Female Child Sexual Offenders—Needs and Challenges for Practice and Research
Reprinted from: *J. Clin. Med.* **2019**, *8*, 401, doi:10.3390/jcm8030401 . . . . **235**

Heiko Graf, Kathrin Malejko, Coraline Danielle Metzger, Martin Walter, Georg Grön and Birgit Abler
Serotonergic, Dopaminergic, and Noradrenergic Modulation of Erotic Stimulus Processing in the Male Human Brain
Reprinted from: *J. Clin. Med.* **2019**, *8*, 363, doi:10.3390/jcm8030363 . . . . **247**

Rubén de Alarcón, Javier I. de la Iglesia, Nerea M. Casado and Angel L. Montejo
Online Porn Addiction: What We Know and What We Don't—A Systematic Review
Reprinted from: *J. Clin. Med.* **2019**, *8*, 91, doi:10.3390/jcm8010091 . . . . **261**

About the Editor

Angel L. Montejo M.D. Ph.D. is a full professor of Psychiatry at the University of Salamanca, head of Community Psychiatry at the University Hospital and head of the Neuroscience Group of the Biomedical Research Institute of Salamanca (IBSAL), Spain. Additionally, he is a Scientific Director of the Spanish Association of Sexuality and Mental Health and former President of the Castellano-Leonesa Association of Psychiatry. He developed the PRSexDQ-Salsex Questionnaire (Psychotropic–Related Sexual Dysfunction Questionnaire (2000)) validated to measure sexual dysfunction related to depression and schizophrenia and translated into English, French, German, Italian, Greek, Polish, Portuguese, Danish, Chinese and Japanese. Professor Montejo earned his medical degree and PhD in Medicine and Surgery at the University of Salamanca, and he completed training in Psychiatry at Maryland (USA), Maudsley Hospital (London), Karolinska Institute (Stockholm), University of Columbia (New York), Massachusetts Gen Hospital (Boston) and others. His main research interests are psychopharmacology, sexuality and psychiatry, psychotropic-related sexual dysfunctions, and the safety and tolerability of psychotropic compounds, such as iatrogenic hyperprolactinaemia. He is highly involved with clinical trials on the development of new compounds for mental diseases such as depression, schizophrenia, anxiety, mild cognitive impairment and dementia. He has been involved as Principal Investigator in 12 competitive public research projects and in 95 international clinical trials about different compounds in Phase I; II; III and IV. Additionally, his research team successfully passed an FDA Inspection on a major depression clinical trial on December 2018. Dr Montejo has participated in several steering and advisory committees in relation to the design of clinical trials and scientific advice on new products from pharmaceutical companies such as Boehringer Ingelheim (duloxetine); Lundbeck (escitalopram); Servier (Agomelatine), Lilly (olanzapine); Astra Zeneca (quetiapine); Bristol Myers Squib (aripiprazole) and Cassen Recordati (cariprazine). He has published more than 200 scientific national and international papers, receiving more than 5400 citations, as well as seven books. Additionally, he is a member of several national and international scientific associations and he participates in the editorial committee of several relevant psychiatric journals, serving as a guest editor of Frontiers in Neurosciences and Journal of Clinical Medicine. His publications, Impact Factor and metrics can be found at: https://scholar.google.es/citations?user=g7wO1tUAAAAJ&hl=es https://www.researchgate.net/profile/Angel_Montejo.

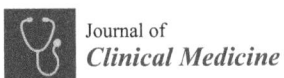

Editorial

Sexuality and Mental Health: The Need for Mutual Development and Research

Angel L. Montejo

University of Salamanca, Psychiatry Service, Clinical Hospital, Faculty of Nursing and Institute of Biomedical Research of Salamanca (IBSAL), Avenue of Donantes de Sangre SN, 37007 Salamanca, Spain; amontejo@usal.es; Tel.: +34-639754620

Received: 21 October 2019; Accepted: 22 October 2019; Published: 26 October 2019

Abstract: Research in the field of sexuality has shown growing scientific development in recent years, although there's a lack of well-trained professionals who could contribute to increasing its benefits. Sexuality continues to be a taboo with different interpretations and difficult delimitation of either normal or pathological behavior. More resources are needed for the understanding of new emerging pathologies, and to increase the research in new models of sexual behavior. All psychiatric diseases include symptoms affecting sexual life, such as impaired desire, arousal, or sexual satisfaction that need to be properly addressed. Health providers and prescribers must detect and prevent iatrogenic sexual dysfunction that can highly deteriorate a patient's sexual life and satisfaction, leading to frequent drop-outs of medication. Approaching and researching aspects of sexual intimacy, life desires, frustrations, and fears undoubtedly constitutes the best mental health care.

Keywords: sexuality; mental health; research; sexual dysfunction

---

Sexuality, understood as a drive and an inherent need for human beings, has unquestionably been part of the occupations and concerns of psychiatrists from the beginning of the century. Not in vain, psychoanalysts theorized about the importance of sexual repression as the origin of a great number of mental diseases. Sexual drive, originally called libido, seemed to be the nucleus of life and its repression or deficiencies a way towards mental suffering. The concept obviously must be extended towards eroticism in a broader sense, not always necessarily coital, and to satisfaction of physical pleasure and intimacy. Over the years, following growth in scientific research, it has become essential to invest increasing interest and more research resources to contribute to the theoretical maxims that could empirically explain the secrets of such important drives.

Fortunately, research in the field of sexuality has shown growing scientific development, leading to the greater interest of researchers [1–8]. The emergence of an increasing number of specific journals focusing on some either large or small sexual issues are symptomatic of our contemporary society's concerns. The great and unexpected role of sexual abuse in the origin or development of some mental illnesses and the boundaries between normal and pathological sexuality, without having so far found satisfactory agreement in this sense, have constituted some of the areas of greatest interest.

However, one of the biggest limitations for the generalization of adequate sexual health is the lack of well-trained professionals who could contribute to increasing its benefits. The training of mental health providers focusing in sexology has not developed accordingly to accompany the population's needs. Sexuality continues to be a taboo, and professionals dealing with its research and treatment remain scarce, even with a large heterogeneous background. The widespread access to continuous, multiple, and often unhealthy sexual content without any ethical filter or prior preparation in our young people has been a new challenge in addressing their understanding. The different interpretations of such a variable concept leads to an extremely difficult delimitation of either normal or pathological sexuality. The easy to use and generalized online access has popularized sexual performance so much that some new unexpected phenomena have recently emerged, such as online shared group rapes or the increased number of "unlinked sexual seekers" looking for some new variate, intense, and prolonged sexual experiences, as well as some novel shocking sensations such as chemsex. More resources are needed to cope with the appearance of these new emerging pathologies, and to increase the research in these new models of sexual behavior. Unfortunately, in most parts of the world, basic training in sexology has not been sufficiently developed as a fundamental part of the scientific growth of our mental health professionals. Sexuality is commonly interpreted as a minor discipline that unfortunately is not included as a part of the basic training to provide adequate support for normal subjects and mental health patients.

It is well known that all psychiatric diseases include some variations in sexual symptoms and difficulties with highly different individual sexual meanings and concerns. Depression, bipolar disorder, anxiety disorders, or even psychosis include symptoms affecting sexual life, such as impaired desire, arousal, or sexual satisfaction that inevitably need to be properly identified and addressed. There are no sexless human beings, and neither are our patients sexless, even if they do not carry out an active sex life.

As a main classification instrument today, the Diagnostic and Statistical Manual of Mental Disorders DSM-5 recognizes certain sexual conditions to which it grants diagnostic criteria, although not without some controversy. It would be very unfortunate if this would be the only approach to bringing the average professional closer to the sexual life and intimacy needs of their patients. These days, hypoactive sexual desire or even aversion to sex (paradoxically frequently iatrogenic after the prescription of a chronic use of serotonergic antidepressants) have reached almost epidemic proportions that remain unnoticed and understudied. Additionally, there is a lack of economic resource investment in their research by the pharmaceutical companies themselves or by public health systems. Generally, a great number of antidepressant prescribers are poorly motivated to detect and prevent iatrogenic sexual dysfunction that can highly deteriorate the patient's sexual life and satisfaction, leading to subsequent emotional deprivation of all those who must endure it in the medium and long term, as serotonergic antidepressants (SSRIs) remain the most prescribed in the Western world.

Taking into account the patients with psychosis, there may be some clinicians who consider that it would be better not to investigate the sexual life of their patients, as this could worsen psychotic symptoms, or simply interpret that the information obtained would be unreliable. Many others may avoid it, because in this way they are not forced to face the side effects of some prescribed antipsychotics that intensely block the dopamine activity and deteriorate sexual functioning. Let us remember that sexuality includes the creation of links and intimacy with another person, which helps patients to fight against the negative symptoms of the disease. Perhaps some clinicians consider that sexual relationships in psychiatric female patients with chronic psychosis mainly involves a risk of pregnancy and the appearance of sexually transmitted diseases. Therefore, implicitly, the absence of any interview about their sexual life and interpersonal relationships, including the needs of intimacy and maternity plans, promotes a silent sterilization. That is, the prescription of an antipsychotic that increases prolactin blood levels is inevitably linked to anovulation and sterility. Can patients then decide on their motherhood? Obviously not, because often those who prescribe these antipsychotics have inappropriately decided for their patients without exchanging a single comment or adequate reflection about their family life project. On the other hand, some HIV-positive patients are severely mentally ill and use prostitution as the only means of obtaining sexual pleasure and intimacy. Most of these patients have limited stable sexual relationships or sex partners, and many of them have none except masturbation, duplicating the general population rates of prostitution and the consequent increased risks of HIV and sexually transmitted diseases. Perhaps some may think that these are issues outside the mental health professional's goal and that they would be much better addressed by other health providers; however, unfortunately, these patients go to a general practitioner infrequently, and rarely establish lasting and close relationships with them. In addition, frequent drop-outs of medication have been reported due to iatrogenic sexual dysfunction associated with the use of hyperprolactinemic antipsychotics, which remains widely underestimated by psychiatrists despite its striking clinical implications in the short, medium, and long term. The abrupt or progressive decline in desire, excitatory, and/or orgasmic function compromises the compliance and makes long-term treatment uncertain in some specific groups, such as young male patients. The emphatic approach to this adverse event by clinicians, through adequate sensitization and training, would prevent catastrophic consequences compromising the clinical evolution of patients with psychosis and, moreover, improve the doctor–patient relationship. Approaching the aspects of intimacy, life desires, frustrations, and fears undoubtedly constitutes real mental health care. As a sample of this, in a recent survey on sexual health in Spain [9] a large number of people were interviewed about their motivation for sexual intercourse. Surprisingly, only a few of them selected sexual pleasure as a fundamental reason (mostly males) or procreation (mostly women). The vast majority pointed out that the main reason was the search for emotional intimacy or to satisfy the need to love and be loved. However, sexual pleasure is once again only a small part of love.

For many of us, it is never too late to regain the study and approach to sexuality and its concerns as something enriching in mental health, and of course in the global existence of our patients. We may not need to be sexologists but recovering sexuality as a basic aspect of mental health must become one of our most current aims. The way forward must be through the incorporation of sexuality as an inseparable part of the human being and its research as an essential instrument in the holistic vision of the existence of our patients.

Conflicts of Interest: The author declares no conflict of interest. Dr. Montejo has received consultancy fees or honoraria/research grants in the last 5 years from Eli Lilly, Forum Pharmaceuticals, Rovi, Servier, Lundbeck, Otsuka, Janssen Cilag, Pfizer, Roche, Instituto de Salud Carlos III, and the Junta de Castilla y León.

References

1. Montejo, A.L.; Montejo, L.; Baldwin, D.S. The impact of severe mental disorders andpsychotropic medications on sexual health and its implications for clinical management. *World Psychiatry* **2018**, *17*, 3–11. [CrossRef] [PubMed]
2. Montejo, A.L.; Prieto, N.; de Alarcón, R.; Casado-Espada, N.; de la Iglesia, J.; Montejo, L. Management Strategies for Antidepressant-Related Sexual Dysfunction: A Clinical Approach. *J. Clin. Med.* **2019**, *7*, 1640. [CrossRef] [PubMed]
3. Clayton, A.H.; Valladares Juarez, E.M. Female Sexual Dysfunction. *Med. Clin. N. Am.* **2019**, *103*, 681–698. [CrossRef] [PubMed]
4. Clayton, A.H.; Kingsberg, S.A.; Goldstein, I. Evaluation and Management of Hypoactive Sexual Desire Disorder. *Sex Med.* **2018**, *6*, 59–74. [CrossRef] [PubMed]
5. Blycker, G.R.; Potenza, M.N. A mindful model of sexual health: A review and implications of the model for the treatment of individuals with compulsive sexual behavior disorder. *J. Behav. Addict.* **2018**, *7*, 917–929. [CrossRef] [PubMed]
6. Parish, S.J.; Hahn, S.R.; Goldstein, S.W.; Giraldi, A.; Kingsberg, S.A.; Larkin, L.; Minkin, M.J.; Brown, V.; Christiansen, K.; Hartzell-Cushanick, R.; et al. The International Society for the Study of Women's Sexual Health Process of Care for the Identification of Sexual Concerns and Problems in Women. *Mayo Clin. Proc.* **2019**, *94*, 842–856. [CrossRef] [PubMed]
7. De Alarcón, R.; de la Iglesia, J.I.; Casado, N.M.; Montejo, A.L. Online Porn Addiction: What We Know and What We Don't-A Systematic Review. *J. Clin. Med.* **2019**, *8*, 91. [CrossRef] [PubMed]
8. Montejo, A.L.; Calama, J.; Rico-Villademoros, F.; Montejo, L.; González-García, N.; Pérez, J.; SALSEX Working Study Group. A Real-World Study on Antidepressant-Associated Sexual Dysfunction in 2144 Outpatients: The SALSEX I Study. *Arch. Sex Behav.* **2019**, *48*, 923–933. [CrossRef] [PubMed]
9. Resultados de la Encuesta Nacional de Salud Sexual 2009. Available online: https://www.ugr.es/~fjjrios/pdf/mi-EncuestaNacionalSaludSexual2009.pdf (accessed on 20 October 2019).

© 2019 by the author. Licensee MDPI, Basel, Switzerland. This article is an open access article distributed under the terms and conditions of the Creative Commons Attribution (CC BY) license (http://creativecommons.org/licenses/by/4.0/).

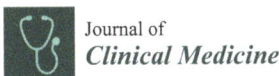

Article

Negative Self-Perception and Self-Attitude of Sexuality Is a Risk Factor for Patient Dissatisfaction Following Penile Surgery with Small Intestinal Submucosa Grafting for the Treatment of Severe Peyronie's Disease

Armin Soave [1,†,‡], Sebastian Laurich [1,†], Roland Dahlem [1,‡], Malte W. Vetterlein [1], Oliver Engel [1], Timo O. Nieder [2], Peer Briken [2], Michael Rink [1], Margit Fisch [1] and Philip Reiss [1,*]

[1] Department of Urology, University Medical Center Hamburg-Eppendorf, 20246 Hamburg, Germany
[2] Institute for Sex Research, Sexual Medicine and Forensic Psychiatry,
University Medical Center Hamburg-Eppendorf, 20246 Hamburg, Germany
* Correspondence: p.reiss@uke.de; Tel.: +49-40-7410-53442; Fax: +49-40-7410-52444
† These authors contributed equally to this work.
‡ Armin Soave, Roland Dahlem are consultants of Boston Scientific.

Received: 31 May 2019; Accepted: 24 July 2019; Published: 28 July 2019

Abstract: Objective: To assess patient satisfaction with surgical outcome, body related self-perceptions, self-attitudes of sexuality, and health related quality of life after penile surgery with small intestinal submucosa (SIS) grafting for the treatment of severe Peyronie's disease (PD). Material and methods: This retrospective study included 82 patients, who were treated with SIS grafting for severe PD between 2009 and 2013 at the University Medical Center Hamburg-Eppendorf. Patients were asked to complete standardized questionnaires including the International Index of Erectile Function Erectile Function domain (IIEF-EF), Short-Form (SF)-8 Health Survey, and Frankfurt Body Concept Scale-Sexuality (FKKS-SEX). Results: Follow-up was available in 58 (69.9%) patients. SIS grafting resulted in subjective straightening of the penis in 53 (91.3%) patients. After a mean follow-up of 28.9 ± 16.5 months, 24 (41.4%) patients were satisfied or very satisfied with surgical outcome. Postoperatively, the mean FKKS-SEX was 23.5 ± 5.9. In total, 36 (62.1%), 18 (31%), and four (6.9%) patients had FKKS-SEX scores corresponding to positive, neutral, and negative self-perception and self-attitude of sexuality, respectively. The mean postoperative SF-8 was 15.2 ± 6.4. Compared to the mean for German controls, patients achieved lower mean scores in the domains social functioning (50.4 ± 7.1), mental health (49.5 ± 9.2), and emotional roles (48.5 ± 6.8). Subjective shortening of the penis (Odds ratio (OR): 2.0), negative body related self-perceptions, and self-attitudes of sexuality (OR: 3.6) as well as IIEF-EF score (OR: 0.9) were risk factors for patient dissatisfaction (p-values ≤ 0.02). Conclusion: A relevant number of patients is not satisfied with surgical outcome after SIS grafting for the treatment of severe PD. Subjective shortening of the penis, negative body related self-perceptions, and self-attitudes of sexuality as well as IIEF-EF score were risk factors for patient dissatisfaction.

Keywords: peyronie's disease; penile induration; sexuality; patient satisfaction

1. Introduction

Peyronie's disease (PD) is a chronic connective tissue disorder of the tunica albuginea of the corpora cavernosa of the penis, and may cause relevant penile pain, penile plaque formation, and loss of penile length, as well as deformity and curvature of the penis [1]. As a consequence, PD may severely impair sexual activity and emotional wellbeing [2]. Up to 54% and 48% of PD patients present with erectile dysfunction (ED) [3] and depression [4], respectively, emphasizing the complexity of symptoms which patients may be affected by.

Surgical treatment is performed to correct penile deformity and penile curvature, with the aim to enable patients to have sexual intercourse. This represents the standard therapy in the stable phase of severe PD [5]. Various surgical procedures have been described, including tunical plication and grafting techniques [6,7]. Currently, xenogenic small intestinal submucosa (SIS) represents one of the most commonly used and widely established grafts for penile surgery in PD patients [5,7]. To date, there have been few published studies on SIS grafting for PD, and these studies have primarily focused on surgical outcome and complications [8–11], whereas patient reported treatment satisfaction has been considered in the minority of studies [12–16]. In addition, patient self-perceptions and attitudes of sexuality following SIS grafting have not been investigated so far.

Thus, the aim of the present study was to analyze body related self-perceptions and self-attitudes of sexuality as well as health-related quality of life following penile surgery with SIS grafting for severe PD, and to identify risk factors for patient dissatisfaction.

2. Patients and Methods

2.1. Patients

We retrospectively collected data of 82 patients with severe PD, who were treated with SIS grafting between 2009 and 2013 at the University Medical Center Hamburg-Eppendorf. Preoperative evaluation included an in-depth history of onset and duration of PD-specific symptoms, prior PD-specific treatment and general medical history. Auto-photographic documentation determined degree, direction, shape, and severity of penile curvature, as described in detail previously [17]. Physical examination and penile ultra-sonography determined location, number, and size of plaques of the tunica albuginea of the penis. Penile length was measured from suprapubic skin to distal glans in the stretched flaccid penis, as described previously [18]. Color duplex Doppler ultra-sonography (CDDU) of the penis combined with intracavernous injection of 20 µg Prostavasin was performed preoperatively according to established standard operating procedures [19].

2.2. Patient Reported Outcome Measure

Patient reported outcomes were assessed using a standardized questionnaire. Firstly, we employed several validated patient reported outcome measures. The validated International Index of Erectile Function Erectile Function domain (IIEF-EF) evaluated erectile function. No ED corresponded to an IIEF-EF score of 26–30, mild ED to a score of 22–25, mild to moderate ED to a score of 17–21, moderate ED to a score of 11–16, and severe ED to a score of 6–10. Health related quality of life was assessed with the validated Short-Form (SF)-8 Health Survey, consisting of eight dimensions including social functioning, mental health, emotional roles, role physical, bodily pain, general health, vitality, and physical functioning [20]. SF-8 physical component score and SF-8 mental component score were calculated weighting each SF-8 item using the norm-based scoring method as described previously [21]. The mean scores in the 8 dimensions were compared to the mean for German controls [22]. A score of 50 is the mean for the German general population, a higher score indicates increased quality of life. Body related self-perceptions and self-attitudes of sexuality were assessed with the Frankfurt Body Concept Scale-Subscale Sexuality (FKKS-SEX), consisting of eight items with six answering options, respectively. The subscale is intended to measure how satisfied patients are with their sexuality, how attractive they consider themselves to potential sexual partners, and how they deal with sexual intimacy. The maximum FKKS-SEX score is 36, the minimum six; a score of 6–18, 19–23 and 24–36 is indicating a negative, neutral, and positive self-perception and self-attitude of sexuality, respectively [23]. Secondly, we included non-validated questions on patient satisfaction, penile paresthesia, and sexual activity. Non-validated questions were assessed using a five-point Likert-scale.

2.3. Follow-Up

Patients were seen at various time points after surgery at the outpatient clinic of our institution and received the standardized questionnaire. In addition, physical examination, penile ultra-sonography, penile length measurement, and CDDU of the penis were performed. There was no preoperative evaluation of health-related quality of life and no preoperative evaluation of self-perception and self-attitude of sexuality. Missing baseline data is denoted in the respective tables of the results section of the manuscript.

2.4. Surgical Procedure and Postoperative Management

Generally, SIS grafting was performed under general anesthesia as described in detail previously [5]. In brief, a circumcision was performed, followed by complete de-gloving of the penis and careful exposure of the dorsal neurovascular bundle. Then, an artificial erection was achieved with intracavernous injection of sodium chloride to identify the maximum convexity of the penile curvature. A transverse incision of the tunica and/or the plaque was performed at the maximum convexity, and the lateral margins of the incision were extended in a Y-formed shape. The length of the Y-shape was chosen depending on the degree of the lateral penile curvature. The size of the SIS graft was chosen depending on the size of the resulting defect of the tunica albuginea of the corpora cavernosa. The Biodesign® four-layer SIS (Cook Medical LLC, Bloomington, IN, USA) was transplanted to the defect and fixed to the tunica albuginea with 3-0 monofil continuous sutures. Then, an artificial erection was provoked again to control for complete straightening of the penis. In cases of remaining slight curvature, a tunical plication was performed according to Yachia's technique [24] at the discretion of the surgeon. After closure of Buck's fascia and skin, a suprapubic catheter was placed, and a compression bandage was put on the penis. Roland Dahlem, Margit Fisch, and Oliver Engel performed all surgical procedures.

Generally, the compression bandage and suprapubic catheter were removed on postoperative day five, and patients were discharged. Patients were advised to perform penile rehabilitation with daily stretching of the penis using a vacuum device plus daily intake of phosphodiesterase-5 inhibitors. Patients were not allowed to have sexual intercourse for six weeks postoperatively.

2.5. Statistical Analysis

All analyses were performed with SPSS 20 (SPSS Inc., IBM Corp., Armonk, NY, USA). All tests were two-sided and a $p < 0.05$ was set to be statistically significant. Differences between continuous variables in one group were assessed using the T-test. Differences between categorical variables were assessed with the Chi square test. Uni-variable binary logistic regression analysis was employed to identify risk factors for patient dissatisfaction. For uni-variable binary logistic regression analysis, patients were grouped as "satisfied" (patients, who responded that they were "satisfied" or "very satisfied" with surgical outcome) and "dissatisfied" (patients, who responded "undecided", "dissatisfied", or "very dissatisfied" with surgical outcome).

3. Results

3.1. Patient Characteristics

Table 1 presents clinical features of the patients. Hypertension, Morbus Dupuytren, and prostatic hyperplasia were the most common comorbidities in 25 (30.5%), 15 (18.3%), and nine (11%) patients, respectively. In total, 11 (13.4%) patients reported previous penile trauma. The mean degree of penile curvature was 65°, and the majority of patients reported dorsal and lateral-left curvature in 51 (62.2%) and 11 (13.4%) patients, respectively.

Table 1. Clinical characteristics of 82 patients treated with small intestinal submucosa grafting for Peyronie's disease.

	All ($n = 82$)
Age (years; mean (95% CI))	56.9 (55.5–58.5)
Body mass index (mean (95% CI)) 6 (7.3%) patients missing	26.6 (25.7–27.4)
Comorbidities (n; %)	
Hypertension	25 (30.5)
Diabetes	7 (8.5)
Depression	5 (6.1)
Morbus Dupuytren	15 (18.3)
Morbus Ledderhose	1 (1.2)
Prostatic hyperplasia	9 (11.0)
Penile trauma	11 (13.4)
Smoking status (n; %)	
Active	45 (54.9)
No	17 (20.7)
Unknown	20 (24.4)
Penile curvature (degree; mean, (95% CI)) 18 (22%) patients missing	64.8 (59.1–70.5)
Direction of penile curvature (n; %)	
Ventral	3 (3.7)
Dorsal	51 (62.2)
Lateral left	11 (13.4)
Lateral right	6 (7.3)
Plaque size (cm; mean, (95% CI)) 44 (53.7%) patients missing	2.9 (1.7–4.2)
Duration of PD-specific symptoms (days; mean (95% CI)) 1 (1.2%) patient missing	343.8 (217.7–469.8)
Previous PD-specific treatments (n; %)	
Potaba	26 (41.3)
Vitamine E	13 (20.6)
Steroids	1 (1.6)
Interferon	1 (1.6)
Verapamil	1 (1.6)
ESWT	1 (1.6)
None	24 (38.1)
Unknown	19 (23.2)
Preoperative Resistance index as measured by CDDU (mean (95% CI)) 29 (35.4%) patients missing	0.87 (0.82–0.93)

Abbreviations: CDDU = Color duplex Doppler ultra-sonography; CI = Confidence interval; ESWT = extracorporal shock wave therapy; PD = Peyronie's disease.

3.2. Patient Reported Outcomes

Follow-up was available in 58 (69.9%) patients. After a mean follow-up of 28.9 ± 16.5 months, complete straightening of the penis was achieved in 53 (91.3%) patients, while five (8.7%) patients reported insufficient straightening. Overall, 41 (70.7%) patients reported paresthesia of the penis, corresponding to hypoesthesia and hyperesthesia in 34 (82.9%) and seven (17.1%) patients, respectively. Penile paresthesia was not bothering in 23 (56.1%) patients. In total, 56 (96.6%) patients reported subjective shortening of the penis. There was no significant difference in measured penile length preoperatively and postoperatively ($p = 0.9$). Postoperatively, 36 (62.1%) patients reported subjective deterioration of erectile function. According to the IIEF-EF score, postoperatively, 22 (37.9%) and

13 (22.4%) patients had severe and moderate ED, respectively, compared to 11 (19.0%) and seven (12.1%) patients with severe and moderate ED preoperatively ($p = 0.041$; Table 2).

Table 2. Change in preoperative and postoperative erectile function in 58 patients treated with small intestinal submucosa grafting for Peyronie's disease.

	Preoperative	Postoperative	Difference	p-Value
IIEF-EF score (mean (95% CI))	12.2 (8.4–15.9) 29 (50%) patients missing	14.5 (12.2–16.9)	2.0 (−4.5–8.5)	0.13 *
Erectile dysfunction according to IIEF-EF (n; %)				
Severe	11 (19.0)	22 (37.9)		
Moderate	7 (12.1)	13 (22.4)		0.041 #
Mild to moderate	4 (6.9)	6 (10.3)		
Mild	3 (5.2)	7 (12.1)		
No	2 (3.4)	10 (17.2)		
Missing	29 (50.0)	0 (0)		

* Paired samples T-test. # Chi square test. Abbreviations: CI = Confidence interval; IIEF-EF = international index of erectile function erectile function domain.

The mean postoperative FKKS-SEX was 23.5 ± 5.9, which corresponds to neutral to positive self-perception and self-attitude of sexuality. In total, 36 (62.1%), 18 (31%), and four (6.9%) patients had FKKS-SEX scores corresponding to positive, neutral, and negative self-perception and self-attitude of sexuality, respectively. The mean postoperative SF-8 was 15.2 ± 6.4. Compared to the mean for German controls, patients achieved lower mean scores in the domains social functioning (50.4 ± 7.1), mental health (49.5 ± 9.2), and emotional roles (48.5 ± 6.8); higher mean scores in the domains role physical (50.0 ± 6.8), bodily pain (54.5 ± 9.1), general health (51.5 ± 7.2), and vitality (51.5 ± 8.1); and equivalent mean scores in the domain physical functioning (49.0 ± 8.2).

3.3. Patient Satisfaction

In total, 24 (41.4%) patients were satisfied or very satisfied with surgical outcome, while 26 (44.8%) patients were dissatisfied or very dissatisfied. Altogether, eight (13.8%) patients were undecided regarding satisfaction with surgical outcome.

In total, 26 (44.8%) of 58 patients with postoperative subjective shortening of the penis were dissatisfied or very dissatisfied with surgical outcome. Overall, 17 (77.3%) patients of 22 patients with severe postoperative ED were dissatisfied or very dissatisfied with surgical outcome. In total, four (100%) patients with low body related self-perceptions and self-attitudes of sexuality were dissatisfied or very dissatisfied with surgical outcome. Of the 26 patients, who were dissatisfied or very dissatisfied with surgical outcome, 19 (73.1%), 19 (73.1%), and four (15.4%) patients had subjective shortening of the penis, subjective deterioration of erectile function, and low body related self-perceptions and self-attitudes of sexuality, respectively.

In uni-variable logistic regression analysis, subjective shortening of the penis, negative body related self-perceptions and self-attitudes of sexuality as well as IIEF-EF score were risk factors for patient dissatisfaction (p-values ≤ 0.02; Table 3).

Table 3. Uni-variable logistic regression of subjective penile shortening, subjective reduced erectile function, negative body related self-perceptions and self-attitudes of sexuality, International Index of Erectile Function Erectile Function domain (IIEF-EF) and Short-Form (SF)-8 score predicting patient dissatisfaction with surgical outcome in 58 patients treated with small intestinal submucosa grafting for Peyronie's disease.

	Odds Ratio	95% CI	p-Value
Subjective loss of penile length	2.026	1.152–3.563	0.014
Subjective reduced erectile function	2.154	0.507–9.147	0.298
Negative body related self-perceptions and self-attitudes of sexuality	3.632	1.231–10.718	0.020
IIEF-EF score	0.870	0.805–0.940	<0.001
SF-8 physical component score	0.963	0.898–1.034	0.299
SF-8 mental component score	0.971	0.920–1.026	0.298

Abbreviations: CI = Confidence interval; IIEF-EF = International index of erectile function erectile function domain; SF-8 = Short-Form-8 Health Survey.

4. Discussion

We found that 41% of patients were satisfied, whereas almost 45% of patients were not satisfied with outcome following surgery, although SIS grafting resulted in complete straightening of the penis in more than 90% of patients. Previously, others have reported inconsistent findings on patient satisfaction with surgical outcome following SIS grafting. Some studies found high satisfaction rates of 82–89% [13–16], while Chung et al. reported that more than 65% of patients were not satisfied with surgical outcome [12]. Variable findings among studies regarding patient satisfaction with surgical outcome may be due to differences in patient characteristics, follow-up, study design, and methods. For example, the prospective study by Sayedahmed et al. included 43 patients, who were recruited from two centers over a time period of eight years. Kovac et al. and Chung et al. included 36 and 46 patients, respectively, who were recruited over a time period of six years and also received dermal and synthetic grafts [12] or dermal and cadaveric pericardial grafts [13], which may render comparison of results difficult. Morgado et al. focused on patient satisfaction with sex life after surgery [16]. Other studies reported less subjective penile shortening in 5–71% of patients [12–16], compared to almost 97% of patients in the present study. Importantly, we could demonstrate that subjective shortening of the penis was a risk factor for patient dissatisfaction, which therefore could be a reason for the observed differences in patient satisfaction. In addition, the present study included a higher proportion of patients with moderate and severe preoperative ED, compared to 7–10% preoperative ED in previous studies [14,15]. It is well established that ED may deteriorate after SIS grafting [5]. We could demonstrate that subjective worsening of erectile function was not a risk factor for patient dissatisfaction. However, higher IIEF-EF postoperative scores significantly reduced the risk of dissatisfaction. Moreover, other studies evaluated patient satisfaction with 5-point scales [12], 4-answering possibilities [15], 3-answering possibilities [13], a modified Erectile Dysfunction Inventory of Treatment Satisfaction [16], or did not report in detail on how patient satisfaction was measured [14], which may contribute to variable results. Finally, we found a higher proportion of patients with penile paresthesia following SIS grafting, compared to previous reports [12–16]. These differences may rely on variable evaluation of penile sensibility among different studies. In addition, circumcision was performed in all patients in the present study and might have contributed to penile paresthesia. Moreover, the type of graft may play a role, although Kovac et al. did not report relevant differences in penile hypoesthesia among patients, who received SIS grafts, dermal grafts or Tutoplast grafts [13]. Finally, the dissection of the dorsal pedicle may also influence sensory changes. The majority of patients in the present study reported that penile paresthesia was not bothering. However, we cannot exclude that this may have contributed to overall dissatisfaction. In the present study, circumcision was performed in all patients during penile surgery, although a case series questioned its need in patients undergoing penile surgery for PD [25]. Although circumcision is in general considered a safe procedure, it may have adverse effects, e.g., hypoesthesia of the glans, as well as negative psychological consequences [26]. Thus, we cannot exclude that circumcision may have added to patient dissatisfaction.

For the first time, the present study incorporated patients' body related self-perceptions and self-attitudes of sexuality, which was assessed with validated FKKS-SEX. Thus far, FKKS-SEX was primarily used in patients with psychiatric disorders, e.g., depression and addiction [23]. We found that the majority of patients had a positive or neutral self-perception and self-attitude of sexuality. Importantly, negative self-perception and self-attitude of sexuality was a risk factor for patient dissatisfaction. Thus, FKKS-SEX may represent a promising tool to preoperatively identify patients, who are at risk for dissatisfaction. At best, it may be helpful in detecting patients with relevant underlying psychological conditions prior surgery. Then, these patients may benefit from rigorous sexological evaluation, support, or intervention in the preoperative and postoperative setting. We used the validated SF-8 to assess health related quality of life, and found that patients had lower social functioning, mental health, and emotional roles compared to the mean for German controls, although neither SF-8 physical component score nor SF-8 mental component score were risk factors for patient dissatisfaction with surgical outcome. Thus far, SF-8 has mainly been used to evaluate patients with other chronic illness, e.g., migraine, depression, and diabetes [20]. Our findings indicate that this questionnaire may be useful in PD patients treated with SIS grafting. However, further prospective studies are needed to confirm the potential of FKKS-SEX and SF-8 in outcome measurement in these patients; and to analyze the possibility of identifying patients with underlying psychological conditions, who may benefit from sexological support or intervention.

We found considerable discrepancy between patients' complaints and objective outcome. First of all, almost 97% of patients reported loss of penile length, whereas measurement revealed no significant change between preoperative and postoperative penile length. This corresponds to findings of other authors, who found that 71% of patients reported subjective loss of penile length, whereas measurement revealed penile shortening in 14% of patients [15]. These findings highlight the importance of thorough preoperative counseling, with the aim to lower patients' unrealistic expectations of SIS grafting, such as restoration of penile length as it was prior disease onset. Second, 62% of patients reported subjective worsening of erectile function. Indeed, postoperatively, more patients reported severe and moderate ED. This corresponds to findings of other authors, who found that 32% of patients reported decreased rigidity, whereas only 18% of patients had IIEF scores corresponding to moderate and severe ED [15]. Compared to the present study, others have previously reported better [13–15] or worse postoperative erectile function [12]. Inconsistent findings regarding postoperative erectile function may be due to differences in methods, follow-up and patient characteristics. For example, other studies used IIEF-5 questionnaire [12–16], had longer [12,14,16] or shorter [13,15] follow-up or did not report on relevant comorbidities [14], which may be associated with ED. Importantly, with longer time from penile surgery, other factors like age and comorbidities may occur and have additional negative impact on erectile function. For example, increasing age is a well-established risk factor for erectile dysfunction [27].

The present study has important limitations, which are first and foremost inherent to the retrospective study design. The number of patients is low, and follow-up was not available in 30% of patients. Therefore, selection bias could have influenced the results both at baseline and at follow-up. In addition, preoperative or postoperative data, e.g., penile length measurement, was not available in a relevant number of patients. Particularly, this may have introduced relevant reporting bias. In addition to validated instruments, the questionnaire included non-validated questions, which renders comparability with results of other studies difficult. Neither FKKS-SEX nor SF-8 have been validated for the use in patients with PD. Moreover, patients did receive the questionnaire at different time points following SIS grafting, which might cause relevant heterogeneity of results. The effect of SIS grafting on health-related quality of life as well as self-perception and self-attitude of sexuality remains uncertain, since preoperative data on SF-8 and FKKS-SEX was not available. The incision of the tunica albuginea of the corpora cavernosa may also have an impact on outcome, especially erectile function, but was not assessed in the present study. Data on treatment of ED after SIS grafting was missing.

Multivariable analysis to identify independent predictors for patient dissatisfaction was not possible, since the number of events was too low. Nevertheless, our data suggest that patient related features as subjective shortening of the penis, negative body related self-perceptions and self-attitudes of sexuality as well as IIEF-EF score were risk factors for patient dissatisfaction. Thus, validation of our results in prospective studies with larger patient cohorts is warranted.

5. Conclusions

A relevant number of patients with severe PD are not satisfied with surgical outcome after SIS grafting. The majority of patients have positive and neutral self-perception and self-attitudes of sexuality. Following SIS grafting, patients have lower social functioning, mental, and emotional health compared to controls. Subjective shortening of the penis, negative body related self-perceptions, and self-attitudes of sexuality as well as IIEF-EF score are risk factors for patient dissatisfaction. Further prospective studies with larger patient cohorts are necessary to validate these findings.

Author Contributions: Conceptualization, A.S., R.D., T.N., P.B. and P.R.; Data curation, S.L., M.W.V. and P.R.; Formal analysis, S.L., T.N., P.B. and P.R.; Investigation, P.R.; Methodology, M.W.V. and P.R.; Project administration, O.E., M.R., M.F. and P.R.; Supervision, R.D., O.E., M.R., M.F. and P.R.; Validation, P.R.; Writing – original draft, A.S. and P.R.; Writing – review & editing, A.S., S.L., R.D., M.W.V., O.E., T.N., P.B., M.R., M.F. and P.R.

Funding: This research received no external funding.

Conflicts of Interest: The authors declare no conflict of interest.

References

1. Al-Thakafi, S.; Al-Hathal, N. Peyronie's disease: A literature review on epidemiology, genetics, pathophysiology, diagnosis and work-up. *Transl. Androl. Urol.* **2016**, *5*, 280–289. [CrossRef] [PubMed]
2. Hellstrom, W.J.; Feldman, R.; Rosen, R.C.; Smith, T.; Kaufman, G.; Tursi, J. Bother and distress associated with Peyronie's disease: Validation of the Peyronie's disease questionnaire. *J. Urol.* **2013**, *190*, 627–634. [CrossRef] [PubMed]
3. Usta, M.F.; Bivalacqua, T.J.; Tokatli, Z.; Rivera, F.; Gulkesen, K.H.; Sikka, S.C.; Hellstron, W.J. Stratification of penile vascular pathologies in patients with Peyronie's disease and in men with erectile dysfunction according to age: A comparative study. *J. Urol.* **2004**, *172*, 259–262. [CrossRef] [PubMed]
4. Nelson, C.J.; Diblasio, C.; Kendirci, M.; Hellstrom, W.; Guhring, P.; Mulhall, J.P. The Chronology of Depression and Distress in Men with Peyronie's Disease. *J. Sex. Med.* **2008**, *5*, 1985–1990. [CrossRef] [PubMed]
5. Hatzichristodoulou, G.; Osmonov, D.; Kübler, H.; Hellstrom, W.J.G.; Yafi, F.A. Contemporary Review of Grafting Techniques for the Surgical Treatment of Peyronie's Disease. *Sex. Med. Rev.* **2017**, *5*, 544–552. [CrossRef] [PubMed]
6. Capoccia, E.; Levine, L.A. Contemporary Review of Peyronie's Disease Treatment. *Curr. Urol. Rep.* **2018**, *19*, 51. [CrossRef]
7. Levine, L.A.; Larsen, S.M. Surgery for Peyronie's disease. *Asian J. Androl.* **2013**, *15*, 27–34. [CrossRef]
8. Breyer, B.N.; Brant, W.O.; Garcia, M.M.; Bella, A.J.; Lue, T.F. Complications of porcine small intestine submucosa graft for Peyronie's disease. *J. Urol.* **2007**, *177*, 589–5891. [CrossRef]
9. Knoll, L.D. Use of small intestinal submucosa graft for the surgical management of Peyronie's disease. *J. Urol.* **2007**, *178*, 2474–2478. [CrossRef]
10. Staerman, F.; Pierrevelcin, J.; Ripert, T.; Menard, J. Medium-term follow-up of plaque incision and porcine small intestinal submucosal grafting for Peyronie's disease. *Int. J. Impot. Res.* **2010**, *22*, 343–348. [CrossRef]
11. Lee, E.W.; Shindel, A.W.; Brandes, S.B. Small intestinal submucosa for patch grafting after plaque incision in the treatment of Peyronie's disease. *Int. Braz. J. Urol. Off. J. Braz. Soc. Urol.* **2008**, *34*, 191–196. [CrossRef] [PubMed]
12. Chung, E.; Clendinning, E.; Lessard, L.; Brock, G. Five-year follow-up of Peyronie's graft surgery: Outcomes and patient satisfaction. *J. Sex. Med.* **2011**, *8*, 594–600. [CrossRef] [PubMed]
13. Kovac, J.R.; Brock, G.B. Surgical outcomes and patient satisfaction after dermal, pericardial, and small intestinal submucosal grafting for Peyronie's disease. *J. Sex. Med.* **2007**, *4*, 1500–1508. [CrossRef] [PubMed]

14. Sayedahmed, K.; Rosenhammer, B.; Spachmann, P.J.; Burger, M.; Aragona, M.; Kaftan, B.T.; Olianas, R.; Frische, H.M. Bicentric prospective evaluation of corporoplasty with porcine small intestinal submucosa (SIS) in patients with severe Peyronie's disease. *World J. Urol.* **2017**, *35*, 1119–1124. [CrossRef] [PubMed]
15. Valente, P.; Gomes, C.; Tomada, N. Small Intestinal Submucosa Grafting for Peyronie Disease: Outcomes and Patient Satisfaction. *Urology* **2017**, *100*, 117–124. [CrossRef]
16. Morgado, A.; Morgado, M.R.; Tomada, N. Penile lengthening with porcine small intestinal submucosa grafting in Peyronie's disease treatment: Long-term surgical outcomes, patients' satisfaction and dissatisfaction predictors. *Andrology* **2018**, *6*, 909–915. [CrossRef] [PubMed]
17. Kelâmi, A. Classification of Congenital and Acquired Penile Deviation. *Urologia Internationalis.* **1983**, *38*, 229–233. [PubMed]
18. Habous, M.; Muir, G.; Soliman, T.; Farag, M.; Williamson, B.; Binsaleh, S.; Elhadek, W.; Mahamoud, S.; Ibrahin, H.; Abdelwahab, O.; et al. Outcomes of variation in technique and variation in accuracy of measurement in penile length measurement. *Int. J. Impot. Res.* **2018**, *30*, 21–26. [CrossRef]
19. Sikka, S.C.; Hellstrom, W.J.; Brock, G.; Morales, A.M. Standardization of vascular assessment of erectile dysfunction: Standard operating procedures for duplex ultrasound. *J. Sex. Med.* **2013**, *10*, 120–129. [CrossRef]
20. Ware, J.E.; Kosinski, M.; Dewey, J.E.; Gandek, B. *How to Score and Interpret Single-Item Health Status Measures: A Manual for Users of the SF-8 Health Survey*; Quality Metric Inc: Lincoln, CA, USA, 2001.
21. Hashine, K.; Kusuhara, Y.; Miura, N.; Shirato, A.; Sumiyoshi, Y.; Kataoka, M. Health-related quality of life using SF-8 and EPIC questionnaires after treatment with radical retropubic prostatectomy and permanent prostate brachytherapy. *Jpn. J. Clin. Oncol.* **2009**, *39*, 502–508. [CrossRef]
22. Ellert, U.; Lampert, T.; Ravens-Sieberer, U. *Messung der Gesundheitsbezogenen Lebensqualität Mit Dem SF-8. Eine Normstichprobe Für Deutschland. Robert Koch-Institut, Epidemiologie Und Gesundheitsberichterstattung*; Springer Medizin Verlag: Berlin, Germany, 2005.
23. Deusinger, I.M. *Die Frankfurter Körperkonzeptskalen: Handanweisung Mit Bericht Über Vielfältige Validierungsstudien*; Hogrefe Verlag Für Psychologie: Göttingen, Germany, 1998.
24. Yachia, D. Our experience with penile deformations: Incidence, operative techniques, and results. *J. Androl.* **1994**, *15*, 63–68.
25. Garaffa, G.; Sacca, A.; Christopher, A.N.; Ralph, D.J. Circumcision is not mandatory in penile surgery. *BJU Int.* **2010**, *105*, 222–224. [CrossRef] [PubMed]
26. Goldman, R. The psychological impact of circumcision. *BJU Int.* **1999**, *83*, 93–102. [CrossRef] [PubMed]
27. Braun, M.; Wassmer, G.; Klotz, T.; Reifenrath, B.; Mathers, M.; Engelmann, U. Epidemiology of erectile dysfunction: Results of the 'cologne male survey'. *Int. J. Impot. Res.* **2000**, *12*, 305–311. [CrossRef]

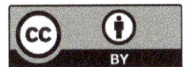

© 2019 by the authors. Licensee MDPI, Basel, Switzerland. This article is an open access article distributed under the terms and conditions of the Creative Commons Attribution (CC BY) license (http://creativecommons.org/licenses/by/4.0/).

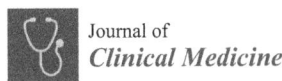

Article

Two Sides of One Coin: A Comparison of Clinical and Neurobiological Characteristics of Convicted and Non-Convicted Pedophilic Child Sexual Offenders

Charlotte Gibbels [1], Christopher Sinke [1], Jonas Kneer [1], Till Amelung [2], Sebastian Mohnke [2], Klaus Michael Beier [2], Henrik Walter [3], Kolja Schiltz [4], Hannah Gerwinn [5], Alexander Pohl [5], Jorge Ponseti [5], Carina Foedisch [6], Inka Ristow [6], Martin Walter [6,7], Christian Kaergel [8], Claudia Massau [8], Boris Schiffer [8] and Tillmann H.C. Kruger [1,*]

1. Division of Clinical Psychology and Sexual Medicine, Department of Psychiatry, Social Psychiatry and Psychotherapy, Hannover Medical School, 30625 Hanover, Germany
2. Institute of Sexology and Sexual Medicine, Charité—Universitätsmedizin Berlin, Corporate Member of Freie Universität Berlin, Humboldt-Universität zu Berlin, and Berlin Institute of Health, 10117 Berlin, Germany
3. Division of Mind and Brain Research, Department of Psychiatry and Psychotherapy, CCM, Charité—Universitätsmedizin Berlin, Corporate Member of Freie Universität Berlin, Humboldt-Universität zu Berlin, and Berlin Institute of Health, 10117 Berlin, Germany
4. Department of Forensic Psychiatry, Ludwig Maximilians University Munich, 80336 Munich, Germany
5. Kiel University, Medical School, Institute of Sexual Medicine and Forensic Psychiatry and Psychotherapy, 24105 Kiel, Germany
6. Department of Psychiatry, Otto-von Guericke-University Magdeburg, 39106 Magdeburg, Germany
7. Department of Psychiatry, University of Tübingen, 72076 Tübingen, Germany
8. Division of Forensic Psychiatry, Department of Psychiatry, Psychotherapy and Preventive Medicine, Ruhr University Bochum, LWL University Hospital, 44791 Bochum, Germany
* Correspondence: krueger.tillmann@mh-hannover.de; Tel.: +49-511-5322-407

Received: 31 May 2019; Accepted: 26 June 2019; Published: 29 June 2019

Abstract: High prevalence of child sexual offending stand in contradiction to low conviction rates (one-tenth at most) of child sexual offenders (CSOs). Little is known about possible differences between convicted and non-convicted pedophilic CSOs and why only some become known to the judicial system. This investigation takes a closer look at the two sides of "child sexual offending" by focusing on clinical and neurobiological characteristics of convicted and non-convicted pedophilic CSOs as presented in the Neural Mechanisms Underlying Pedophilia and sexual offending against children (NeMUP)*-study. Seventy-nine male pedophilic CSOs were examined, 48 of them convicted. All participants received a thorough clinical examination including the structured clinical interview (SCID), intelligence, empathy, impulsivity, and criminal history. Sixty-one participants (38 convicted) underwent an inhibition performance task (Go/No-go paradigm) combined with functional magnetic resonance imaging (fMRI). Convicted and non-convicted pedophilic CSOs revealed similar clinical characteristics, inhibition performances, and neuronal activation. However, convicted subjects' age preference was lower (i.e., higher interest in prepubescent children) and they had committed a significantly higher number of sexual offenses against children compared to non-convicted subjects. In conclusion, sexual age preference may represent one of the major driving forces for elevated rates of sexual offenses against children in this sample, and careful clinical assessment thereof should be incorporated in every preventive approach.

Keywords: NeMUP; child sexual offending; child sexual abuse; pedophilia; fMRI; SCID

1. Introduction

With a prevalence of 12.7%, child sexual offenses occur across most ethnic, religious and socioeconomic groups all over the world [1]. This is especially devastating since the effects on children's wellbeing and development are tremendous and might persist until adulthood [2–4]. The high prevalence in comparison to the low conviction rate of child sexual offenders (CSOs) [2] suggests that the majority of CSOs may never get caught. The reasons for the low conviction rate remain unclear but could originate from three different circumstances: (1) Characteristics of the victim (e.g., age), (2) characteristics of the offender (e.g., being better at hiding the crime due to intelligence), and (3) circumstances of the crime (e.g., abuse by an intimate person). One of the most frequently described risk-factors concerning child sexual offending is a pedophilic preference which has been described in about 50% of convicted CSOs [5,6]. The International Classification of Diseases, tenth edition (ICD-10) [7] defines diagnostic criteria of pedophilia as a sexual preference for children—boys or girls or both—usually of prepubertal or early pubertal age including the following criteria: "(A) The general criteria for F65 disorders of sexual preference must be met (G1. Recurrent intense sexual urges and fantasies involving unusual objects or activities. G2. Acts on the urges or is markedly distressed by them. G3. The preference has been present for at least six months). (B) A persistent or a predominant preference for sexual activity with a prepubescent child or children. (C) The person is at least 16 years old and at least five years older than the child or children" [7].

Pedophilia has often been linked to higher psychiatric comorbidities [8–10] as well as neurobiological and neuropsychological alterations (e.g., [11]). These results correspond to Krueger and Schiffer [12], who showed that convicted pedophiles serving prison sentences in a forensic treatment facility performed lower on all subtests of a shortened IQ test than a control group except for completing images. Multiple studies showed coherence between pedophilic CSOs and impairment in behavioral inhibition [13–15]. Nevertheless, Gerwinn et al. [10] were one of the first revealing an effect of offender status but not of pedophilia on intelligence and other measures in their subgroups. Furthermore, it was shown that essential alterations of brain structure and function—which were assumed to be pedophilia-specific—were predominantly associated with child sexual offending rather than with the pedophilic preference [16–19]. Most importantly, Kärgel et al. [17] even found non-offending pedophiles to perform significantly better in a behavioral inhibition task (go/nogo paradigm). This leads to the hypothesis that behavioral inhibition potentially secures non-offending pedophiles from acting upon their urges in comparison to sexually offending pedophiles.

Alternatively, there may be effects such as the number of the victims and age of the offender that can lead to imprisonment. Neutze et al. [20] found an age difference between detected and undetected pedophilic CSOs with the detected CSOs being older. Hence, it might be possible that being convicted is just a matter of time. The authors [20] conclude that two sets of factors are associated with detection status: (1) "preceding" ones that might influence whether an individual is detected (e.g., age or education) and (2) "resulting" ones which may either be a response to detection (e.g., emotion-oriented coping, childhood sexual victimization) or reflect a bias in self-report measures (e.g., sexual self-regulation problems, paraphilic interests) in order to avoid negative consequences (e.g., severe punishment) [20].

In the last years, research on neurobiological underpinnings of pedophilia has gained some attention. Unfortunately, the majority of the few studies focusing on child sexual offending and pedophilia mainly examined convicted CSOs. Some studies did not even take sexual preference into consideration at all when comparing groups of offenders and non-offenders. For that reason, results cannot be seen as representative for pedophilia in general, and findings are restricted to the particular group of convicted CSOs [15]. Subsequently, it must be considered that there could be an offender effect rather than an effect of pedophilia itself. Hence, when investigating characteristics due to a pedophilic preference, it is crucial to distinguish between convicted pedophiles, non-convicted pedophiles, and convicted CSOs who are not pedophilic.

Throughout the last years, the research consortium NeMUP, which is the acronym for "neural mechanisms underlying pedophilia and sexual offending against children", discriminated between pedophilia and child sexual offending by using a two by two factorial design (offender status/pedophilia). Results of the NeMUP consortium showed increased levels of psychiatric comorbidities, sexual dysfunctions, and adverse childhood experiences among pedophiles as well as child sexual offenders [10]. Additionally, regression analyses were more powerful in segregating offender status than sexual preference (mean classification accuracy: 76% versus 68%). In summary, results of the NeMUP consortium showed that executive dysfunctions in CSOs are rather small and may be independent of pedophilic preferences. Neurobiological assessment showed changes in brain structure, metabolism [21] and function, which were particularly associated with the offending status but not with pedophilic preference [16–19].

Regarding the characteristics of victims that might differentiate between convicted and non-convicted CSOs, it is important to acknowledge that the authors have no intention to blame victims of sexual offenses. Nevertheless, some victim related factors might decrease the likelihood of incarceration of the offenders. It has been shown that children who were older, came from incestuous families, felt greater responsibility for the abuse, and feared negative consequences of disclosure took longer to disclose a crime [22]. Additionally, the sex of the victim could possibly discriminate between convicted and non-convicted CSOs. Since it could be shown that reports of female victims are twice as frequent as of male victims [1] it is also possible that males are victimized equally often but report sexual offenses less frequently [23]. This might be caused by more intense feelings of shame and guilt [24]. Finally, another factor that might differentiate between convicted and non-convicted CSOs may be the quality of the relationship between offender and victim. Whereas it is more probable that sexual offenses against children are committed by a relative or a good friend of the family [25,26] this could also lead to a dilemma concerning a complaint to the police.

While the current investigation did not put an emphasis on victims' characteristics, it was designed to carefully analyze clinical, neuropsychological and neurobiological features of convicted and non-convicted CSOs in order to unravel possible factors that might increase or decrease the probability to be convicted.

2. Method

2.1. Participants

Participants of the study were recruited by research associates and practicing psychotherapists as part of the multi-site research project "Neural Mechanisms Underlying Pedophilia and Sexual Offending against Children" (NeMUP, www.nemup.de) which includes five collaborative research sites from (forensic) psychiatry or sexual medicine located in Berlin, Bochum/Essen, Hanover, Kiel and Magdeburg. Most sites of the project were involved in the prevention project "Don't offend" (www.dont-offend.org) for self-identified pedophiles seeking therapy [27]. Additionally, some subjects were recruited in prisons or during fulfilment of a suspended sentence. Moreover, the official "NeMUP"-website (www.nemup.de) as well as various German internet forums were used to inform self-identified pedophilic men and child sex offenders without pedophilia about the study [10]. For a detailed description of recruitment and collection of the whole NeMUP data, the reader is kindly asked to take a look at Gerwin et al. [10]. The present study only included the NeMUP sample of pedophiles who committed child sexual offenses in the analysis. This group (CSO) contains men who fulfill the criteria of being pedophile/hebephile and have committed at least one "hands-on" [10] delict against children under the age of 14. All participants provided written informed consent before participating, and all local ethics committees located in Berlin, Bochum/Essen, Hanover, Kiel, and Magdeburg approved the study (approval code 6048).

While pedophilia is a sexual preference for prepubescent children and teleiophilia is a sexual responsiveness to adults [10], hebephilia is defined as a sexual preference for children in early pubertal stages. The hebephilic group was subsumed under the label of pedophilia according to ICD-10 that defines pedophilia as a "sexual preference for children ... of pre-pubertal or early pubertal stage" (ICD 10).

"Hands-on" delicts were defined as sexual acts that involved touching or manipulating the child's naked body or genitals (manually or orally) by the offender with the intention of sexually stimulating himself, penetrating the child (anally or vaginally) or forcing the child to (anally or vaginally) penetrate or touch/manipulate the offenders' genitals [10]. Pedophiles who had not committed such a "hands-on" offense and/or who were currently or historically consumers of material that shows the sexual exploitation of children or so-called indicative pictures (e.g., fully clothed children in erotic poses) were not assigned into this group. This procedure does in no way indicate to degrade such behavior as "non-criminal", it was used to differentiate between pedophiles who were or were not able to refrain from direct sexual behavior towards children.

In the present study, the group of CSOs was divided into two different subgroups. The first subgroup (non-convicted CSOs) contained men who had not been convicted for their sexual offenses against children, hence pedophiles in the so-called "dark field". The other group (convicted CSOs) included men that had been convicted for their crimes. Men belonging to the non-convicted CSOs were mainly recruited within the "Don't Offend" project in Germany [27] and various German internet forums. Participants who were categorized into the subgroup of convicted CSOs were recruited in prisons or during fulfillment of suspended sentences. Exclusion criteria were acute psychiatric or neurological disorders others than pedophilia, acute episodes of alcohol or drug abuse as well as past dependencies and current medication related to sexual functioning. Overall, 31 non-convicted CSOs and 48 convicted CSOs were incorporated into data analysis.

2.2. Procedure

Data were collected in two different sessions over two days. The first session included the survey of interviews and diagnostic data, whereas during the second session the magnetic resonance imaging (MRI) assessment was performed.

Structured clinical interview for DSM (SCID) [28] enabled to screen for DSM Axis I and Axis II disorders.

Semi-structured interview was performed in order to gain information about the participants' sexual interaction interest(s), child pornography consumption, history of offenses in general and biographical information (e.g., age of first coitus, psychiatric disorders in family, own children).

Sexual gender and age orientation was measured by a modification of the Kinsey Scale [29] where participants were asked to indicate range and peak for the age and sex of their preferred sexual partner using the Tanner stages I to V [10]. In case of uncertainty concerning the age preference legal information (if available) and individual case conferences were utilized to ensure a valid clinical diagnosis.

Intelligence was estimated by the German version of the Wechsler Adult Intelligence Scale (WAIS-IV) [30]. Global intelligence was assessed by means of four subtests ("Similarities", "Vocabulary", "Block Design", and "Matrix Reasoning") [30]. All assessments were carried out by experienced research associates, trained to use these instruments.

Childhood trauma questionnaire (CTQ) [31] was given to the participants to estimate the burden of self-experienced abuse and neglect. The questionnaire screens for a history of five different types of maltreatment (sexual abuse, physical abuse, emotional abuse, physical neglect and emotional neglect). Moreover, an assessment of psychiatric and criminal history of both parents was included in the semi-structured interview for assessing other relevant clinical variables. In the current paper, the difference between the five different types of maltreatment for each group was used to describe differences in experienced childhood trauma. Thresholds for severe childhood trauma can be found at Glaesmer et al. [32].

Empathy was measured using the multifaceted empathy test (MET) [33]. The MET consists of 26 photographs, mostly depicting people in emotionally charged situations. The test assesses cognitive empathy by requiring subjects to deduce mental states of the individuals shown in the photographs. In order to address emotional empathy participants also rate their own emotional reaction in response to the pictures. Unfortunately, no cut-off values for the MET can be found in the literature. However, since the paper focuses on the differentiation between two groups the differences between both groups were used to describe differences in empathy.

Barratt impulsiveness scale (BIS-11) [34] was used to measure self-reported impulsiveness. The questionnaire consists of 30 items and is designed to assess three facets of impulsiveness: (1) attentional impulsiveness, defined as the (in-)ability to concentrate or focus attention, (2) motor impulsiveness, the propensity to act without thinking, and (3) non-planning impulsiveness, or the lack of planning the future and forethought. In the current paper, the difference between the total score for each group was used to describe differences in impulsiveness. For an overview of different clinical scores of BIS-11 the reader is kindly asked to look at Stanford et al. [35].

2.3. Imaging Parameters and Processing

Since not all participants fulfilled the criteria to be examined with MRI (e.g., because of claustrophobia or having a pacemaker) only subgroups of the sample were included in the measurements. Therefore, the analysis of the Go/No-go paradigm included 23 non-convicted CSOs and 38 CSOs convicted participants instead of the overall 31 non-convicted CSOs and 48 convicted CSOs.

The MRI images were acquired at five separate 3T MRI scanners that were equipped with 32 channel head coils: 2× Siemens Skyra, 2× Siemens Trio and 1× Phillips Achiva. T1 images were created by means of MPRAGE sequence (slices = 192, FoV = 256 mm, voxel size = $1 \times 1 \times 1$ mm, TR = 2.500 ms, TE = 4.37 ms, flip angle = 7, distance factor = 50%). T2 weighted images were gained using an echo planar imaging (EPI) sequence (slices = 38, field of view = 240 mm, voxel size = $2.3 \times 2.3 \times 3$ mm, time of repetition = 2.400 ms, echo time 30 ms, flip angle = 80, distance factor = 10%). MRI phantom stability measures [36] were accompanied to prevent signal fluctuations across all sites. For functional imaging analysis, the Statistical Parametric Mapping Software (SPM 12) [37] was used. The first five images were discarded to account for T1 relaxation effects. Before statistical analysis, functional volumes were (1) slice time corrected using the middle slice as reference, (2) realigned and unwarped, (3) co-registered to the according T1 image, (4) spatially normalized into Montreal Neurological Institute (MNI) space utilizing the individual T1 image and (5) smoothed with an isotropic Gaussian kernel (full width half maximum of 8 mm).

Go/nogo task: As a measure of impulse control and behavioral inhibition participants performed an event-related go/nogo task preceded by an alertness task of go-trials. The alertness task was applied to allow the participant to familiarize with the MRI environment as well as to provide a baseline measure for reaction time to a simple target stimulus. The projection screen was localized either in front (Hanover) or behind the magnet bore (Berlin, Essen, Kiel). At first, an instruction was presented which informed the participants to respond as fast as possible to any presented stimulus indicated by "X". Afterwards, the stimulus presentation of 50 alertness trials was initiated. Next, a second instruction screen followed introducing the go/nogo condition containing 150 trials. Participants were asked to respond as fast as possible to frequently presented go-trials (80% indicated by "X") and withhold the response to infrequently presented no-go trials (20% indicated by "+"). Stimuli were presented using Presentation Software package (Neurobehavioral Systems, Berkeley, CA, USA) and were shown in a pseudo-randomized order, precluding the occurrence of two repeatedly presented no-go stimuli. Stimuli were presented 200 ms with an inter-stimulus-interval (ISI) of 1500–2500 ms. Before scanning, participants were instructed to respond with the right forefinger to the response box. The number of commission errors of no-go trials as well as the reaction times of alertness were used for further statistical analysis to provide a behavioral measure of response inhibition. Outliers differing more than threefold from the distance between the 25% and 75% percentile of the distribution were excluded from analysis. Visual impairments were corrected by a goggle system that was compatible with MR.

2.4. Statistical Analysis

Behavioral analysis: SPSS version 24 [38] was used for statistical analysis. To distinguish effects between non-convicted CSOs and convicted CSOs with respect to intelligence, clinical characteristics, empathy, impulsiveness, childhood trauma, victim characteristics, and biographical information, t-tests were used for interval data and Chi^2 tests for dichotomous data. Since the study is part of the NeMUP project there was no specialized sample size calculation for this particular paper. However, the sample size for the whole NeMUP research was calculated for each of the four groups that were included in research (pedophiles with child sexual abuse, pedophiles without child sexual abuse. child sexual abusers without pedophilia and controls). For group one which was included in the current paper, there was a sample size calculation of 60 participants to ensure MRI results were measurable. Concerning non-convicted pedophiles, there are only to papers known by the authors that integrated non-convicted pedophiles into their research. Beier et al. [27] included 53 pedophiles and 22 control participants in his design. Engel et al. [28] included 35 treated pedophiles and 51 treatment refusers in his analysis. For that reason, the sample size of the current paper stands in line with other research published on this topic.

In order to correct for multiple testing, Bonferroni–Holm correction was implemented for different subgroups. Subgroups were: Characteristics of the offender, clinical information, experienced childhood trauma, characteristics of the victims, delict specifics, history of delicts (except hands-on delicts) as well as sexual problems and paraphilias. In order to determine if the number of delicts could be associated with other (sexual) characteristics of the offender, correlations between sexual age preference, sexual gender preference, and quantity of sexual child offenses were included in the analysis. In Table 1 subgroups are described in more detail as well as their descriptive statistic parameters.

For behavioral data of go/nogo paradigm, reaction time, error rate and error quote were analyzed using two sample t-tests.

Table 1. Characteristics of non-convicted and convicted child sexual offenders (CSOs).

	Non-Convicted CSOs (n = 31)				Convicted CSOs (n = 43)				T
	M	SD	Minimum	Maximum	M	SD	Minimum	Maximum	
Offender characteristics									
Age	40.4	10.8	20	59	39.8	9.0	24	62	0.27
Intelligence (WAIS)									
Estimated general IQ	100.26	18.51	62	140	98.27	18.95	66	166	0.46
Estimated verbal IQ	95.00	21.52	54	137	92.14	17.45	57	129	0.65
Estimated performance IQ	106.87	19.41	78.00	143.0	103.31	17.29	63.00	149.00	0.85
Empathy (MET)									
Emotional	5.11	1.25	2.65	7.44	5.33	1.74	1.44	8.11	−0.57
Cognitive	6.98	1.02	4.63	9.00	7.10	1.04	3.88	8.50	−0.49
Impulsiveness (BIS-11)	64.46	9.86	47.00	81.00	63.49	8.59	46.00	88.00	0.44
Family background									
Experienced childhood trauma (CTQ)									
Emotional abuse	11.20	4.90	5.00	23.00	10.24	5.41	5.00	25.00	0.79
Sexual abuse	7.00	2.45	5.00	14.00	9.48	6.34	5.00	25.00	−2.40
Physical abuse	7.70	3.37	5.00	20.00	8.43	4.71	5.00	22.00	−0.74
Emotional neglect	13.20	4.91	5.00	25.00	12.37	4.57	5.00	25.00	0.75
Physical neglect	7.60	2.90	5.00	17.00	7.85	3.05	5.00	20.00	−0.35
Information about the victims									
Age (mean)									
Female victim	10.50	3.19	5.0	15.5	8.68	2.31	5.0	13.0	2.15
Male victim	11.28	2.59	6.0	15.0	10.18	2.48	3.0	14.5	−0.25
History of Delicts (except hands-on Delicts)									
Quantity of violent offense	0.13	0.43	0	2	0.66	1.23	0	2	0.125
Quantity of other offenses	0.83	1.23	0	5	0.55	1.23	0	7	−0.28
Delict specifics									
Quantity of child sexual offenses	1.94	1.41	1	7	4.53	3.91	1	17	−4.23 ***
Number of victims	2.35	2.53	1	11	5.08	8.71	1	60	0.39
Number of female victims	1.58	2.59	0	11	1.33	2.13	0	10	0.48
Number of male victims	0.77	1.43	0	7	3.76	8.81	0	60	−2.32

Table 1. Cont.

	Non-Convicted CSOs ($n = 31$)				Convicted CSOs ($n = 43$)				T
	M	SD	Minimum	Maximum	M	SD	Minimum	Maximum	
	n [a]				n [a]				χ^2
Clinical diagnoses									
SCID I disorders									
Affective disorders	13				16				0.40
Anxiety disorders	8				9				0.63
Sexual disorders	0				0				1.60
Obsessive compulsive disorders	1				1				0.11
Substance disorders	6				12				0.29
Eating disorders	0				1				0.64
ADHD	1				0				1.60
SCID II disorders									0.91
Cluster A	2				3				0.00
Cluster B	11				10				2.22
Cluster C	6				12				0.29
Sexual age orientation									14.00 *
Hebephile	1				3				
Pedophile	5				19				
Mixed pedophile and teleiophile	5				11				
Mixed hebephile and teleiophile	11				3				
Mixed pedophile and hebephile	5				5				
Mixed pedophile, hebephile and teleiophile	4				8				
Sexual gender orientation									4.01
Heterosexual	17				17				
Homosexual	8				23				
Bisexual	6				9				
Intrafamilial (incest) delicts	7				6				1.49
Extrafamilial delicts	24				43				1.49

M: Mean, SD: standard deviation, [a] number of participants fulfilling the criteria, * $p \leq 0.05$, *** $p \leq 0.001$.

fMRI analysis: SPM12 was used to analyze functional volumes. For first-level analysis the following events were included as regressors in the design matrix: (1) alertness, (2) hits to go-trials, (3) false responses to no-go trials, (4) false responses to no-go trials (commission errors), (5) movement as regressors of no interest. Event-related responses were convolved with the canonical hemodynamic response (HRF), and separate linear contrast images (vectors for each condition) were built. For assessing group differences, contrast images were analyzed using two-sided t-tests (non-convicted CSOs vs. convicted CSOs) between groups for the different regressors of interest: (1) alertness, (2) go-trials, (3) successfully inhibited no-go trials and (4) false responses to no-go trials (commission errors). Groups neither differed in age nor IQ so these variables were of no interest for further analysis. The threshold for all analyses was set to $p = 0.05$, familywise error (FWE) corrected for multiple comparisons.

3. Results

3.1. Characteristics of the Offender

As shown in Table 1, no significant differences could be found which distinguished between the two offender groups concerning age or intelligence (neither in relation to general, verbal nor performance intelligence). Moreover, measurements for empathy or impulsiveness did not separate between non-convicted and convicted CSOs. No correlation between sexual age preference, sexual gender preference, and quantity of sexual child offenses was seen.

3.2. Sexuality

Non-convicted and convicted CSOs differed in sexual age orientation χ^2 (1, $n = 79$) = 14.00, $p = 0.03$. Convicted CSOs were more often pedophilic ($n = 19$ convicted, $n = 5$ non-convicted) or mixed pedophilic/teleiophilic ($n = 11$ convicted, $n = 5$ non-convicted), whereas non-convicted CSOs showed an age preference more often than mixed hebephilic/teleiophilic ($n = 3$ convicted, $n = 11$ non-convicted). There was no difference in sexual gender orientation χ^2 (1, $n = 79$) = 4.01, $p = 0.135$).

3.3. Experienced Childhood Trauma

There were no significant differences in self-experienced childhood traumatization as assessed by the CTQ questionnaire between non-convicted and convicted CSOs. A more detailed overview of the data can be found in Table 1.

3.4. Clinical Information

As can be seen in Table 1, no significant difference was found between the two groups concerning any clinical features.

3.5. Delinquency

CSO delicts: Non-convicted CSOs and convicted CSOs differed in the quantity of their sexual child offenses ($t(78) = -4.23, p < 0.001$), but not in the number of victims or in the number of victims by gender. A marginal significance for a difference in the number of male victims was evident ($t(78) = -2.32, p = 0.06$). There was neither a correlation between sexual age preference and quantity of sexual child offenses nor between sexual gender preference and quantity of sexual child offenses.

Non-CSO delicts: As can be seen in Table 1, the two groups did not differ concerning delicts other than child sexual offending.

3.6. Victims' Characteristics

The groups showed a marginal significance in the difference of age of female victims ($t(78) = -2.51, p = 0.06$).

3.7. Go/No-Go Task

Non-convicted and convicted CSOs did not significantly differ in this task, neither in post-error slowing nor in reaction times to commission errors. For detailed information see Table 2.

Table 2. Inhibited response to no-go trials for both groups.

	Non-Convicted CSOs ($n = 31$)	Convicted CSOs ($n = 49$)	Statistics (t-Value)
RT Alertness in ms, M (SD)	263.009 (58.269)	273.540 (47.545)	$t(78) = -0.74; p = 0.46$
RT Go in ms, M (SD)	388.062 (43.298)	400.053 (54.644)	$t(78) = -0.85; p = 0.40$
Global Error Rate, M (SD)	0.0598 (0.043)	0.0532 (0.0394)	$t(78) = 0.61; p = 0.54$
Global Error Quote, M (SD)	11.455 (8.830)	10.632 (7.875)	$t(78) = 0.37; p = 0.71$

Coordinates are denoted by x, y, z in mm according to the MNI-space (Montreal Neurological Institute).

3.8. fMRI Analysis

Successful response-inhibition activated clusters in the anterior cingulate cortex, supplemental motor cortex, insula and middle temporal gyrus (FWE corrected on voxel level, see Table 3) for both groups. No differences were found between both groups.

Table 3. Go/No-Go task performance.

Location (AAL)	Hemisphere	x	y	z	Size	t-Value
Inhibited response to no-go trials for both groups, FWE peak level						
Insula	L	−22	24	8	18	6.28
ACC	L	−4	34	22	76	6.15
Middle temporal gyrus	R	46	−42	−8	28	6.03
Middle temporal gyrus	L	−54	−22	−14	16	5.99
Supplemental motor area	R	2	24	46	12	5.43

4. Discussion

Overall, only subtle differences between non-convicted and convicted CSOs were identified. Thus, most of the initial hypotheses of the authors concerning differences between convicted and non-convicted pedophilic offenders could not be supported. Data shows that non-convicted CSOs were neither more intelligent nor less impulsive nor suffered less from psychiatric disorders than convicted CSOs in this study. Additionally, no differences could be found concerning their age, the number of victims or the level of empathy. Interestingly, convicted CSOs committed more delicts than non-convicted CSOs. Furthermore, non-convicted and convicted CSOs differed in sexual age orientation. Moreover, all hypotheses except age and gender preference concerning characteristics of victims could not be supported in the present study. However, there was a marginal significance concerning the number of male victims and the age of female victims.

Our data shows that the risk of being caught increases with the number of victims. First, it is likely that with an increasing number of delicts it becomes more probable that one victim is able to identify the offender or to confide in another person about the crime. Second, more frequent delicts of child sexual offending may increase hubris of the offender and lead to carelessness concerning the crime scene, which may finally lead to the offender's incarceration.

Since convicted CSOs were more often exclusively pedophilic or mixed pedophilic/teleiophilic it is possible that harming a child might lead more often to incarceration than harming an adolescent. This might be due to the social perspective that harming adolescents might be less harmful. Additionally, there is an ongoing debate about whether or not hebephilia is relevant for psychopathology [39]. This debate has been consistent with the evolutionary psychology position that emphasizing the adaptive partner-preference is for fecund females (although females are actually subfecund for one to two years after menarche) [39,40]. Hence it is possible, that mixed hebephilic/teleiphilic preference—which has been shown more often in the group of non-convicted CSOs—will be longer "below radar level" than pedophilic preference. However, since the following data is cross-sectional no causal connections are possible.

The present data suggest that incarceration effects are not as prominent as often stated in criticisms about research with convicted subjects. The general criticism that it is difficult or even impossible to interpret data gained by imprisoned groups exclusively can subsequently be put into another perspective. Nonetheless, it is important to keep incarceration effects, environmental effects, and the effect of critical life events such as being convicted in mind.

Relating to the aim of the study to find differences between both groups which might help to decrease the number of CSOs and—more importantly—undetected CSOs, the difference in the number of delicts between non-convicted CSOs and convicted CSOs actually is of high relevance. However, it is important not to interpret the results as a causal relationship between the number of delicts that would lead to incarceration or not.

The presented data is in line with findings from Neutze et al. [20], showing more group similarities than differences between detected and undetected offenders altogether.

Additionally, the present study compared 'resulting' factors of convicted CSOs and non-convicted CSOs. "Preceding" factors are defined as the ones that might influence whether an individual is detected (e.g., age or education) whereas (2) "resulting" ones may either be a response to detection (e.g., emotion-oriented coping, childhood sexual victimization) or reflect a bias in self-report measures (e.g., sexual self-regulation problems, paraphilic interests) in order to avoid negative consequences (e.g., severe punishment). Differences which have been described between convicted and non-convicted CSOs concerning age and education in the study of Neutze et al. [20] (non-convicted CSOs were younger) [20], were not replicated in the present study. Furthermore, the report of suffering more from own childhood victimization in the group of convicted CSO [20] was observable as a marginal significance in the present study. Therefore, the two different sets of factors, proposed by Neutze et al. [20], that are associated with detection status were not observed in the present study. Overall, future research should address these factors.

The consequences of child sexual offending are, as already mentioned, fatal and costly for society (the estimated lifetime economic burden of CSO is approximately $9.3 billion in the US [20]) as well as for children's wellbeing and development [2–4]. Additionally, the devastating effect may persist until adulthood. Thus, emphasis should be laid on preventing offenses. Due to a lack of confidentiality regulations in many countries, offering therapy is only possible after incarceration, i.e., after the crime has not to be concealed anymore. Since therapy may decrease the risk of committing another crime by focusing on dynamic risk factors of offending [27], offering a therapeutic concept to non-convicted CSOs may not only decrease the number of delicts, but it may also reduce the socioeconomic burden and increase the well-being of children. Future research should focus on how preventive approaches may help to reduce the number of offenses.

However, to go one step further offering therapy to non-convicted CSOs might raise the concern that treating this group could lead to better "skills" in hiding crimes and criminal behavior. By working on topics such as behavioral control, social skills, and empathy, non-convicted CSOs might not only learn how to hide a crime better, they may also be able to get better in contacting children and—if so—therapy of non-convicted CSOs might theoretically actively exaggerate the risk of (re)offending. Furthermore, there is a wide discussion in society whether or not offender treatment does more harm than good [41,42]. However, since it is shown in the present study that non-convicted CSOs and convicted CSOs seem to suffer from comparable psychiatric burdens and difficulties, it is unlikely that they will learn skills which may increase their risk of offending. Regarding the fact that detected and undetected CSOs do not differ in clinical characteristics, there is no reason for withholding therapy from undetected CSOs. Moreover, Beier et al. [27] showed that therapy in the German "Dunkelfeld" (dark field) project altered dynamic risk factors for child sexual offending and reduced related behaviors. This knowledge is fundamental to ensure the protection and wellbeing of children and to uncover child sexual abuse as early as possible.

5. Limitations

First of all, participants were recruited as part of the multi-site research project NeMUP, which includes five collaborative research sites from (forensic) psychiatry or sexual medicine located in Berlin, Bochum/Essen, Hanover, Kiel and Magdeburg and did not only include convicted and non-convicted CSOs but also healthy controls and "hands-off" pedophiles who have not committed a crime yet. There were several exclusion criteria which were important for other investigations in the NeMUP consortium but might limit generalizing the results of this study. Those were an intellectual disability, psychotic disorder, current severe major depressive disorder (score greater than 15 on the Hamilton Depression Scale) or anxiety disorder (score greater than 25 in the Hamilton Anxiety Scale), clinically predominant substance misuse or dependence and any psychotropic medication. Subsequently, it is possible that differences between CSOs and non-convicted CSOs vanished not because differences did not exist but because of the early exclusion of offenders with a high psychiatric burden. Future research should include participants with current mental disorders and a high psychiatric burden to ensure differences are not disappearing due to strict inclusion and exclusion criteria. Additionally, the questions asked on recruitment might lead to possible bias such as not detecting pedophiles who are ashamed of "coming out" with their sexual preference or not integrating participants with a high psychiatric burden due to exclusion criteria. Since a large number of participants has been recruited within the "Don't offend"-network this might represent another bias because these subjects are all motivated to undergo psychotherapy.

Another difficulty in the study is the missing detailed data about the crime itself and the crime scene. Due to our quantitative approach, we were not able to include this data as well. However, it is indeed possible that circumstances of the crime and the crime scene are a certain factor for leading to conviction or non-conviction. Circumstances such as sadism or threatening the victim were not included in the analysis. These factors may be important not only for the likelihood of reporting the crime but also for the effort of engaged third parties such as social workers and/or the police. The topic of circumstances of the crime should be taken into consideration for future research. The following paper focuses on the characteristics of the offenders and only a few characteristics of the victims. Since each and every crime has its own characteristics and specifics, it is difficult to investigate the circumstances of a crime by using quantitative research. Concerning alterations in the characteristics of convicted in comparison to non-convicted CSOs, the study only included pedophilic CSOs who are either known by the judicial system, and therefore, convicted or are in the so-called "dark field".

Moreover, the reliance on self-report concerning detection status of non-convicted CSOs might be a problem for analysis. Future research has to find a way of limiting the risk of false-negative responses by the participants due to the possible withholding of information in virtue of shame for being detected. Another limitation is the confinement of the study sample to individuals who applied voluntarily. For that reason, it is possible that differences or similarities between help-seeking offenders and those not seeking help—independent of detection status—may not have been targeted.

Nevertheless, the study design is cross-sectional, and causal connections are therefore prohibited.

Finally, including measurements for socially desirable responding to the procedure of collecting data would be appreciated.

6. Concluding Remark

The study shows effects on a marginally significant level for the number of victims, number of male victims, age of female victims, and self-reported sexual abuse. Additionally, a significant effect for the number of sexual offenses was shown. Hence, convicted CSOs may represent a specific subsample with higher risk and a greater burden of adverse life events though differences appear to be smaller than commonly perceived. The main strength of this study is that it is one of the first focusing on differences between detected and undetected CSOs. Until now, there is only one other study [20] known by the authors that tried to understand which factors may play an important role in the incarceration of CSOs. Because of its design, the study was able to examine differences between those groups.

Author Contributions: Conceptualization, C.G., C.S. and T.H.C.K.; Methodology, C.G., C.S.; Software, C.S.; Validation, C.S., K.M.B., H.W., K.S., J.P., M.W., B.S. and T.H.C.K.; Formal Analysis, C.G., C.S.; Investigation, J.K., T.A., S.M., H.G., A.P., C.F., I.R., C.K., C.M.; Resources, C.G., J.K., T.A., S.M., H.G., A.P., C.F., I.R., C.K., C.M., C.S., K.M.B., H.W., K.S., J.P., M.W., B.S. and T.H.C.K.; Data Curation, C.G.; Writing-Original Draft Preparation, C.G.; Writing-Review & Editing, C.G., C.S., J.K., T.A., S.M., H.G., A.P., C.F., I.R., C.K., C.M., K.M.B., H.W., K.S., J.P., M.W., B.S. and T.H.C.K.; Visualization, C.G. and C.S.; Supervision, C.S., K.M.B., H.W., K.S., J.P., M.W., B.S. and T.H.C.K.; Project Administration, K.M.B., H.W., K.S., J.P., M.W., B.S. and T.H.C.K.; Funding Acquisition, K.M.B., H.W., K.S., J.P., M.W., B.S. and T.H.C.K.

Funding: This research was funded by the Federal Ministry of Education and Research (BMBF). Grant number 01KR1205 to B.S., M.W., K.M.B., H.W., J.P. and T.H.C.K. Parts of the study were also funded by the German Research Foundation (DFG): Schi 1034/3-1 to B.S.

Conflicts of Interest: The authors declare no conflict of interest.

References

1. Stoltenborgh, M.; Van Ijzendoorn, M.H.; Euser, E.M.; Bakermans-Kranenburg, M.J. A global perspective on child sexual abuse: Meta-analysis of prevalence around the world. *Child. Maltreat.* **2011**, *16*, 79–101. [CrossRef]
2. Kessler, R.C.; McLaughlin, K.A.; Green, J.G.; Gruber, M.J.; Sampson, N.A.; Zaslavsky, A.M.; Benjet, C. Childhood adversities and adult psychopathology in the WHO world mental health surveys. *Br. J. Psychiatry.* **2010**, *197*, 378–385. [CrossRef]
3. Tomoda, M.H.; Navalata, A.; Polcary, C.P.; Sadato, A.; Teicher, N. Childhood sexual abuse is associated with reduced gray matter volume in visual cortex of young women. *Biol. Psychiatry* **2009**, *66*, 642–648. [CrossRef]
4. Heim, C.M.; Mayberg, H.S.; Mletzko, T.; Nemeroff, C.B.; Pruessner, J.C. Decreased cortical representation of genital somatosensory field after childhood sexual abuse. *Am. J. Psychiatry* **2013**, *170*, 616–623. [CrossRef]

5. Seto, M.M. *Pedophilia and Sexual Offending Against Children: Theory, Assessment, and Intervention*; American Psychological Association: Washington, DC, USA, 2008.
6. Whitaker, D.J.; Le, B.; Hanson, R.K.; Baker, C.K.; McMahon, P.M.; Ryan, G.; Rice, D.D. Child abuse neglect risk factors for the perpetration of child sexual abuse: A review and meta-analysis. *Child. Abuse Negl.* **2008**, *32*, 529–548. [CrossRef]
7. World Health Organization. *The ICD-10 Classification of Mental and Behavioural Disorders: Clinical Descriptions and Diagnostic Guidelines*; World Health Organization: Geneva, Switzerland, 1992.
8. Dunsieth, N.W., Jr.; Nelson, E.B.; Brusman-Lovins, L.A.; Holcomb, J.L.; Beckman, D.; Welge, J.A.; McElroy, S.L. Psychiatric and legal features of 113 men convicted of sexual offenses. *J. Clin. Psychiatry* **2010**, *65*, 293–300. [CrossRef]
9. Eher, R.; Neuwirth, W.; Fruehwald, S.; Frottier, P. Sexualization and lifestyle impulsivity: Clinically valid discriminators in sexual offenders. *Int. J. Offender Ther. Comp. Criminol.* **2003**, *47*, 452–467. [CrossRef]
10. Gerwinn, H.; Weiß, S.; Tenbergen, G.; Amelung, T.; Födisch, C.; Pohl, A.; Wittfoth, M. Clinical characteristics associated with paedophilia and child sex offending–Differentiating sexual preference from offence status. *Eur. Psychiatry* **2018**, *51*, 74–85. [CrossRef]
11. Cantor, J.M.; Lafaille, S.; Soh, D.W.; Moayedi, M.; Mikulis, D.J.; Girard, T.A. Diffusion tensor imaging of pedophilia. *Arch. Sex. Behav.* **2015**, *44*, 2161–2172. [CrossRef]
12. Kruger, T.H.; Schiffer, B. Neurocognitive and personality factors in homo- and heterosexual pedophiles and controls. *J. Sex. Med.* **2011**, *8*, 1650–1659. [CrossRef]
13. Schiffer, B.; Vonlaufen, C. Executive dysfunctions in pedophilic and nonpedophilic child molesters. *J. Sex. Med.* **2011**, *8*, 1975–1984. [CrossRef]
14. Suchy, Y.; Eastvold, A.D.; Strassberg, D.S.; Franchow, E.I. Understanding processing speed weaknesses among pedophilic child molesters: Response style vs. neuropathology. *J. Abnorm. Psychol.* **2014**, *123*, 273–285. [CrossRef]
15. Mohnke, S.; Mueller, S.; Amelung, T.; Krueger, T.H.; Ponseti, J.; Schiffer, B.; Walter, H. Brain alterations in paedophilia: A critical review. *Prog. Neurobiol.* **2014**, *122*, 1–23. [CrossRef]
16. Kärgel, C.; Massau, C.; Weiß, S.; Walter, M.; Kruger, T.H.; Schiffer, B. Diminished functional connectivity on the road to child sexual abuse in pedophilia. *J. Sex. Med.* **2015**, *12*, 783–795. [CrossRef]
17. Kärgel, C.; Massau, C.; Weiß, S.; Walter, M.; Borchardt, V.; Krueger, T.H.; Gerwinn, H. Evidence for superior neurobiological and behavioral inhibitory control abilities in non-offending as compared to offending pedophiles. *Hum. Brain Mapp.* **2017**, *38*, 1092–1104. [CrossRef]
18. Massau, C.; Tenbergen, G.; Kärgel, C.; Weiß, S.; Gerwinn, H.; Pohl, A.; Ristow, I. Executive functioning in pedophilia and child sexual offending. *J. Int. Neuropsychol. Soc.* **2017**, *23*, 460–470. [CrossRef]
19. Schiffer, B.; Amelung, T.; Pohl, A.; Kaergel, C.; Tenbergen, G.; Gerwinn, H.; Marr, V. Gray matter anomalies in pedophiles with and without a history of child sexual offending. *Transl. Psychiatry* **2017**, *7*, e1129. [CrossRef]
20. Neutze, J.; Grundmann, D.; Scherner, G.; Beier, K.M. Undetected and detected child sexual. *Int. J. Law Psychiatry* **2012**, *35*, 168–175. [CrossRef]
21. Kruger, T.H.; Sinke, C.; Kneer, J.; Tenbergen, G.; Khan, A.Q.; Burkert, A.; Pohl, A. Child sexual offenders show prenatal and epigenetic alterations of the androgen system. *Transl. Psychiatry* **2019**, *9*, 28. [CrossRef]
22. Goodman-Brown, T.B.; Edelstein, R.S.; Goodman, G.S.; Jones, D.P.; Gordon, D.S. Why children tell: A model of children's disclosure of sexual abuse. *Child. Abuse Negl.* **2003**, *27*, 525–540. [CrossRef]
23. Holmes, G.R.; Offen, L.; Waller, G. See no evil, hear no evil, speak no evil: Why do relatively few male victims of childhood sexual abuse receive help for abuse-related issues in adulthood? *Clin. Psychol. Rev.* **1997**, *17*, 69–88. [CrossRef]
24. University of Michigan. *Male Survivors of Sexual Assault*; Sexual Assault Prevention and Awareness Center: Ann Arbor, MI, USA, 2018.
25. Wetzels, P. *Gewalterfahrungen in der Kindheit: Sexueller Missbrauch, Körperliche Misshandlung und Deren langfristige Konsequenzen*; Verlagsgesellschaft: Baden-Baden, Germany, 1997.
26. Stadler, L.; Bieneck, S.; Pfeiffer, C. *Repräsentativbefragung Sexueller Missbrauch 2011*; Kriminologisches Forschungsinstitut: Hannover, Germany, 2012.
27. Beier, K.M.; Grundmann, D.; Kuhle, L.F.; Scherner, G.; Konrad, A.; Amelung, T. The German dunkelfeld project: A pilot study to prevent child sexual abuse and the use of child abusive images. *J. Sex. Med.* **2015**, *12*, 529–542. [CrossRef]

28. Wittchen, H.-U.; Zaudig, M.; Fydrich, T. *SKID. Strukturiertes Klinisches Interview für DSM-IV. Achse I und II. Handanweisung*; Hogrefe Publishing Group: Göttingen, Germany, 1997; p. 3.
29. Martin, N.G.; Kirk, K.; Dunne, M.P.; Bailey, J.M. Measurement models for sexual orientation in a large Australian twin sample. *Behav. Genet.* **1998**, *28*, 475–476.
30. Wechsler, D. *Wechsler Adult Intelligence Scale–Fourth Edition (WAIS–IV)*; The Psychological Corporation: San Antonio, TX, USA, 2008.
31. Wingenfeld, K.; Spitzer, C.; Mensebach, C.; Grabe, H.J.; Hill, A.; Gast, U.; Driessen, M. Die deutsche version des childhood trauma questionnaire (CTQ): Erste befunde zu den psychometrischen Kennwerten. *Psychother. Psychosom. Medizinische Psychol.* **2010**, *60*, 442–450. [CrossRef]
32. Glaesmer, H.; Schulz, A.; Häuser, W.; Freyberger, H.J.; Brähler, E.; Grabe, H.J. Der childhood trauma screener (CTS)-Entwicklung und validierung von Schwellenwerten zur Klassifikation. *Psychiatr. Prax.* **2013**, *40*, 220–226. [CrossRef]
33. Dziobek, I.; Rogers, K.; Fleck, S.; Bahnemann, M.; Heekeren, H.R.; Wolf, O.T.; Convit, A. Dissociation of cognitive and emotional empathy in adults with asperger syndrome using the multifaceted empathy test (MET). *J. Autism Dev. Disord.* **2008**, *38*, 464–473. [CrossRef]
34. Patton, J.H.; Stanford, M.S.; Barratt, E.S. Factor structure of the barratt impulsiveness scale. *J. Clin. Psychol.* **1995**, *51*, 768–774. [CrossRef]
35. Stanford, M.S.; Mathias, C.W.; Dougherty, D.M.; Lake, S.L.; Anderson, N.E.; Patton, J.H. Fifty years of the barratt impulsiveness scale: An update and review. *Pers. Individ. Dif.* **2009**, *47*, 385–395. [CrossRef]
36. Hellerbach, A. *Phantomentwicklung und Einführung einer systematischen Qualitätssicherung bei multizentrischen Magnetresonanztomographie-Untersuchungen*; Philipps-Universität: Marburg, Germany, 2013.
37. Ashburner, J.; Barnes, G.; Chen, C.; Daunizeau, J.; Flandin, G.; Friston, K.; Penny, W. *SPM12 Manual*; The FIL Methods Group: London, UK, 2013.
38. IBM Corp. *IBM SPSS Statistics for Windows, Version 24.0*; IBM Corp.: Armonk, NY, USA, 2016.
39. Blanchard, R.; Lykins, A.D.; Wherrett, D.; Kuban, M.E.; Cantor, J.M.; Blak, T.; Klassen, P.E. Pedophilia, Hebephilia, and the DSM-V. *Arch. Sex. Behav.* **2009**, *38*, 335–350. [CrossRef]
40. Wood, J.W. *Dynamics of Human Reproduction*, 1st ed.; Routledge: New York, NY, USA, 1994.
41. Wolf, C. Was bringt die Therapie von Sexualstraftätern? *Spektrum.* 2018. Available online: https://www.spektrum.de/news/was-bringt-die-therapie-von-sexualstraftaetern/1605646 (accessed on 13 February 2019).
42. Friedrichsen, G. Strafjustiz: Noch gefährlicher durch Therapie. *Der Spiegel.* 2002. Available online: http://www.spiegel.de/spiegel/print/d-25554388.html (accessed on 13 February 2019).

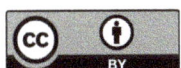

© 2019 by the authors. Licensee MDPI, Basel, Switzerland. This article is an open access article distributed under the terms and conditions of the Creative Commons Attribution (CC BY) license (http://creativecommons.org/licenses/by/4.0/).

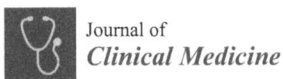

Article

Frequency of Sexual Dysfunction in Patients Treated with Desvenlafaxine: A Prospective Naturalistic Study

Angel L. Montejo [1,2,*], Joemir Becker [2], Gloria Bueno [3], Raquel Fernández-Ovejero [4], María T. Gallego [2], Nerea González [5], Adrián Juanes [6], Laura Montejo [7], Antonio Pérez-Urdániz [2,3], Nieves Prieto [2,3] and José L. Villegas [2]

1. Nursing School E.U.E.F., University of Salamanca, 37004 Salamanca, Spain
2. Instituto de Investigación Biomédica de Salamanca, Servicio de Psiquiatría, Hospital Universitario de Salamanca, 37007 IBSAL, Spain; jbecker@saludcastillayleon.es (J.B.); mtgallego@saludcastillayleon.es (M.T.G.); perurdan@ono.com (A.P.-U.); nprietom@saludcastillayleon.es (N.P.); jlvillegas@saludcastillayleon.es (J.L.V.)
3. Departamento de Psiquiatría, Universidad de Salamanca, 37004 Salamanca, Spain; gloriabueno@usal.es
4. Servicio Navarro de Salud, 31008 Osasunbidea, Spain; rqfo25@gmail.com
5. Departamento de Estadística, Universidad de Salamanca, 37004 Salamanca, Spain; nerea_gonzalez_garcia@usal.es
6. Atención Primaria de Salamanca, 37900 SACYL, Spain; ajuanesd@yahoo.es
7. Barcelona Bipolar and Depressive Disorders Program, Institute of Neurosciences, University of Barcelona, IDIBAPS, CIBERSAM, Hospital Clinic of Barcelona, 08401 Catalonia, Spain; laumonteg@gmail.com
* Correspondence: amontejo@usal.es; Tel.: +34-639-754-620

Received: 29 March 2019; Accepted: 16 May 2019; Published: 21 May 2019

Abstract: Despite being clinically underestimated, sexual dysfunction (SD) is one of the most frequent and lasting adverse effects associated with antidepressants. Desvenlafaxine is an antidepressant (AD) with noradrenergic and serotonergic action that can cause a lower SD than other serotonergic ADs although there are still few studies on this subject. Objective: To check the frequency of SD in two groups of depressive patients: one group was desvenlafaxine-naïve; the other was made up of patients switched to desvenlafaxine from another AD due to iatrogenic sexual dysfunction. A naturalistic, multicenter, and prospective study of patients receiving desvenlafaxine (50–100 mg/day) was carried out on 72 patients who met the inclusion criteria (>18 years old and sexually active), who had received desvenlafaxine for the first time ($n = 27$) or had switched to desvenlafaxine due to SD with another AD ($n = 45$). Patients with previous SD, receiving either drugs or presenting a concomitant pathology that interfered with their sexual life and/or patients who abused alcohol and/or drugs were excluded. We used the validated Psychotropic-Related Sexual Dysfunction Questionnaire (PRSexDQ-SALSEX) to measure AD-related sexual dysfunction and the Clinical Global Impression Scale for psychiatric disease (CGI-S) and for sexual dysfunction (CGI-SD) at two points in time: baseline and three months after the commencement of desvenlafaxine treatment. Results: In desvenlafaxine-naïve patients, 59.2% of the sample showed moderate/severe sexual dysfunction at baseline, which was reduced to 44% at follow-up. The PSexDQ-SALSEX questionnaire total score showed a significant improvement in sexual desire and sexual arousal without changes in orgasmic function at follow-up ($p < 0.01$). In the group switched to desvenlafaxine, the frequency of moderate/severe SD at baseline (93.3%) was reduced to 75.6% at follow-up visit. Additionally, SD significantly improved in three out of four items of the SALSEX: low desire, delayed orgasm, and anorgasmia at follow-up ($p < 0.01$), but there was no significant improvement in arousal difficulties. The frequency of severe SD was reduced from 73% at baseline to 35% at follow-up. The CGI for psychiatric disease and for sexual dysfunction improved significantly in both groups ($p < 0.01$). There was a poor tolerability with risk of treatment noncompliance in 26.7% of patients with sexual dysfunction due to another AD, this significantly reduced to 11.1% in those who switched to desvenlafaxine ($p = 0.004$). Conclusion: Sexual dysfunction improved significantly in depressed patients who initiated treatment with desvenlafaxine and in those who switched from another AD to desvenlafaxine, despite this, desvenlafaxine treatment is not completely devoid of sexual adverse effects. This switching strategy could be highly relevant in clinical practice due to the significant improvement in moderate/severe and poorly tolerated SD, while maintaining the AD efficacy.

Keywords: desvenlafaxine; sexual dysfunction; antidepressant; treatment; prsexdq-salsex questionnaire; switching strategy

1. Introduction

Sexual dysfunction (SD) is one of the most frequent and lasting adverse effects caused by serotonergic antidepressants (ADs). However, unfortunately, it is underestimated in the data elaborated by pharmaceutical companies in post-registration studies, where frequencies of 2–16% are reflected [1,2], much lower than those found in specific case series studies [3–5], systematic reviews [6,7], and meta-analyses [8]. The reasons for this underestimation could be that the frequency of SD is obtained from clinical trials designed to find efficacy; these are usually unreliable short-term studies because they can include either sexually inactive patients or lack specific sexual dysfunction questionnaires, counting only spontaneous communications of sexual adverse events.

The real prevalence of SD secondary to treatment with ADs calculated in clinical practice is much higher, as has been demonstrated in studies including long series of patients [9,10]. Using specific questionnaires such as the Psychotropic-Related Sexual Dysfunction Questionnaire (PRSexDQ-SALSEX) [11,12] or the Changes in Sexual Function Questionnaire (CSFQ) [13], a prevalence of SD secondary to Selective Serotonin Reuptake Inhibitors (SSRI) of between 50–79% in sexually active patients has been shown [14–17], increasing to more than 80% in healthy volunteers who received SSRI for at least eight weeks [18,19].

In a recent study using the PRSexDQ-SALSEX to evaluate the frequency and tolerance of sexual dysfunction in the majority of ADs approved for the treatment of depression, such as SSRI, serotonin-noradrenaline reuptake inhibitors (SNRIs), clomipramine, agomelatine, bupropion, and mirtazapine, 79% patients showed sexual dysfunction, as indicated by a total score ≥3 on the PRSexDQ-SALSEX; 64% showed moderate-severe sexual dysfunction, with no differences between men and women on these outcomes [5]. Sexual dysfunction is extremely common in patients receiving ADs, especially serotonergic ones, with a significantly lower frequency of SD associated with non-serotonergic ADs such as mirtazapine, agomelatine, and bupropion. The consequences of this adverse side effect range from the deterioration of the quality of life to quitting treatment due to the sexual dysfunction which occurs in 20–35% of patients [15,20], with the consequent risk of relapse and other negative repercussions related to depression [21,22].

The most common symptoms of SD are a decrease in desire and a delay in achieving orgasm. Erectile dysfunction is less common, although paroxetine, citalopram, and venlafaxine produce it in about 30–40% of patients at usual therapeutic doses [1,5,13,20]. Anorgasmia or lack of ejaculation is the worst side effect tolerated by patients [15]. Unfortunately, SDs are rarely examined routinely by physicians and only 15–40% of patients report it spontaneously, despite the high frequency observed in those treated with AD [1,5,13,15] and with antipsychotics [23,24]. Therefore, it is necessary to use specific questionnaires to detect SDs and its influence on the quality of life of the patient and his/her partner in the short, medium, and long term. This feature of sexual tolerability should be considered carefully in the selection of an AD [25].

Other ADs, with non-serotonergic mechanisms of action (agomelatine, mirtazapine, bupropion) have been shown to produce little deterioration in the sexuality of patients in controlled studies compared to serotonergic ADs in medium- and long-term case series [26–29]. However, it might be possible that the clinical effect of non-serotonergic compounds was insufficient in some groups of patients in need for a serotonergic effect to deal with symptoms such as obsessive-compulsive behavior or in severely depressed patients.

Dual SNRIs, mixed inhibitors of the reuptake of serotonin and noradrenaline (duloxetine and desvenlafaxine), may have a lower frequency of SD, although there are contradictory data regarding this in several studies with varying designs [15,30]. The evidence for mirtazapine having an advantage over selective serotonin reuptake inhibitors (SSRIs) is lacking and there are currently not sufficient data as regards the effects of desvenlafaxine. Usually, sexual function data come from clinical trials on efficacy which include moderately depressed patients and do not select the trial population according to inclusion and exclusion criteria in terms of prior activity and sexual satisfaction.

Well-designed comparative studies of present ADs with a direct assessment of sexual side effects as the primary outcome measure are scarce [31]. On the other hand, ADs can improve sexual function in depressed patients. There is less frequency of SD in patients who respond better to treatment compared to those who do not significantly improve in the medium and long term [15]. With respect to this, the effect of duloxetine on the patient's sexual life seems to be linked to the AD effect. SD is more frequent in populations that show a lower response to ADs compared to those that respond adequately [32]. On the other hand, vortioxetine, with a serotonergic, noradrenergic, and dopaminergic multimodal mechanism of action, seems to be associated with lower SD according to the data derived from clinical registration trials [33,34] and a specific study of switching to vortioxetine due to sexual dysfunction [35]; however, additional data obtained with naturalistic designs in real clinical practice are needed to corroborate this.

The SD managing approach includes dose reduction, the addition of an antidote, such as an inhibitor of phosphodiesterase type 5 (IPD5) if there is erectile dysfunction, AD withdrawal for 24–48 h before intercourse in the case of anorgasmia, and a change of treatment to another non-serotonergic AD [5,36–38]. None of these methods are free from risk, which can include relapses or the appearance of new adverse side effects concomitant to the change of treatment. Therefore, it is necessary to adequately clarify the role that different ADs play in the appearance of SD and the deterioration of the quality of life that they can produce in the patient. To start with, drugs that do not have deteriorating effects on sexual life in sexually active patients should always be taken into account in patients with depression. On the other hand, given that SD is more frequent with some ADs, it should always be considered in the investigation of new molecules, seeking better tolerability profiles in the medium and long term [39].

There are still few studies that specifically analyze the influence of desvenlafaxine on the sexual function of patients. The risk of SD associated with desvenlafaxine treatment has been studied in a post-hoc analysis of a clinical trial compared to placebo using the ASEX. After 12 weeks, orgasm delay was observed at a higher rate than placebo in men, but not in women. Other sexual functions such as desire and arousal were not affected [40]. In another randomized double-blind study, no differences were found between desvenlafaxine (50–100 mg) and placebo [41]. The data suggest that there could be higher SD with 100 mg/day, but these data were not conclusive since no statistically significant differences were obtained. After an integrated analysis of short-term, randomized, double-blind, placebo-controlled registration studies for major depressive disorder (50–400 mg/day) with desvenlafaxine vs. placebo for eight weeks, very few adverse sexual effects were found with desvenlafaxine: erectile dysfunction in men (7% vs. 1% with placebo) and anorgasmia in women (1% vs. 0%) [42]. This low frequency of SD data does not seem to be in line with what was expected of a drug with a serotonergic mechanism of action. This could be due to the fact that these studies were not specifically designed to find differences in sexual function with samples properly selected using inclusion and exclusion criteria, or because only spontaneous communications were taken into account over a short period of eight weeks.

Until now, there have been hardly any naturalistic studies specifically designed to evaluate the SD associated with desvenlafaxine under the conditions of usual clinical practice. The methodology, to obtain adequate results, should include patients with a previous active sexual life and lack of another pathology or concomitant medication that might affect sexual function, in order to determine the causality that the drug (and not other associated factors) plays in the possible dysfunction of sexual life.

In a recent study with a naturalistic design in patients with depression or anxiety disorder treated with fluoxetine, mirtazapine, escitalopram, sertraline, and desvenlafaxine, the sexual function of 209 patients was evaluated using the PRSexDQ-SALSEX questionnaire at baseline and at six weeks. Twenty-one percent showed sexual dysfunction at the beginning of treatment and this increased to 41% in week 6. With regard to individual questionnaire items, by week 6, sexual desire improved, but erectile and ejaculatory function in men and orgasmic function in women worsened. Fluoxetine and sertraline were associated with impaired sexual function, whereas mirtazapine was associated with favorable sexual function. At week 2, mirtazapine and desvenlafaxine were predictors of favorable sexual outcome. Additionally, sexual dysfunction was more frequent in men than in women [43].

The main goal of this study is to evaluate the frequency of SD in patients treated with desvenlafaxine under usual clinical practice conditions using two independent groups: the first one with new patients, desvenlafaxine-naïve, defined as patients who never before received an AD treatment, and the second group with patients who were changed to desvenlafaxine due to experiencing SD secondary to another AD.

2. Experimental Section

A naturalistic, multicenter, prospective study was conducted in patients treated with desvenlafaxine (at a dose as recommended by the data sheet and usual clinical practice of 50–100 mg/day) or another AD. We included 72 patients who met the inclusion and exclusion criteria into two groups: group A, desvenlafaxine-naïve, with 27 patients receiving desvenlafaxine for the first time, and group B, with 45 patients switched to desvenlafaxine for presenting SD caused by another AD.

2.1. Study Population

Inclusion and exclusion criteria were used to guarantee the validity of the sample, avoiding possible confounding factors. Patients were consecutively included if they fulfilled the following inclusion criteria for group A (desvenlafaxine-naïve): over 18 years old, sexually active (defined as at least one sexual activity in the last six months), who started treatment with desvenlafaxine 50–100 mg/day according to usual clinical practice. The following inclusion criteria were used for group B (switched to desvenlafaxine): over 18 years old, receiving treatment with AD for at least eight weeks prior, a history of self-reported normal sexual functioning before the prescription of the AD, excluding a mildly impaired libido (libido impairment is part of the depressive symptoms). Exclusion criteria: patient receiving more than one AD or requiring concomitant treatment that may influence sexual activity (antipsychotics, antihypertensives, beta-blockers, sex hormones, opiates), alcohol and/or drug abuse and serious medical illness that could cause sexual dysfunction. Patients were allowed to receive treatment with benzodiazepines. In the baseline visit, information on patient demographics, psychiatric history, and the treatments that the patient was receiving were recorded.

2.2. Measurement Scales

Sexual function was evaluated with the Psychotropic-Related Sexual Dysfunction Questionnaire (PRSexDQ-SALSEX), which has shown good psychometric properties both in patients with depression [9] and in patients with schizophrenia [10]. In patients with depression, the PRSexDQ-SALSEX has shown adequate internal consistency, with a Cronbach's alpha value of 0.93, and adequate construct validity [9]. As may be expected, the PRSexDQ-SALSEX showed a high correlation with the Clinical Global Impression Scale for sexual dysfunction ($r = 0.79$) and a moderate correlation with Hamilton Depression Rating Scale scores ($r = 0.63$). The PRSexDQ-SALSEX also showed good discrimination between naïve and pretreated depressed or dysthymic patients, with statistically significant differences between those groups of patients. In brief, the PRSexDQ-SALSEX has seven questions, and is hetero-applied by the evaluator. The first two questions use a yes/no format to record whether patients have noticed any change in their sexual function since they initiated treatment and whether the sexual dysfunction was spontaneously reported. The next four questions (items 1 to 4) employ a four-point scale, from no problem to severe problem, to assess the presence and severity of decreased libido, delayed ejaculation/orgasm, lack of ejaculation/orgasm, and difficulties with having or maintaining erection/lubrication. The last question (item 5) evaluates the tolerability of the changes in sexual functioning on a four point scale: 0, No sexual dysfunction; 1, Well, no problem due to this reason; 2, Fair, the dysfunction bothers him or her, although he or she has not considered discontinuing the treatment for this reason, or it interferes with the couple's relationship; 3, Poor, the dysfunction presents an important problem, and he or she has considered discontinuing treatment because of it, or it seriously interferes with the couple's relationship. These five latter items (i.e., items 1 to 5) account for the total score of the PRSexDQ-SALSEX, which ranges from 0 to 15. According to this total score, patients may be categorized as having no sexual dysfunction (a score of 0 or the item 1 (libido) scoring 1 and the item 5 (tolerability) scoring 1), or having mild (total score of 3–5) dysfunction, provided that no item scores ≥ 2 (i.e., provided that the patient does not have moderate sexual dysfunction in a specific dimension), moderate (total score of 6–10 or an item scoring 2, provided that no item scores 3 (i.e., provided that the patient does not have severe sexual dysfunction in a specific dimension)) or severe (total score of 11–15 or an item scoring 3) sexual dysfunction.

The severity of the psychiatric disorder was evaluated at baseline with the 7-point Clinical Global Impression of Severity Scale (CGI) [44], as well as the CGI of Sexual Dysfunction (CGI-SD), which is a clinician-rated instrument identical to the CGI used for the assessment of psychopathology. Additionally, a 7-point CGI of Change scale was used for psychiatric severity (CGI-CS) [44] and for sexual dysfunction (CGI-CSD) in the follow-up visit, three months after the baseline visit. The research team consisted of eight researchers previously trained in the application of SALSEX belonging to the Department of psychiatry of the University Hospital of Salamanca (seven psychiatrists) and the Primary Care Service of Salamanca (one general practitioner) between June 2015 and June 2016.

2.3. Ethical Aspects

The protocol was favorably evaluated by the Research Ethics Committee of Salamanca (CEIC) in November 2014. It was classified by the Spanish Agency for Medicines and Healthcare Products (AEMPS) as a post-authorization study with prospective follow-up (EPA-SP study) and was authorized later by the General Directorate of Public Health of Castilla y León, dated February 2015, with the code AMG-DES-2014-01. All patients signed an informed consent following the international norms and procedures of medical research in humans using the declaration of Helsinki of the World Medical Association of 1964.

2.4. Sample Size

There are no specific published data so far to estimate the sample size based on the effect size. There is only a post-hoc analysis of a pivotal clinical trial in which desvenlafaxine did not show any significant difference vs. placebo in the mean change of ASEX scale at endpoint (12 weeks of treatment), with a mean reduction in ASEX of -1.13 (SD = 0.47) in the males group and -1.93 (SD = 0.37) in the females group treated with desvenlafaxine [40]. This is not a study primarily designed to evaluate sexual functioning and its design presents relevant differences to the design of our study, so the values needed to calculate sample size are not available. We have therefore considered this as a pilot study to evaluate the changes in sexual functioning assessed with the PRSexDQ-SALSEX questionnaire, with mean change global score as the main outcome, estimating a sample size of 50 subjects (25 per group) to detect differences in sexual functioning after three months of treatment with desvenlafaxine. A study withdrawal rate of 15% was assumed.

2.5. Statistical Analysis

Valid data were analyzed from the database which was created ad-hoc. The main variable "mean change in PRSexDQ-SALSEX global score from baseline to follow-up visit" and secondary variables "mean change in PRSexDQ-SALSEX global score at follow-up visit", "mean change in each item of PRSexDQ-SALSEX score at follow-up visit", and "mean change in all CGIs" were analyzed. The distribution of the quantitative variables was examined using the Kolmogorov–Smirnov test. Later, they were described using mean and standard deviation (mean ± standard deviation (sd)) in the case of data that followed the normal distribution, otherwise, median and interquartile range (the first quartile subtracted from the third quartile) (median ± IQR) were used. The differences between independent groups of quantitative variables were evaluated using the Student's t-test for data of normal distribution, or otherwise using the non-parametric Mann–Whitney U test. The differences in the response to quantitative variables between paired groups were examined using the Student's t-test for paired data (for normally distributed variables) or the Wilcoxon test (for non-parametric data). The descriptive analysis of categorical qualitative variables was carried out through frequencies and percentages. Chi-square test and Fisher's exact test were used to analyze the association of qualitative variables. The statistical package SPSS, version 22.0, (IBM Corporation, Armonk, NY, USA) was used for the statistical analysis, with strict quality control procedures. The results were considered significant if $p < 0.05$.

3. Results

3.1. Study Population

Initially, 109 patients were included, of whom 37 did not attend the follow-up visit (nine in group A and 28 in group B, 10 men and 27 women), so they were lost for the study. Finally, 72 patients were included (52 women and 20 men) with a mean age of 43.4 ± 11.8 diagnosed with affective pathology (major depression, single episode, 47.2%, recurrent major depression, 12.5%, anxious depressive disorder, 8.3%, dysthymia, 13.9%, adaptive disorder, 8.3% and others, 9.8%). They were diagnosed following the International Classification of Diseases 10th Revision (ICD-10) criteria [45]. Of the total of patients who completed the study, 37.5% were from group A (desvenlafaxine-naïve) and the remaining 62.5% were from group B (changed to desvenlafaxine from a different AD). Group A consisted of 27 patients (22 women and 5 men, average age 42.7 ± 10.9) and group B of 45 patients (30 women and 15 men, average age 43.87 ± 12.34). The patients switched to desvenlafaxine coming from other previous treatments consisted of 16 patients with escitalopram (36%), 10 duloxetine (22%); 6 venlafaxine (13%); 5 sertraline (11%); 4 paroxetine (9%); 4 Fluoxetine (9%). In 52.3% of the cases, a gradual change was made, and in the rest of the cases, a sudden change was made to clinical criteria without using a washout period.

3.2. SALSEX Questionnaire

The spontaneous communication of SD (item B of SALSEX) occurred in 27.3% of patients in group A and in 35% of group B. The overall SALSEX results for group A and B are shown in Table 1.

In group A, an overall global SALSEX score was obtained at the baseline visit of 5.4 ± 4.3 (with 0 = no SD and 15 = maximum dysfunction), indicating a degree of mild/moderate initial SD in the sample of desvenlafaxine-naïve patients. The overall score on the SALSEX scale between the baseline (5.4 ± 4.3) and follow-up visit (3.9 ± 3.6) was reduced in a highly significant way ($p = 0.007$) (Figure 1), showing a clinical improvement in the sexual function of patients who started treatment with desvenlafaxine at follow-up. In the desvenlafaxine-naïve group, the intensity of the SD was reduced by 28%.

Table 1. Descriptive statistics of SALSEX questionnaire of groups A and B. Baseline vs. follow-up visit.

	Group A. Desvenlafaxine-Naïve			Group B. Switched to Desvenlafaxine		
	Baseline	Follow-Up Visit	*p*-Value	Baseline	Follow-Up Visit	*p*-Value
SALSEX total	5.4 (4.3)	3.9 (3.6)	0.007 **	9.6 (3.6)	6.8 (3.9)	0.000 **
Libido Decreased	1 (2)	1 (1)	0.039 *	3 (2)	2 (2)	0.000 **
Orgasm delayed	0 (2)	0 (1)	0.429	2 (1)	2 (1)	0.001 **
Anorgasmia	1 (2)	1 (1)	0.206	2 (1.5)	1 (1.5)	0.000 **
Arousal problems	1 (2)	0 (2)	0.004 **	2 (1)	1 (2)	0.069
Tolerability of SD	1 (2)	1 (2)	0.003 **	2 (1)	1 (1)	0.002 **

** = highly significant *p*-value (<0.01); * = significant *p*-value (<0.05).

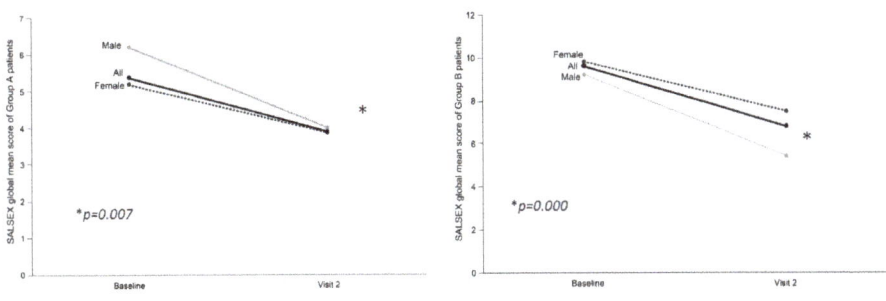

Group A (desvenlafaxine-naïve patients). Group B (patients switched from another antidepressant).

Figure 1. Differences in overall sexual function from baseline at three months in patients treated with desvenlafaxine.

Patients in group B (changed to desvenlafaxine) obtained a global average score on the SALSEX scale at the baseline visit of 9.6 ± 3.6 and 6.8 ± 3.9 in the follow-up visit, resulting in this highly significant difference ($p = 0.000$) (Figure 1). The improvement in overall sexual function measured with total SALSEX was greater in group B (all patients suffered from SD secondary to previous treatment) as their initial SD was reduced by 36% in the second visit.

Taking into account the total score of the SALSEX, the severity of the SD was distributed into several groups: mild (Salsex = 1–5 points); moderate (Salsex = 6–10 or any item = 2); and intense (Salsex = 11–15 or any item = 3). Desvenlafaxine-naïve patients showed a significant decrease in severe SD at follow-up (11 patients in baseline vs. 5 patients in the follow-up visit) ($p < 0.05$) (Figure 2). In group B of patients changed to desvenlafaxine, there was a decrease in the group of intense SD from the baseline visit (32 patients in the baseline vs. 17 in the follow-up visit) ($p < 0.05$).

The overall frequency of baseline SD (defined as SALSEX score ≥3) was 74% of 27 patients in group A desvenlafaxine-naïve (14.8% mild, 18.5% moderate, and 40.7% intense) and 70.3% at follow-up (mild 25.9%, moderate 25.9%, and intense 18.5%). In desvenlafaxine-naïve patients, 59.2% of the sample showed clinically relevant (moderate/severe) sexual dysfunction at baseline that was reduced to 44% at follow-up. A similar global frequency was observed in SD from the beginning but with a significant decrease in intensity ($p = 0.045$), reducing the percentage of cases with severe SD. In group B, the overall frequency of SD was 100% at baseline (6.7% mild, 22.2% moderate, and 71.1% intense), decreasing to 91.2% at follow-up (15.6% mild, 37.8% moderate, and 37.8% intense). In this group, the frequency of clinically relevant (moderate/severe) SD at baseline (93.3%) was reduced to 75.6% at follow-up. A significant reduction in the intensity of SD after switching to desvenlafaxine was observed ($p = 0.011$).

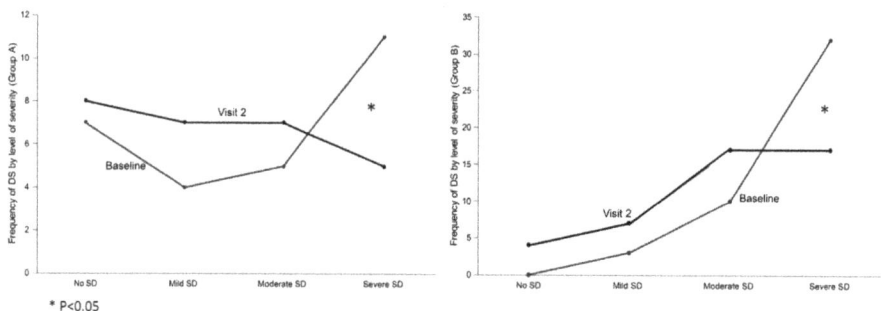

Figure 2. Differences in sexual level of severity from baseline at three months in patients treated with desvenlafaxine.

3.2.1. Gender Differences

Analyzing the differences between men and women, significant improvements were found in the overall SALSEX scale in both men and women for the two treatment groups (Table 2 and Figure 3). The overall improvement was more intense in men of both groups (a 38% improvement in group A in the follow-up visit and 41.3% in group B), although it is necessary to take into account that the sample of men is much lower in the study and this can influence the results (52 females vs. 20 males).

Table 2. Gender differences. Global SALSEX score of groups A and B, at baseline and follow-up.

	SALSEX TOTAL Score		
	Baseline Median (IR)	Follow-Up Visit Median (IR)	p-Value
Group A			
Male ($n = 5$)	8 (10.5)	4 (6)	0.000 **
Female ($n = 22$)	6 (8.25)	3 (7)	0.043 *
Group B			
Male ($n = 15$)	10 (8)	5 (9)	0.000 **
Female ($n = 30$)	11 (3.25)	8 (5.25)	0.001 **

** = highly significant p-value (<0.01); * = significant p-value (<0.05).

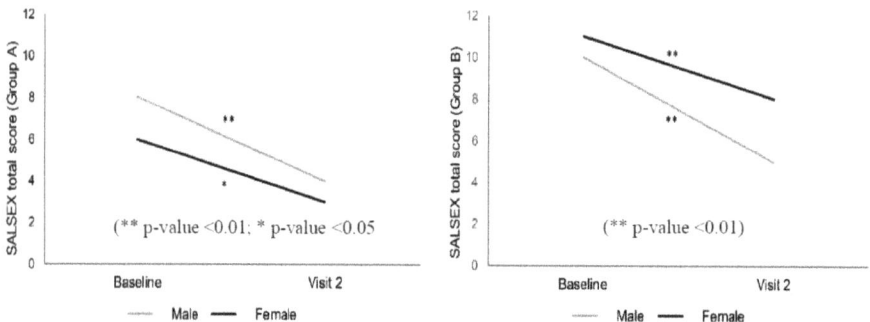

Figure 3. Gender differences in overall sexual function from baseline at three months in patients treated with desvenlafaxine.

3.2.2. Differences by Dose

The patients in the study mostly received doses of 50 mg/day and 100 mg/day of desvenlafaxine. The mean dose of group A was 53.7 ± 13.3 mg/day at the baseline visit and 63.7 ± 24.7 at follow-up. Patients in group B received doses of 62.5 ± 22.1 mg/day of desvenlafaxine at the baseline visit and 63.44 ± 26.39 mg/day at follow-up. In group A, 92.6% ($n = 25$) of them received a dose of 50 mg/day and the remaining 7.4% ($n = 2$), a dose of 100 mg/day at the baseline visit; while in the follow-up visit 66.7% ($n = 18$) and 29.6% ($n = 8$) of them received doses of 50 and 100 mg, respectively. In the case of patients in group B, at the baseline visit, 75% of patients ($n = 18$) received a dose of 50 mg/day and the remaining 25% ($n = 6$), a dose of 100 mg/day. At follow-up, 60% of patients ($n = 27$) received a dose of 50 mg/day, while only 28.9% ($n = 13$) received a dose of 100 mg/day. The possible association between desvenlafaxine dose and PRSexDQ-SALSEX global score was examined. In this sense, there were no statistically significant differences in the overall PRSexDQ-SALSEX scale score in the baseline visit or in the follow-up visit between those who received a dose of 50 mg/day and those who received a dose of 100 mg/day in any of the two groups of patients. At the descriptive level, overall SALSEX scores were lower in those patients who received a higher dose of desvenlafaxine, although the percentage of cases that received a dose of 100 mg/day of desvenlafaxine was very small and conclusive results cannot be extracted regarding this.

3.2.3. Analysis of the PRSexDQ-SALSEX Dimensions

The analysis of the individual items in the desvenlafaxine-naïve group showed that no worsening was observed in any of the items in the follow-up visit compared with the baseline visit. On the contrary, there was a significant improvement in desire ($p = 0.039$) and in sexual arousal ($p = 0.004$) without significant change in orgasm, so we can say that sexual affectation by desvenlafaxine in the studied sample is scarce (Figure 4).

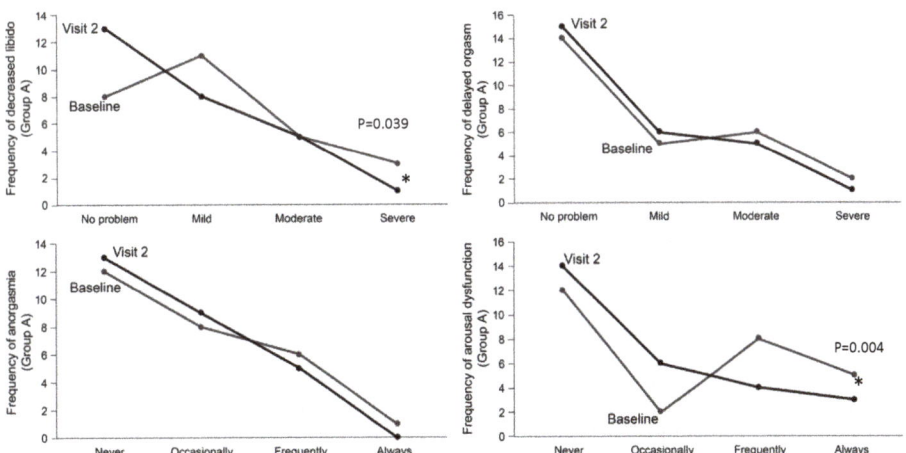

Figure 4. Group A. Desvenlafaxine-naïve patients. Changes in sexual functioning at follow-up.

In patients that switched to desvenlafaxine, significant improvements in sexual desire, delayed orgasm, and anorgasmia appear in the follow-up visit ($p = 0.001$). Regarding the item of arousal difficulty (erection in males and vaginal lubrication in women), no significant differences were found ($p = 0.69$) (Figure 5).

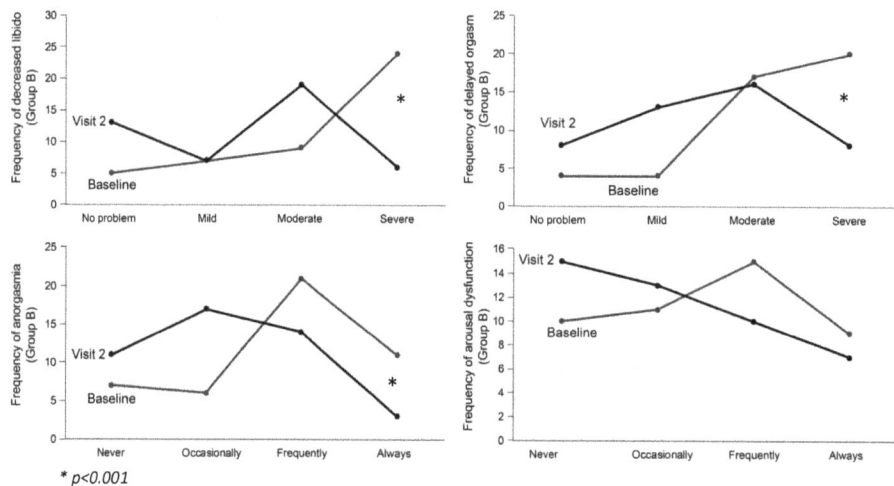

Figure 5. Group B. Patients switched to desvenlafaxine. Changes in sexual functioning at follow-up.

3.2.4. Tolerability of Sexual Dysfunction

Item 5 of the SALSEX measures the tolerability and patient acceptance of SD by means of an intensity scale in which "1 = Tolerates the SD well", "2 = Tolerates the SD with some difficulties although has not thought of dropping out of the treatment for this reason" and "3 = Tolerates the SD poorly, with it affecting his/her relationship with partner and/or has considered dropping out of the treatment for this reason". Regarding the patients who tolerated the SD poorly and who were at risk of noncompliance (item 5 = 3) in the two groups, an improvement in the tolerability of the SD at the baseline visit was observed compared with the follow-up visit ($p = 0.002$) (18.5% of baseline poor tolerability vs. 0% in the follow-up visit in desvenlafaxine-naïve group), significantly decreasing the risk of dropouts for this reason. Similarly, patients switched to desvenlafaxine showed poor tolerability with a risk of dropout at baseline in 26.7% of cases, which significantly reduced to 11.1% at the follow-up visit ($p = 0.004$).

3.3. Clinical Global Impression Scales

In the scale of severity of psychiatric pathology (CGI), significant improvements were observed in both groups (group A: $p = 0.000$, group B: $p = 0.003$). Therefore, it can be considered that patients treated with desvenlafaxine showed a significant improvement in clinical situation, both when used as a starting treatment or when switching from another AD. The CGI scale of SD intensity (CGI-SD), coinciding with the results of PRSexDQ-SALSEX, showed no changes in the desvenlafaxine-naïve group but a significant improvement in the intensity of SD in patients switched to desvenlafaxine due to SD ($p = 0.000$); therefore, it can be deduced that the improvement in SD is also accompanied by improvements in the clinical situation (Table 3).

Table 3. Clinical Global Impression of Severity Scale (CGI) scores of groups A and B, comparing baseline and follow-up visit values.

	Group A. Desvenlafaxine-Naïve			Group B. Switched to Desvenlafaxine		
	Baseline	Follow-Up Visit	*p*-Value	Baseline	Follow-Up Visit	*p*-Value
CGI Depression	4 (1.3)	1 (1)	0.000 **	3 (1)	2 (2)	0.003 **
CGI Sexual Dysfunction	3 (3)	3 (2)	0.539	5 (1)	3 (1.8)	0.000 **

** = highly significant *p*-value (<0.01).

4. Discussion

The results of this naturalistic and prospective study show that sexual functioning improved in both patient groups (desvelafaxine-naïve patients and those switched to desvenlafaxine from another AD) measured by the overall score of the SALSEX scale. Contrary to what usually occurs in patients treated with serotonergic drugs who present a high frequency of SD, treatment with desvenlafaxine, which has a dual serotonergic and noradrenergic mechanism of action, was associated with a moderate/severe deterioration (clinically significant) in sexual functioning in 44.4% of sexually active patients who started treatment with desvenlafaxine. It is interesting that in contrast to the figures obtained in a recent study carried out with the same methodology using the PRSexDQ-SALSEX, the frequency of moderate/severe SD was higher (66% with SSRI and 75% with SNRIs (venlafaxine, and duloxetine)) [15]. In this study, desvenlafaxine presents a much more favorable profile associated with SD in desvenlafaxine-naïve patients (44.4%) despite having a mechanism of mixed serotonergic and noradrenergic action and so being considered in the group of dual ADs.

This lower deterioration of sexual function compared with other studies on serotonergic ADs that impair sexual function (as is widely described in the literature [13,19,21]) can be very relevant when choosing a drug with dual effects but with a lower ability to influence sexual functioning. In contrast to venlafaxine, which has shown a high frequency of sexual dysfunction in comparative studies including series of cases measured with the same PRSexDQ-SALSEX questionnaire [13,15], desvenlafaxine, the primary metabolite of venlafaxine, has a much lower frequency of sexual dysfunction, which could be due to the fact that desvenlafaxine is also a relatively low potency 5-HT and NE reuptake inhibitor. The lower pharmacodynamic potency in the reuptake of serotonin compared to venlafaxine might be linked to the lower effect in the dopaminergic brake, mediated by serotonin, associated with sexual dysfunction. Recently, it has been shown that paroxetine, a potent inhibitor of serotonin reuptake, influences the mechanism of AD-related sexual dysfunction through the inhibition of tyrosine hydroxylase in dopaminergic neurons related to sexual areas such as substantia nigra, pars compacta, and the ventral tegmental area but not with agomelatine in male rats [46].

In the group of patients switched to desvenlafaxine, with previous SD secondary to treatment with another AD (SSRI or SNRI), an improvement in the frequency of moderate/severe SD was observed, going from 93.3% to 75.6%. In this group in which most had severe dysfunction (and taking into account that desvenlafaxine was not devoid of sexual dysfunction in the follow-up visit), there was a significant decrease in baseline values, indicating a clinical improvement in these patients. In addition, a significant decrease was seen in those who initially showed deterioration in desire and orgasmic dysfunction without there being an improvement in sexual arousal. On the other hand, analyzing a very important aspect from the clinical point of view, the poor tolerability for patients with previous sexual dysfunction also improved significantly, decreasing from 26% to 11% in those who tolerate the SD badly (where it significantly affects the quality of life and/or the couple's relationship and/or the patient has thought about dropping out of the treatment).

Some studies that have focused on the relationship between compliance and SD indicate that between 20–35% of patients receiving AD present a risk of dropout [13,15,19,24]. An observational study showed that the most frequent adverse effect related to the noncompliance of treatment three months after the start of an AD was sexual dysfunction (47%), followed by weight changes, gastrointestinal discomfort, and insomnia [47]. The improvement in the risk of noncompliance with the switch to desvenlafaxine could undoubtedly have very relevant implications to the medium- and long-term results, avoiding relapses and reducing the deterioration in the quality of life.

Regarding the possible differences between men and women, in our study, significant improvements were found in the overall SALSEX scale in both men and women for the two treatment groups ($p < 0.05$), with more evident improvements in males switched to desvenlafaxine. These data coincide with previous examples with large sample sizes where a higher frequency of SD was observed in females taking AD [13,15]. There are data on the generalization of SD in the general population through extensive surveys in different countries, noting that among women between 40 and 80 years old, there are frequent problems related to desire, anorgasmia, and sexual arousal, while erectile dysfunction is the most common sexual problem among males, obviously increasing with age [48,49]. Gender differences play a fundamental role in sexual activity, with males generally showing more interest in sexual activity and staying active for longer. At least 38% of males remain interested in sexuality when above 75 years old vs. 16% in females [50]. The elderly male population is of great interest, because a group of them receiving ADs which impair sexual functioning are more likely to show a worse acceptance than younger males after the appearance of SD [1,13,15].

The spontaneous communication of SD (item B of SALSEX) was found in 27.3% of patients in group A and in 35% of group B that had previously received AD. Recent findings show the high frequency of SD after AD use (78% for men and 80% for women) [15], which surpass the figures found in the general population, contrasting with the scarcity of spontaneous communications. Nevertheless, spontaneous communication has increased over the years using the SALSEX questionnaire, from 14% in 1997 [1] to 20% in 2001 [13], reaching up to 44% in 2019 [15]. This increase in spontaneous communication is possibly due to the greater knowledge and sensitivity regarding this problem in the general population, with psychiatrists, AD prescribers, and general practitioners. One factor that undoubtedly contributes to this limited communication is related to the low frequency with which prescribers systematically interview patients about the presence of SD, this seeming to be relevant to both doctors and nurses [51,52].

In relation to possible differences between the frequency of SD with 50 and 100 mg/day, the Mann–Whitney U test revealed no statistically significant differences ($p > 0.05$) in the overall score of the SALSEX scale at follow-up in any of the groups; this is possibly due to the small number of patients taking 100 mg/day. The data from this study partially confirm those obtained in pre-registration clinical trials conducted with desvenlafaxine, which indicated a better profile of sexual tolerability compared with other serotonergic ADs [42]; however, in our sample, desvenlafaxine is not exempt from sexual dysfunction at the average doses used of 63.44 mg/day (±26.39). In one of the trials on placebo-controlled desvenlafaxine using the ASEX at 12 weeks, orgasm retardation was superior to placebo in males, but not in females, without affecting desire or sexual arousal [38]. There seems to be a difference in the sexual effects when taking into account the dose used being 50 mg similar to placebo, although the studies were not carried out considering inclusion and exclusion criteria on sexual activity and the factors that may influence it. Thus, in another clinical trial designed to measure functionality, male and female outpatients with major depression were randomly assigned 12 weeks of double-blind treatment with desvenlafaxine at 50 mg/day or placebo, sexual functioning scores, measured with the ASEX, were comparable between groups [53]. In another randomized study, no differences were found in SD with desvenlafaxine at 50 mg/day, 100 mg/day, and placebo but there were suggestions that there could be higher SD in the 100 mg group although statistical significance was not achieved [39]. The existing information on the frequency of desvenlafaxine-associated SD comes from a post-hoc analysis of three double-blind and short-term clinical trials (two months) using the self-administered ASEX Scale in outpatients with depression using doses of 50–100 mg. The results indicate that SD rates were 54%, 47%, and 49% for 50 mg/day, 100 mg/day, and placebo, respectively, with adjusted odds ratios (95% confidence interval) vs. placebo of 1205 (0.928, 1.564) and 1129 (0.795,

1.604), respectively [54]. These results partially coincide with the SD figures found in our study with 44% of moderate/severe SD at three months in desvenlafaxine-naïve patients; however, the frequency was much higher (76%) in patients switched to desvenlafaxine due to previous AD-related sexual dysfunction after following the course for three months.

To our knowledge, this is the first study carried out in patients switched to desvenlafaxine due to SD secondary to the use of another AD (mainly SSRIs and SRNIs) so it is not possible to compare the frequency found here with previous studies. Given the characteristics of this group containing 45 patients with previous sexual dysfunction (most of them poorly tolerated) and who met inclusion and exclusion criteria to avoid the most common confounders (sexual dysfunction prior to taking the AD, previous active and satisfactory sexual life, and the absence of concomitant treatments and medical pathologies that could affect sexual function), it is possible that there were other confounding factors that contributed to the presence of sexual dysfunction, since in 75.6% of patients, SD remained at three month follow-up visit. However, the improvement in the frequency and intensity of SD was significant after the change to desvenlafaxine, followed by an improvement of three of four SALSEX items in the follow-up visit ($p < 0.01$), such as low desire, delayed orgasm, and anorgasmia, but it was not significant in arousal difficulties. Additionally, the SD intensity decreased significantly in each of the items and the frequency of severe SD was reduced from 73% at baseline to 35% at follow-up.

The Clinical Global Impression (CGI) scores for psychiatric disease (CGI-S) and for sexual dysfunction (CGI-SD) improved significantly in both groups ($p < 0.01$) at follow-up, indicating an improvement both in the previous psychiatric pathology (mainly affective disorder) and in the subjective impression of the patient on the previous SD. The patient's CGI scales are very relevant in naturalistic studies because they indicate the subjective perception of the patient independently of the absolute value of a scale designed to measure an adverse effect. These improvements in the CGI scales coincide with the improvement in the tolerability of SD in both groups, decreasing the risk of treatment dropouts and ameliorating the quality of life.

One of the factors that may influence the sexual improvement observed in the patients switched to desvenlafaxine could well be a subjective effect underlying the patient's decision to participate in a study to improve sexual function and compliance with their expectations of improvement, perhaps increasing sexual frequency. However, other studies with the same methodology using the SALSEX scale have shown that the change to another serotonergic AD (paroxetine) was not followed by a significant decrease in the frequency of SD (100% at baseline versus 89% at six months), but a clear improvement was found after switching to another non-serotonergic AD (amineptine) from 100% at baseline to 55% at six months. This finding suggests that the effect of the treatment itself is more powerful than the subjective effect on the patient [55]. Another dual AD with a similar mechanism of action to desvenlafaxine such as milnacipran [56] has also been shown in a prospective randomized study to improve the initial SD in parallel with the AD effect in patients from some different cultural backgrounds, such as Brazil and Europe [57]. Duloxetine, a dual-action AD, has shown lower SD scores than SSRI (23% vs. 28%), although not significant, associated with greater clinical improvement in the CGI severity after six months [30,32].

There are few studies of patients who switch to non-serotonergic drugs. One of them with a similar naturalistic and uncontrolled methodology, designed to change from fluoxetine to bupropion due to sexual dysfunction, demonstrated an important improvement in sexual function maintaining the AD response after eight weeks of follow-up [58].

Finally, the clinical improvement in this study of the change to desvenlafaxine group is of great interest, since no dropouts or relapses were observed due to lack of AD efficacy. In a similar study of switching to amineptine vs. paroxetine, 7.5% of the amineptine group had depressive relapses during the following six months of follow-up compared with none in the paroxetine group [52]. This feature is very relevant for clinical practice because the recommendations for managing AD-related SD include a change of AD to another one with a different mechanism of action as a first option. However, the clinical efficacy and risk of noncompliance or relapse related to this have not been discussed in the literature [15]. Although possibly useful in some patients receiving serotonergic AD, a reduction in the dose is not supported by convincing results and is associated with a risk of relapse.

Our study has several limitations. We did not record information on potentially confounding factors that are considered to be risk factors for the occurrence of sexual dysfunction, such as educational background, marital status, or employment status. On the other hand, patients were informed of the objectives of the study including the evaluation of sexual functioning before participating in the study. It is, therefore, possible that patients who were more motivated to participate in the study, showed better results after switching to desvenlafaxine. Additionally, since it is a naturalistic design in real-life clinical practice, there was no control group of patients who continued with the same treatment as previously, so a comparison of both groups is not possible. Despite the fact that our study was conducted under clinical practice conditions, the exclusion of some patients limited the external validity of our results. Finally, some aspects of sexual functioning, such as subjective satisfaction and sexual pain, were not evaluated, since they are not included in the PRSexDQ-SALSEX Questionnaire, but could be taken into consideration in further studies [59]. Being a naturalistic study, patients could take benzodiazepines according to usual clinical practice and these could have some effect on sexual dysfunction [60,61]; however, the doses used were low and only lasted a short time (3–6 weeks).

5. Conclusions

Sexual dysfunction improved significantly in depressed patients who initiated treatment with desvenlafaxine and in those that switched from another AD to desvenlafaxine; however, it was not completely devoid of sexual adverse effects. This switching strategy could be highly relevant in clinical practice due to the significant improvement of moderate/severe and poorly tolerated sexual dysfunction accompanied by the maintenance of AD efficacy. The change to desvenlafaxine can be a useful alternative in AD switching strategies to help fight iatrogenic sexual dysfunction while maintaining the efficacy of the previous drug and without the risk of dropout or relapse associated with switching to other non-serotonergic compounds. Additional ADs that do not adversely impact sexual function are needed as well as further research into how to manage this side effect in men and women. Finally, as a result of the scarcity of studies conducted in real clinical practice on the usefulness of different switching methods to combat iatrogenic SD, additional research is needed to generate new and strong evidence on the management of this important adverse event in daily clinical practice, which influences compliance, affects medium- and long-term outcomes, and deteriorates the quality of life of the patients.

Author Contributions: Conceptualization A.L.M.; methodology, A.L.M., L.M. and N.G., formal analysis, N.G.; investigation, J.B., G.B., R.F.-O., M.T.G., A.J., A.P.-U., N.P. and J.L.V.; resources, A.L.M.; data curation, N.G., A.P.-U. and A.L.M.; writing original A.L.M.; draft preparation, A.L.M., N.G.; writing—review and editing, A.P.-U. and A.L.M.; funding acquisition, A.L.M.

Funding: This study was financed by Pfizer USA by an unrestricted medical grant.

Conflicts of Interest: Angel L. Montejo has received consultancy fees or honoraria/research grants in the last 5 years from Eli Lilly, Forum Pharmaceuticals, Rovi, Servier, Lundbeck, Otsuka, Janssen Cilag, Pfizer, Roche, Instituto de Salud Carlos III, and the Junta de Castilla y León. The rests of the authors declare no conflict of interest. The funders had no role in the design of the study; in the collection, analyses, or interpretation of data; in the writing of the manuscript, or in the decision to publish the results.

References

1. U.S. Food and Drug Administration FDA. Paroxetine Hydrochloride Prescribing Information. Available online: https://www.accessdata.fda.gov/drugsatfda_docs/label/2012/020031s067,020710s031.pdf (accessed on 23 April 2019).
2. Prozac (Fluoxetine Hydrochloride) Capsules Label—FDA. Available online: https://www.accessdata.fda.gov/drugsatfda_docs/label/2011/018936s091lbl.pdf (accessed on 23 April 2019).

3. Montejo, A.L.; Llorca, G.; Izquierdo, J.A.; Ledesma, A.; Bousoo, M.; Calcedo, A.; Carrasco, J.L.; Ciudad, J.; Daniel, E.; De la Gandara, J. SSRI-induced sexual dysfunction: Fluoxetine, paroxetine, sertraline, and fluvoxamine in a prospective, multicenter, and descriptive clinical study of 344 patients. *J. Sex Marital Ther.* **1997**, *23*, 176–194. [CrossRef] [PubMed]
4. Lee, K.U.; Lee, Y.M.; Nam, J.M.; Lee, H.K.; Kweon, Y.S.; Lee, C.T.; Jun, T.Y. Induced Sexual Dysfunction among Newer AD in a Naturalistic Setting. *Psychiatry Investig.* **2010**, *7*, 55–59. [CrossRef] [PubMed]
5. Williams, V.S.; Edin, H.M.; Hogue, S.L.; Fehnel, S.E.; Baldwin, D.S. Prevalence and impact of -associated sexual dysfunction in three European countries: Replication in a cross-sectional patient survey. *J. Psychopharmacol.* **2010**, *24*, 489–496. [CrossRef] [PubMed]
6. Reichenpfader, U.; Gartlehner, G.; Morgan, L.C.; Greenblatt, A.; Nussbaumer, B.; Hansen, R.A.; Van Noord, M.; Lux, L.; Gaynes, B.N. Sexual dysfunction associated with second-generation antidepressants in patients with major depressive disorder: Results from a systematic review with network meta-analysis. *Drug Saf.* **2014**, *37*, 19–31. [CrossRef]
7. Montejo, A.L.; Montejo, L.; Baldwin, D.S. The impact of severe mental disorders and psychotropic medications on sexual health and its implications for clinical management. *World Psychiatry* **2018**, *17*, 3–11. [CrossRef]
8. Serretti, A.; Chiesa, A. Treatment-emergent sexual dysfunction related to antidepressants: A meta-analysis. *J. Clin. Psychopharmacol.* **2009**, *29*, 259–266. [CrossRef]
9. Laumann, E.O.; Paik, A.; Rosen, R.C. Sexual dysfunction in the United States: Prevalence and predictors. *JAMA* **1999**, *281*, 537–544. [CrossRef]
10. Bonierbale, M.; Lancon, C.; Tignol, J. The ELIXIR study: Evaluation of sexual dysfunction in 4557 depressed patients in France. *Curr. Med. Res. Opin.* **2003**, *19*, 114–124. [CrossRef]
11. Montejo, A.L.; García, M.; Espada, M.; Rico-Villademoros, F.; Llorca, G.; Izquierdo, J.A. Psychometric characteristics of the psychotropic-related sexual dysfunction questionnaire. Spanish work group for the study of psychotropic-related sexual dysfunctions. *Actas Esp. Psiquiatr.* **2000**, *28*, 141–150.
12. Montejo, A.L.; Rico-Villademoros, F. Psychometric properties of the Psychotropic-Related Sexual Dysfunction Questionnaire (PRSexDQ-SALSEX) in patients with schizophrenia and other psychotic disorders. *J. Sex Marital Ther.* **2008**, *34*, 227–239. [CrossRef]
13. Clayton, A.H.; McGarvey, E.L.; Clavet, G.J. The Changes in Sexual Functioning Questionnaire (CSFQ): Development, reliability, and validity. *Psychopharmacol. Bull.* **1997**, *33*, 731–745. [PubMed]
14. Montejo, A.I. Llorca, G.; Izquierdo, J.A.; Ledesma, A.; Bousoño, M.; Calcedo, A.; Carrasco, J.L.; Daniel, E.; de Dios, A.; de la Gándara, J.; et al. Sexual dysfunction secondary to SSRIs. A comparative analysis in 308 patients. *Actas Luso-Esp. Neurol. Psiquiatr. Cienc. Afines* **1996**, *24*, 311–321. [PubMed]
15. Montejo, A.L.; Llorca, G.; Izquierdo, J.A.; Rico-Villademoros, F. Incidence of sexual dysfunction associated with antidepressant agents: A prospective multicenter study of 1022 outpatients. Spanish Working Group for the Study of Psychotropic-Related Sexual Dysfunction. *J. Clin. Psychiatry* **2001**, *62* (Suppl. 3), 10–21. [PubMed]
16. Fava, M.; Rankin, M. Sexual functioning and SSRI. *J. Clin. Psychiatry* **2002**, *63* (Suppl. 5), 13–16. [PubMed]
17. Montejo, A.L.; Calama, J.; Rico-Villademoros, F.; Montejo, L.; González-García, N.; Pérez, J.; SALSEX Working Study Group. A Real-World Study on Antidepressant-Associated Sexual Dysfunction in 2144 Outpatients: The SALSEX I Study. *Arch. Sex Behav.* **2019**. [CrossRef]
18. Montejo, A.L.; Prieto, N.; Terleira, A.; Matias, J.; Alonso, S.; Paniagua, G.; Naval, S.; Parra, D.G.; Gabriel, C.; Mocaër, E.; et al. Better sexual acceptability of agomelatine (25 and 50 mg) compared with paroxetine (20 mg) in healthy male volunteers. An 8-week, placebo-controlled study using the PRSEXDQ-SALSEX scale. *J. Psychopharmacol.* **2010**, *24*, 111–120. [CrossRef] [PubMed]
19. Montejo, A.L.; Deakin, J.F.W.; Gaillard, R.; Harmer, C.; Meyniel, F.; Jabourian, A.; Gabriel, C.; Gruget, C.; Klinge, C.; MacFayden, C.; et al. Better sexual acceptability of agomelatine (25 and 50 mg) compared to escitalopram (20 mg) in healthy volunteers. A 9-week, placebo-controlled study using the PRSexDQ scale. *J. Psychopharmacol.* **2015**, *29*, 1119–1128. [CrossRef]
20. Clayton, A.H.; Montejo, A.L. Major depressive disorder, antidepressants, and sexual dysfunction. *J. Clin. Psychiatry* **2006**, *67* (Suppl. 6), 33–37.
21. Clayton, A.H.; Pradko, J.F.; Croft, H.A.; Montano, C.B.; Leadbetter, R.A.; Bolden-Watson, C.; Bass, K.I.; Donahue, R.M.; Jamerson, B.D.; Metz, A. Prevalence of sexual dysfunction among newer antidepressants. *J. Clin. Psychiatry* **2002**, *63*, 357–366. [CrossRef]

22. Clayton, A.H.; Alkis, A.R.; Parikh, N.B.; Votta, J.G. Sexual Dysfunction Due to Psychotropic Medications. *Psychiatr. Clin. N. Am.* **2016**, *39*, 427–463. [CrossRef]
23. Serretti, A.; Chiesa, A. A meta-analysis of sexual dysfunction in psychiatric patients taking antipsychotics. *Int. Clin. Psychopharmacol.* **2011**, *26*, 130–140. [CrossRef] [PubMed]
24. Montejo, A.L.; Rico-Villademoros, F.; Spanish Working Group for the Study of Psychotropic-Related Sexual Dysfunction. Changes in sexual function for outpatients with schizophrenia or other psychotic disorders treated with ziprasidone in clinical practice settings: A 3-month prospective, observational study. *J. Clin. Psychopharmacol.* **2008**, *28*, 568–570. [CrossRef]
25. Baldwin, D.S.; Manson, C.; Nowak, M. Impact of Antidepressant Drugs on Sexual Function and Satisfaction. *CNS Drugs* **2015**, *29*, 905–913. [CrossRef]
26. Kennedy, S.H.; Rizvi, S.; Fulton, K.; Rasmussen, J. A double-blind comparison of sexual functioning, efficacy, and tolerability between agomelatine and venlafaxine XR. *J. Clin. Psychopharmacol.* **2008**, *28*, 329–333. [CrossRef]
27. Montejo, A.; Majadas, S.; Rizvi, S.J.; Kennedy, S.H. The effects of agomelatine on sexual function in depressed patients and healthy volunteers. *Hum. Psychopharmacol.* **2011**, *26*, 537–542. [CrossRef]
28. Kennedy, S.H.; Fulton, K.A.; Bagby, R.M.; Greene, A.L.; Cohen, N.L.; Rafi-Tari, S. Sexual function during bupropion or paroxetine treatment of major depressive disorder. *Can. J. Psychiatry* **2006**, *51*, 234–242. [CrossRef] [PubMed]
29. Abler, B.; Seeringer, A.; Hartmann, A.; Grön, G.; Metzger, C.; Walter, M.; Stingl, J. Neural correlates of antidepressant-related sexual dysfunction: A placebo-controlled fMRI study on healthy males under sub chronic paroxetine and bupropion. *Neuropsychopharmacology* **2011**, *36*, 1837–1847. [CrossRef] [PubMed]
30. Dueñas, H.; Lee, A.; Brnabic, A.J.; Chung, K.F.; Lai, C.H.; Badr, M.G.; Uy-Ponio, T.; Ruiz, J.R.; Varrey, P.; Jian, H.; et al. Frequency of treatment-emergent sexual dysfunction and treatment effectiveness during SSRI or duloxetine therapy: 8-week data from a 6-month observational study. *Int. J. Psychiatry Clin. Pract.* **2011**, *15*, 80–90. [CrossRef] [PubMed]
31. Schweitzer, I.; Maguire, K.; Ng, C. Sexual side-effects of contemporary antidepressants: Review. *Aust. N. Z. J. Psychiatry* **2009**, *43*, 795–808. [CrossRef]
32. Dueñas, H.; Brnabic, A.J.; Lee, A.; Montejo, A.L.; Prakash, S.; Casimiro-Querubin, M.L.S.; Khaled, M.; Dossenbach, M.; Raskin, J. Treatment-emergent sexual dysfunction with SSRIs and duloxetine: Effectiveness and functional outcomes over a 6-month observational period. *Int. J. Psychiatry Clin. Pract.* **2011**, *15*, 242–254. [CrossRef]
33. Mahableshwarkar, A.R.; Jacobsen, P.L.; Serenko, M.; Chen, Y.; Trivedi, M.H. A randomized, double-blind, placebo-controlled study of the efficacy and safety of 2 doses of vortioxetine in adults with major depressive disorder. *J. Clin. Psychiatry* **2015**, *76*, 583–591. [CrossRef]
34. Alam, M.Y.; Jacobsen, P.L.; Chen, Y.; Serenko, M.; Mahableshwarkar, A.R. Safety, tolerability, and efficacy of vortioxetine (Lu AA21004) in major depressive disorder: Results of an open-label, flexible-dose, 52-week extension study. *Int. Clin. Psychopharmacol.* **2014**, *29*, 36–44. [CrossRef]
35. Jacobsen, P.L.; Mahableshwarkar, A.R.; Chen, Y.; Chrones, L.; Clayton, A.H. Effect of Vortioxetine vs. Escitalopram on Sexual Functioning in Adults with Well-Treated Major Depressive Disorder Experiencing SSRI-Induced Sexual Dysfunction. *J. Sex Med.* **2015**, *12*, 2036–2048. [CrossRef]
36. O'Mullan, C.; Doherty, M.; Coates, R.; Tilley, P.J. Searching for answers and validation: Australian women's experiences of coping with the adverse sexual effects of antidepressants. *Aust. J. Prim. Health* **2015**, *21*, 305–309. [CrossRef]
37. Taylor, M.J.; Rudkin, L.; Bullemor-Day, P.; Lubin, J.; Chukwujekwu, C.; Hawton, K. Strategies for managing sexual dysfunction induced by antidepressant medication. *Cochrane Database Syst. Rev.* **2013**, CD003382. [CrossRef]
38. Rizvi, S.J.; Kennedy, S.H. Management strategies for SSRI-induced sexual dysfunction. *J. Psychiatry Neurosci.* **2013**, *38*, E27–E28. [CrossRef]
39. Baldwin, D.S.; Palazzo, M.C.; Masdrakis, V.G. Reduced treatment-emergent sexual dysfunction as a potential target in the development of new antidepressants. *Depress Res. Treat.* **2013**, *2013*, 256841. [CrossRef]
40. Clayton, A.H.; Reddy, S.; Focht, K.; Musgnung, J.; Fayyad, R. An evaluation of sexual functioning in employed outpatients with major depressive disorder treated with desvenlafaxine 50 mg or placebo. *J. Sex Med.* **2013**, *10*, 768–776. [CrossRef] [PubMed]

41. Clayton, A.H.; Tourian, K.A.; Focht, K.; Hwang, E.; Cheng, R.F.; Thase, M.E. Desvenlafaxine 50 and 100 mg/d versus placebo for the treatment of major depressive disorder: A phase 4, randomized controlled trial. *J. Clin. Psychiatry* **2015**, *76*, 562–569. [CrossRef] [PubMed]
42. Clayton, A.H.; Kornstein, S.G.; Rosas, G.; Guico-Pabia, C.; Tourian, K.A. An integrated analysis of the safety and tolerability of desvenlafaxine compared with placebo in the treatment of major depressive disorder. *CNS Spectr.* **2009**, *14*, 183–195. [CrossRef] [PubMed]
43. Preeti, S.; Jayaram, S.D.; Chittaranjan, A. Sexual Dysfunction in Patients with Antidepressant-treated Anxiety or Depressive Disorders: A Pragmatic Multivariable Longitudinal Study. *East Asian Arch. Psychiatry* **2018**, *28*, 9–16.
44. Guy, W. Clinical global impressions. In *ECDEU Assessment Manual for Psychopharmacology, Revised*; National Institute of Mental Health: Rockville, MD, USA, 1976; pp. 218–222.
45. World Health Organization. Available online: https://www.who.int/classifications/icd/icdonlineversions/en/ (accessed on 23 April 2019).
46. Santana, Y.; Montejo, A.L.; Martín, J.; LLorca, G.; Bueno, G.; Blázquez, J.L. Understanding the Mechanism of Antidepressant-Related Sexual Dysfunction: Inhibition of Tyrosine Hydroxylase in Dopaminergic Neurons after Treatment with Paroxetine but Not with Agomelatine in Male Rats. *J. Clin. Med.* **2019**, *8*, 133. [CrossRef]
47. Goethe, J.W.; Woolley, S.B.; Cardoni, A.A.; Woznicki, B.A.; Piez, D.A. Selective serotonin reuptake inhibitor discontinuation: Side effects and other factors that influence medication adherence. *J. Clin. Psychopharmacol.* **2007**, *27*, 451–458. [CrossRef] [PubMed]
48. Nicolosi, A.; Laumann, E.O.; Glasser, D.B.; Moreira, E.D., Jr.; Paik, A.; Gingell, C. Sexual behavior and sexual dysfunctions after age 40: The global study of sexual attitudes and behaviors. *Urology* **2004**, *64*, 991–997. [CrossRef] [PubMed]
49. Laumann, E.O.; Nicolosi, A.; Glasser, D.B.; Paik, A.; Gingell, C.; Moreira, E.; Wang, T. Sexual problems among women and men aged 40–80 y: Prevalence and correlates identified in the Global Study of Sexual Attitudes and Behaviors. *Int. J. Impot. Res.* **2005**, *17*, 39–57. [CrossRef]
50. Lindau, S.T.; Gavrilova, N. Sex, health, and years of sexually active life gained due to good health: Evidence from two US population based cross sectional surveys of ageing. *BMJ* **2010**, *340*, c810. [CrossRef] [PubMed]
51. Quinn, C.; Happell, B.; Browne, G. Talking or avoiding? Mental health nurses' views about discussing sexual health with consumers. *Int. J. Ment. Health Nurs.* **2011**, *20*, 21–28. [CrossRef]
52. Higgins, A.; Barker, P.; Begley, C.M. Iatrogenic sexual dysfunction and the protective withholding of information: In whose best interest? *J. Psychiatr. Ment. Health Nurs.* **2006**, *13*, 437–446. [CrossRef]
53. Dunlop, B.W.; Reddy, S.; Yang, L.; Lubaczewski, S.; Focht, K.; Guico-Pabia, C.J. Symptomatic and functional improvement in employed depressed patients: A double-blind clinical trial of desvenlafaxine versus placebo. *J. Clin. Psychopharmacol.* **2011**, *31*, 569–576. [CrossRef]
54. Clayton, A.H.; Hwang, E.; Kornstein, S.G.; Tourian, K.A.; Cheng, R.F.; Abraham, L.; Mele, L.; Boucher, M. Effects of 50 and 100 mg desvenlafaxine versus placebo on sexual function in patients with major depressive disorder: A meta-analysis. *Int. Clin. Psychopharmacol.* **2015**, *30*, 307–315. [CrossRef] [PubMed]
55. Montejo, A.L.; Llorca, G.; Izquierdo, J.A.; Carrasco, J.L.; Daniel, E.; Pérez-Sola, V.; Vicens, E.; Bousoño, M.; Sánchez-Iglesias, S.; Franco, M.; et al. Sexual dysfunction with antidepressive agents. Effect of the change to amineptine in patients with sexual dysfunction secondary to SSRI. *Actas Esp. Psiquiatr.* **1999**, *27*, 23–34. [PubMed]
56. Mandrioli, R.; Protti, M.; Mercolini, L. New-Generation, non-SSRI Antidepressants: Therapeutic Drug Monitoring and Pharmacological Interactions. Part 1: SNRIs, SMSs, SARIs. *Curr. Med. Chem.* **2017**. [CrossRef] [PubMed]
57. Baldwin, D.; Moreno, R.A.; Briley, M. Resolution of sexual dysfunction during acute treatment of major depression with milnacipran. *Hum. Psychopharmacol.* **2008**, *23*, 527–532. [CrossRef] [PubMed]
58. Walker, P.W.; Cole, J.O.; Gardner, E.A.; Hughes, A.R.; Johnston, J.A.; Batey, S.R.; Lineberry, C.G. Improvement in fluoxetine-associated sexual dysfunction in patients switched to bupropion. *J. Clin. Psychiatry* **1993**, *54*, 459–465.
59. Isidori, A.M.; Pozza, C.; Esposito, K.; Giugliano, D.; Morano, S.; Vignozzi, L.; Corona, G.; Lenzi, A.; Jannini, E.A. Development and validation of a 6-item version of the female sexual function index (FSFI) as a diagnostic tool for female sexual dysfunction. *J. Sex Med.* **2010**, *7*, 1139–1146. [CrossRef] [PubMed]

60. Kupelian, V.; Hall, S.A.; McKinlay, J.B. Common prescription medication use and erectile dysfunction: Results from the Boston Area Community Health (BACH) survey. *BJU Int.* **2013**, *112*, 1178–1187. [CrossRef]
61. Mazzilli, R.; Angeletti, G.; Olana, S.; Delfino, M.; Zamponi, V.; Rapinesi, C.; Del Casale, A.; Kotzalidis, G.D.; Elia, J.; Callovini, G.; et al. Erectile dysfunction in patients taking psychotropic drugs and treated with phosphodiesterase-5 inhibitors. *Arch. Ital. Urol. Androl.* **2018**, *90*, 44–48. [CrossRef] [PubMed]

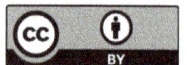

© 2019 by the authors. Licensee MDPI, Basel, Switzerland. This article is an open access article distributed under the terms and conditions of the Creative Commons Attribution (CC BY) license (http://creativecommons.org/licenses/by/4.0/).

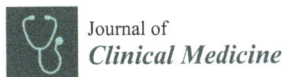

Article

(Don't) Look at Me! How the Assumed Consensual or Non-Consensual Distribution Affects Perception and Evaluation of Sexting Images

Arne Dekker [1,*,†], Frederike Wenzlaff [1,†], Anne Daubmann [2], Hans O. Pinnschmidt [2] and Peer Briken [1]

1. Institute for Sex Research and Forensic Psychiatry, University Medical Center Hamburg-Eppendorf, 20246 Hamburg, Germany; f.wenzlaff@gmail.com (F.W.); briken@uke.de (P.B.)
2. Institute of Medical Biometry and Epidemiology, University Medical Center Hamburg-Eppendorf, 20246 Hamburg, Germany; a.daubmann@uke.de (A.D.); h.pinnschmidt@uke.de (H.O.P)
* Correspondence: dekker@uke.de
† These authors contributed equally to this work.

Received: 8 April 2019; Accepted: 13 May 2019; Published: 17 May 2019

Abstract: The non-consensual sharing of an intimate image is a serious breach of a person's right to privacy and can lead to severe psychosocial consequences. However, little research has been conducted on the reasons for consuming intimate pictures that have been shared non-consensually. This study aims to investigate how the supposed consensual or non-consensual distribution of sexting images affects the perception and evaluation of these images. Participants were randomly assigned to one of two groups. The same intimate images were shown to all participants. However, one group assumed that the photos were shared voluntarily, whereas the other group were told that the photos were distributed non-consensually. While the participants completed several tasks such as rating the sexual attractiveness of the depicted person, their eye-movements were being tracked. The results from this study show that viewing behavior and the evaluation of sexting images are influenced by the supposed way of distribution. In line with objectification theory men who assumed that the pictures were distributed non-consensually spent more time looking at the body of the depicted person. This so-called 'objectifying gaze' was also more pronounced in participants with higher tendencies to accept myths about sexual aggression or general tendencies to objectify others. In conclusion, these results suggest that prevention campaigns promoting 'sexting abstinence' and thus attributing responsibility for non-consensual distribution of such images to the depicted persons are insufficient. Rather, it is necessary to emphasize the illegitimacy of the non-consensual distribution of sexting images, especially among male consumers of the material.

Keywords: eye tracking; non-consensual image sharing; intimate images; objectification; objectifying gaze; rape myth acceptance; sexting

1. Introduction

Sexting, the sending of intimate or explicit personal pictures, videos, or texts [1], has become common practice within different age groups [2–5]. Definitions vary, and the confusion of consensual and non-consensual sexting proves to be a central conceptual problem. [6,7]. While consensual sexting refers to the purposeful, active, and often pleasurable sending of one's own images, the non-consensual sharing of sexting images happens against the will or without the knowledge of the person depicted [8]. This non-consensual sharing is one of the most frequently discussed risks in the context of sexting [9–18]. If sexting images are forwarded against the will of the person depicted (e.g., in their circle of friends) or published on the internet, this poses a serious risk to mental health. Situations in which victims are exposed to public humiliation and online bullying can lead to grave psychosocial consequences, in some cases even suicide [3,7].

Not only in the public debate but also in 'sexting abstinence' campaigns [19], sexting, in general, is deemed dangerous [20]. Not differentiating between consensual and non-consensual sexting can lead to victim blaming if the depicted producers of the images are held responsible for the unintended dissemination [7]. This mechanism has been criticized in the theoretical context of 'rape culture' [21–23] and linked to the broader concepts of 'sexual objectification' [24–27] and 'rape myth acceptance' [26,28,29]. Objectification theory postulates that in western societies women are sexually objectified, treated as objects and are only considered worthy to the extent that their bodies give pleasure to others [29] (for reviews [28,30]). Sexual objectification can be seen as a continuum ranging from acts of violence to subtler acts such as objectifying gazes [30,31]. These gazes, conceptualized as visually inspecting (sexual) body parts, have been empirically demonstrated using eye-tracking technology [32]. Additionally, people who sexually objectify others have been shown to be more likely to accept rape myths [24,25], which serve to normalize sexual violence, e.g., through victim blaming (for reviews [27,33]). These subtle myths have been conceptualized as cognitive schemes [34] and demonstrated to influence eye movements [35,36].

Although research has evolved around non-consensual sexting and its correlates [7,9,20], little effort has been conducted to investigate reasons for consuming such images. The question arises why people consume non-consensual sexting material when mere comparisons with consensual material do not reveal apparent differences in image content. Is there a specific attraction in the non-consensuality itself, at least for some of the consumers? Against this background, we experimentally investigate the question of how the supposed way of distribution (consensual vs. non-consensual) influences the perception of sexting images. Thus, the study promises important findings for future prevention efforts.

In accordance with the objectification theory we expect differences in evaluation and perception of sexting images depending on their supposedly consensual or non-consensual forwarding. In line with previous research, we argue that increased objectification is associated with higher attractiveness ratings of the objectified person [37] and a more pronounced objectifying gaze [32]. We further hypothesize that supposedly non-consensually forwarded images are considered as more intimate and their further distribution as more unpleasant. Overall tendencies for other objectification and higher rape-myth acceptance are also expected to increase objectification.

A large part of the scientific literature on sexting focuses on the behavior of adolescents. This may reflect widespread societal fears, but, in fact, sexting experience is significantly higher among adults than among adolescents. In a current systematic review [3] the prevalence estimate of studies of adolescents sending messages containing sexually suggestive texts or photos was found to be 10.2% (95% CI (1.77–18.63)), while the estimated mean prevalence of studies of adults was 53.31% (95% CI (49.57–57.07)). Against this background, and also because the present experimental study does not focus on a representative image of the user population, we have decided to examine a sample of adults. We assume that the mechanisms shown are comparable in adolescents, but this must be demonstrated by future research.

2. Materials and Methods

2.1. Participants

A total of 76 participants (57% female, $M_{age} = 31.99$, $SD_{age} = 10.28$) were recruited via university newsletters. They were informed about the tasks and the stimulus content but were kept naïve to the full purpose of the experiment. Participants provided written consent to study participation. No compensation was given. The ethics committee of the state chamber of psychotherapists of Hamburg (Psychotherapeutenkammer Hamburg) approved the study protocol of the present study (03/2015-PTK-HH).

2.2. Stimuli and Apparatus

Volunteers personally known to the authors but unknown to the study participants provided 14 semi-nude sexting images [38]. One additional image per gender was obtained from freely available internet sources for public presentation purposes, resulting in a set of 16 pictures (50% female).

Stimulus presentation and data collection were conducted on a 22-inch widescreen monitor (1680 × 1050 pixels) using SensoMotoric Instruments (SMI GmbH, Teltow, Germany) software ExperimentCenter™. A remote eye tracker (SMI, RED system) recorded eye movements at 120 Hz from 50 cm viewing distance using a head-chin rest.

2.3. Questionnaires

Individuals' objectification of others was assessed using a German translation of the modified version of the Self-Objectification Questionnaire [39] for other objectification (Other Objectification Scale, OOS [40]). The scale consists of 10 body attributes, five competence-based (i.e., strength) and five are appearance-based (i.e., physical attractiveness). Participants were asked to rank how important they perceive each attribute (10 = "most important"; 1 = "least important") separately for men and women. Possible scores range from −25 to 25 with higher scores indicating higher levels of objectification.

Participants further completed an 11-item short version of the German Acceptance of Modern Myths About Sexual Aggression Scale (AMMSA) [41] which had been used successfully in other eye tracking studies already [35,36]. Each item was rated on a 7-point scale (1 = "completely disagree"; 7 = "completely agree").

2.4. Procedure

Participants read an introductory text stating that the study aimed to understand more about the evaluation of sexting images. Depending on the condition, picture distribution was either described as voluntary (consensual condition) or as unwanted, against the will of the depicted person (non-consensual condition). The manipulation was strengthened by asking participants to state three feelings the image distribution could have evoked in the depicted persons. Following, participants saw the images three times with different tasks. Pictures were randomized within blocks, starting with the male images. Pictures were presented individually on full screen for 5 seconds, preceded by a black fixation cross on the left side shown for 1 second. The first task was to freely view the pictures. Second, participants rated the sexual attractiveness of the depicted person. For the third task, participants were asked to evaluate how intimate they considered the image content and how unpleasant further picture distribution would be for the depicted person (ranging from 1 = "not at all ... "; 7 = "very ... "). After completion of the sociodemographic information, and the questionnaires, participants were thanked and debriefed.

2.5. Data Reduction and Data Analysis

To account for repeated measures made on the same subject, a mixed model approach was employed. We examined the fixed effects of the independent variables condition (consensual vs. non-consensual distribution), gender (women vs. men), image gender (female vs. male images), of their three and two-way interactions and of the OOS score and AMMSA score on the ratings of (1) sexual attractiveness, (2) intimacy of image content, and (3) perceived unpleasantness of picture distribution. Random intercepts were assumed for participants. We report the marginal means and their 95%-confidence intervals. We report the results of the final models after a backward elimination of the non-significant effects according to Kleinbaum et al. [42]. All statistical tests were two-tailed ($\alpha = 0.05$).

The eye tracking data were analyzed using the same model as described above with the objectifying gaze as the dependent variable. The objectifying gaze was operationalized as the relative time spent looking at the body compared to the time spent looking at faces [32]. We created two areas of interest

(AOI) on each image, one containing the head and the other containing all the rest of the body. The total dwell time for both AOIs, i.e., the overall time viewing the person depicted, was set to 100%. For the following analysis, we focus on the percentage of that time directed at the body. Accordingly, an increase in viewing time on the body always results in a decrease of dwell time on the face, since both values always add up to 100%. So a stronger objectifying gaze refers to relatively longer viewing time on the body and shorter viewing time on the face.

Computations were done using the GENLINMIXED (Generalized linear mixed model) routine of SPSS version 22 (IBM Corporation, Armonk, NY, USA) and eye tracking data reduction was realized using the standard settings of BeGaze^{TM} (SMI, Teltow, Germany), providing gaze information such as duration (dwell time).

3. Results

3.1. Participants

Prior to data analysis participants were excluded due to poor recordings ($n = 5$), non-heterosexual orientation ($n = 3$), or due to inadequate responses to the manipulation check ($n = 10$) as rated by four independent raters. A total of 58 participants (57% female, $M_{age} = 31.45$, $SD_{age} = 10.18$) remained for data analysis (see Table 1). Table 1 also shows the means of participants' AMMSA and OOS scores. In this context, it is particularly important that the mean values of the two study groups do not differ.

Table 1. Participant characteristics and questionnaire data.

	Condition	
	Consensual [a]	Non-Consensual [b]
Female (%)	52%	61%
Age (M, SD)	32.20 (11.75)	31.42 (9.16)
Age (Range)	21–68	19–59
AMMSA score (M, SD)	2.96 (1.33)	2.44 (0.90)
OOS score (of Women; M, SD)	4.58 (10.86) [c]	−0.44 (10.16)
OOS score (of Men; M, SD)	0.67 (8.42)	−0.94 (9.67)

The means do not significantly differ between conditions ($p > 0.08$). OOS score = Scores on the Other Objectification Scale (Strelan and Hargreaves, 2005) separately for the objectification of women and of men; the possible range is from −25 (low objectification) to 25 (high objectification). AMMSA score = Scores on the 11-item short version of the Acceptance of Modern Myths About Sexual Aggression scale (Gerger et al., 2007); the possible range is from 1 (low acceptance) to 7 (high acceptance). [a] $n = 25$. [b] $n = 33$. [c] $n = 24$.

3.2. Ratings

Separate models were conducted for each of the three explicit ratings, namely sexual attractiveness of the person depicted, perceived intimacy of the image content, and unpleasantness of further distribution. Only the significant effects of the final models are reported here.

For attractiveness ratings, we did not find that condition (consensual vs. non-consensual distribution; see Table 2) had any effect. We did, however, find that gender had an effect as well as an interaction effect between participant gender and image gender. Overall, men rated the images of men as more attractive (M = 4.17, SE = 0.32) than women did (M = 3.02, SE = 0.31; $t(924) = 3.25$, $p < 0.001$). Women also rated the images of men as less attractive than images of women (M = 4.46, SE = 0.32, $t(924) = 9.36$, $p < 0.001$). No other effects reached significance.

Concerning the intimacy ratings, we found an interaction effect between condition and gender ($p = 0.008$, see Table 2). Pairwise contrasts revealed that women who assumed non-consensual distribution regarded the images as more intimate (M = 4.86, SE = 0.25) than women who assumed consensual distribution (M = 4.56, SE = 0.26; $t(924) = 2.58$, $p = 0.01$).

Analyzing influences on how unpleasant further distribution was considered for the depicted person, we found that condition (consensual vs. non-consensual distribution; $p < 0.001$) had a highly significant effect (see Table 2). Pairwise contrasts revealed that participants assuming non-consensual sharing considered further distribution as more unpleasant (M = 4.63, SE = 0.28) than participants who assumed consensual sharing (M = 4.26, SE = 0.28; $t(924) = 3.74$, $p < .001$). We also found an interaction effect between gender and image gender. Women rated the unpleasantness of further distribution lower for images of men (M = 4.08, SE = 0.40) than male participants did (M = 4.41, SE = 0.40; $t(924) = 2.50$, $p = 0.013$). Furthermore, the AMMSA score reached significance (coefficient = −0.13, $p = 0.002$), indicating that the higher participants scored on the AMMSA-scale, the less unpleasant they considered picture distribution for the depicted person.

Table 2. Final models of the influences on ratings of sexual attractiveness, intimacy, and presumed unpleasantness of further distribution.

Dependent Variable	Independent Variable	F	p Value	Coefficient [a]	95% Confidence Interval	
					Lower Limit	Upper Limit
Sexual Attractiveness	Gender	50.82	<0.001	−1.15	−1.39	−0.91
	Image Gender	4.34	0.038	0.38	−0.50	1.26
	Gender × Image Gender	36.89	<0.001	1.06	0.72	1.40
Intimacy	Condition	0.610	0.435	0.16	−0.09	0.42
	Gender	0.025	0.874	0.22	−0.01	0.45
	Group × Gender	7.029	0.008	−0.46	−0.80	−0.12
Unpleasantness	Condition	14.02	<0.001	−0.37	−0.56	−0.18
	Gender	1.47	0.225	−0.34	−0.60	−0.07
	Image Gender	0.52	0.473	0.18	−0.93	1.28
	Gender × Image Gender	5.41	0.020	0.44	0.07	0.82
	AMMSA score	9.48	0.002	−0.13	−0.22	−0.049

Fixed effects ($df1 = 1$, $df2 = 924$). AMMSA score = Scores on the 11-item short version of the Acceptance of Modern Myths About Sexual Aggression scale (Gerger et al., 2007). [a] The coefficient value indicates the increase of the rating per score-increase of 1 (e.g., unpleasantness rating decrease of −0.13 per AMMSA score increase of 1).

3.3. Eye Tracking Analysis

Regarding eye movements, we were interested in the objectifying gaze, operationalized as the relative time viewing the body. We found a significant interaction of condition and gender ($F(1,834) = 8.36$, $p < 0.001$). Men in the non-consensual condition demonstrated a stronger objectifying gaze as they looked significantly longer at bodies (M = 54.37, SE = 8.99) than men in the consensual condition (M = 46.52, SE = 9.01; $t(834) = 4.25$, $p < 0.001$) (see Figure 1). Within the non-consensual condition, men also demonstrated the objectifying gaze more than women did, spending more time looking at bodies than women did (M = 49.53, SE = 8.97; $t(834) = 3.07$, $p = 0.002$). Notably, there was no such gender difference within the consensual condition ($p > 0.05$).

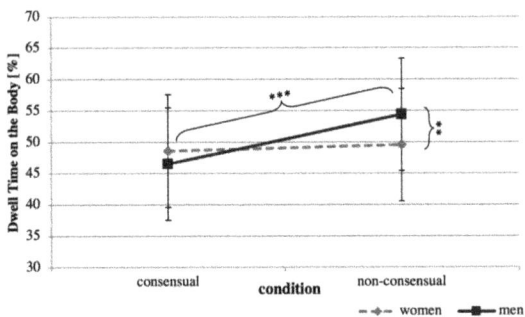

Figure 1. Estimates of the mean proportion (and standard error) of dwell time spent on the body by condition and gender. *** $p < 0.001$; ** $p < 0.01$.

The effects of the OOS score and the AMMSA score were significant ($p < 0.001$), indicating that relative dwell time on the body increases for higher scores. In other words, this reveals a more pronounced objectifying gaze for higher tendencies to objectify and accept myths about sexual aggression (see Table 3).

Table 3. Influences on the proportion of dwell time spent looking at the body.

Independent Variable	F	p Value	Coefficient [a]	95% Confidence Interval	
				Lower Limit	Upper Limit
Condition	12.45	<0.001	−7.85	−11.48	−4.22
Gender	1.34	0.247	−4.84	−7.94	−1.74
Gender × Condition	8.36	0.004	6.92	2.22	11.61
OOS score	23.90	<0.001	0.30	0.18	0.42
AMMSA score	31.06	<0.001	2.96	1.92	4.00

Fixed effects ($df1 = 1$, $df2 = 834$). OOS score = Scores on the Other-Objectification questionnaire (Strelan and Hargreaves, 2005). AMMSA score = Scores on the 11-item short version of the Acceptance of Modern Myths About Sexual Aggression scale (Gerger et al., 2007). [a] The coefficient value indicates the increase of dwell time on the body per score-increase of 1 (e.g., dwell time increase of 2.96 per AMMSA score increase of 1).

4. Discussion

We demonstrate that not only explicit ratings but also the implicit viewing behavior are influenced by the assumed consensual or non-consensual distribution of sexting images.

4.1. Image Evaluations

Participants who assumed the non-consensual distribution of a sexting image, namely the sharing against the will of the person depicted, rated the further distribution of the images as more unpleasant. This finding demonstrates that not only the picture content itself or personal feelings about sexting but also the surrounding information is considered when estimating the unpleasantness of further picture distribution. Interestingly, women rated the unpleasantness of distribution lower for images of men than male participants did. Seeing images of other men, the risk saliency of becoming a victim and having one's images shared non-consensually might have increased for men, leading to higher ratings of unpleasantness. Due to the common stories of non-consensual sexting involving women, female participants might be aware of personal risks at any time independent of the condition. As the potential consequences of forwarding are more severe for women [43,44], female participants might consider further forwarding as less unpleasant because of the less severe consequences for men. However, it is important to note that the images of men and women should not be compared directly with each other in this study as picture compositions varied. Men were usually posing less sexually than women, which is due to the naturalistic creation of the images, but likely influences the ratings of unpleasantness.

Overall, higher general rape myth acceptance led to lower ratings of perceived unpleasantness of further distribution in both conditions. Higher endorsement of rape myths is indicative of a higher likelihood of victim blaming, which is in line with the common risk discourses on sexting [7,12,22,45]. Accordingly, considering non-consensual sharing a risk inherent in sexting allows minimizing the expected level of unpleasantness of further distribution. The depicted person is deemed responsible for having taken the image to begin with and hence either stupid or reckless. In other words, the estimated unpleasantness decreases when victim blaming increases. This is crucial as this pattern is not only typical for cases of revenge pornography [46] but also for other forms of sexual harassment [26,47] and has even found its way into 'sexting abstinence' campaigns [20]. Concerning the perceived intimacy of the images, women assuming non-consensual distribution rated the images as more intimate for both genders than women assuming consensual sharing. Men, however, did not differ between the consensual or non-consensual distribution of images of either men or women. This could be attributed to the fact that women are more likely to be victims of non-consensual sexting [3] and to be victimized in general in most forms of online gender-based violence [19,48]. Being aware of the potential personal risk might make women more sensitive to the intentions of the depicted person and violations of privacy.

Unlike expected, the assumed way of distribution did not affect how participants rated the sexual attractiveness. Previous research linking objectification and attractiveness ratings presented women in casual wear and the same women in bikinis [46]. Such a strong manipulation allows for large differences between conditions. Using the same semi-nude images in both conditions as done in our study might not have been a strong enough manipulation to affect explicit attractiveness ratings. The exhibited interaction effect between gender and image gender, more precisely higher ratings of male images by men, is likely due to factors inherent in the images and not the context. Therefore, we do not consider them as relevant for this study.

4.2. The Objectifying Gaze

The objectifying gaze, defined as the relative amount of time looking at the body, was influenced by condition and participant gender. Men assuming non-consensual distribution displayed the objectifying gaze more than assuming voluntary sharing and more than women assuming either manner of distribution. Hence, we were able to demonstrate for the first time that the supposed way of distribution influences how participants look at images and how strongly they display the objectifying gaze. Previous research suggests that especially women are sexually objectified in the media [26,49,50] and during interpersonal interactions [51,52]. The objectifying gaze has been linked to negative social perceptions, dehumanization, and self-objectification [53–55]. While an appearance-focus in women has been linked to negative social perceptions [54,55] and severe mental health problems [55], no comparable research on men exists.

Although mostly discussed for men, women are thought to have internalized the objectifying gaze so much that they demonstrate it toward other women as well [56]. However, in our study, only men assuming non-consensual distribution differed from the other participant groups, albeit unaffected by the gender of the depicted person. Unlike other studies [57–60], we did not find systematic influences of image gender on viewing behavior. We suggest that our manipulation might have evoked other task demands that resulted in viewing patterns different from free viewing conditions, possibly covering influences of image gender [61]. In line with previous research, higher general tendencies to objectify others, as well as higher acceptance of rape myths, were related to a more pronounced objectifying gaze [35]. Numerous gender-specific functions and consequences have been reported for rape myths acceptance (for a review see [62]). Still, due to cultural changes, rape myths and sexist beliefs have become increasingly subtle as taken into consideration and measured by the acceptance of modern myth about sexual aggression scale applied here [63]. This study is the first to consider the influences of both biases on eye movements and suggests that subtle attitudes indeed affect viewing behavior. These influences and their implications should be further investigated in the context of sexual aggression.

4.3. Limitations and Future Research

Our study was conducted in the laboratory with well educated, heterosexual participants viewing images of young, attractive adults who were semi-nude, unlike in most severe cases of non-consensual image sharing [64]. Accordingly, the generalizability of our results needs further investigation. Future research has to take intersectional influences (e.g., skin color or age) into account, as these factors are relevant in the context of objectification [50]. Concerning participants, intersectionality is also important, as cultural influences regarding eye-movements [65], sexual objectification [66], and sexual harassment [67,68] have been found. Other reasons for fixating more on bodies (e.g., social comparison) or avoiding faces (e.g., shame) should be explored as well.

As mentioned above, in this study we have focused on adult participants for two main reasons: First, the prevalence of sexting among adults is actually higher than among adolescents. Secondly, we were not interested in a representative image of the user population, but in an experimental comparison of two equivalent groups. Nevertheless, it is possible that the correlations shown do not exist among adolescent users. For this reason, a replication of the present study with adolescent participants would be desirable.

Although we demonstrated that the supposed manner of distribution affects the perception of sexting images, qualitative research asking consumers of non-consensual sexting for their motives seems like an important step to further identify the beliefs behind such behavior, (e.g., the enjoyment of power) [69]. Another aspect is the perceived agency of the depicted person that might be decreased by non-consensual forwarding, which in turn could facilitate objectification. This idea needs further investigation.

Since everyday sexual objectification is common [70], it is crucial to examine and develop theories regarding possible outcomes and further explore the similarities between sexual assault and non-consensual pornography, or technology-facilitated violence in general.

As rapid changes of the technological landscape routinely link new types of specific behavior (e.g., non-consensual sexting) to existing theory (e.g., on sexual objectification) they can inform the creation of prevention programs [46,71]. The well-researched theory of 'sexual double standards' suggests that women's sexuality is often perceived as pure and damageable through active desire, holding women responsible for protecting themselves from aggressive male sexuality [72,73]. This leads to the paradoxical position for women of experiencing social and cultural pressure to be sexy while simultaneously risking negative social consequences when portraying themselves in such manner online [74,75]. Considering the sexual double standard allows us to understand nonconsensual sexting as reaffirming stereotypical gender roles that place women under the control of men [53,55]. As girls are more likely to engage in sexualized self-presentations on social network sites and more attention is paid to their physical appearance than that of boys [76], gendered aspects need to be considered [17,77]. While arguments have been made to consider sexting as an empowering (social) media production [78,79] and to frame sexy appearance as a feminist act to counter the negative effects of objectification [80], this positive reframing carries the potential negative effect of normalizing unwanted sexual attention, which may outweigh the possible benefits of individual self-preservation [71].

5. Conclusions

In conclusion, we demonstrated that viewing behavior and evaluation of sexting images are influenced by their supposed consensual or non-consensual distribution. In line with objectification theory, an 'objectifying gaze' was more pronounced in men who assumed non-consensual picture distribution, meaning they spent a relatively longer time looking at the body of a depicted person. This 'objectifying gaze' was also more pronounced for participants with higher tendencies to accept myths about sexual aggression or general tendencies to objectify others. The results suggest that prevention campaigns that focus on a general message of sexting abstinence and thus attribute responsibility for non-consensual distribution of such images to the persons depicted are insufficient. Rather, it is necessary to emphasize the illegitimacy of the non-consensual distribution of sexting images, especially among male consumers of the material. This can be done, for example, in the context of school educational events, but there is also at least one example of an appropriate public prevention campaign: http://notyourstoshare.scot/. Only with these or comparable measures can the serious psychological consequences of public humiliation and online bullying be prevented in the long term.

Author Contributions: Conceptualization, A.D. (Arne Dekker), F.W., and P.B.; methodology, A.D. (Arne Dekker), F.W.; software, not applicable; formal analysis, F.W., A.D. (Anne Daubmann), H.O.P.; investigation, F.W.; resources, A.D. (Arne Dekker), P.B.; data curation, F.W.; writing—original draft preparation, A.D. (Arne Dekker), F.W.; writing—review and editing, A.D. (Arne Dekker), F.W., P.B.; visualization, F.W.; supervision, P.B.; project administration, A.D. (Arne Dekker); funding acquisition, P.B.

Funding: This research was funded by the German Federal Ministry of Education and Research (Bundesministerium für Bildung und Forschung, BMBF, 01SR1602).

Acknowledgments: We would like to thank all volunteers for providing their images.

Conflicts of Interest: The authors declare no conflict of interest.

References

1. Chalfen, R. "It's only a picture": Sexting, "smutty" snapshots and felony charges. *Vis. Stud.* **2009**, *24*, 258–268. [CrossRef]
2. Albury, K.; Crawford, K. Sexting, consent and young people's ethics: Beyond Megan's Story. *Continuum* **2012**, *26*, 463–473. [CrossRef]
3. Klettke, B.; Hallford, D.J.; Mellor, D.J. Sexting prevalence and correlates: A systematic literature review. *Clin. Psychol. Rev.* **2014**, *34*, 44–53. [CrossRef]
4. Strassberg, D.S.; McKinnon, R.K.; Sustaíta, M.A.; Rullo, J. Sexting by High School Students: An Exploratory and Descriptive Study. *Arch. Sex. Behav.* **2013**, *42*, 15–21. [CrossRef] [PubMed]
5. Van Ouytsel, J.; Walrave, M.; Ponnet, K.; Heirman, W. The Association Between Adolescent Sexting, Psychosocial Difficulties, and Risk Behavior: Integrative Review. *J. Sch. Nurs.* **2015**, *31*, 54–69. [CrossRef] [PubMed]
6. Agustina, J.R.; Gómez-Durán, E.L. Sexting: Research Criteria of a Globalized Social Phenomenon. *Arch. Sex. Behav.* **2012**, *41*, 1325–1328. [CrossRef] [PubMed]
7. Krieger, M.A. Unpacking "Sexting": A Systematic Review of Nonconsensual Sexting in Legal, Educational, and Psychological Literatures. *Trauma Violence Abuse* **2017**, *18*, 593–601. [CrossRef]
8. Stokes, J.K. The Indecent Internet: Resisting Unwarranted Internet Exceptionalism Combating Revenge Porn. *Berkeley Technol. Law J.* **2014**, *29*, 929–952.
9. Walker, K.; Sleath, E. A systematic review of the current knowledge regarding revenge pornography and non-consensual sharing of sexually explicit media. *Aggress. Violent Behav.* **2017**, *36*, 9–24. [CrossRef]
10. Baumgartner, S.E.; Valkenburg, P.M.; Peter, J. Unwanted online sexual solicitation and risky sexual online behavior across the lifespan. *J. Appl. Dev. Psychol.* **2010**, *31*, 439–447. [CrossRef]
11. Citron, D.K.; Franks, M.A. Criminalizing revenge porn. *Wake Forest Law Rev.* **2014**, *49*, 345–391.
12. Döring, N. Consensual sexting among adolescents: Risk prevention through abstinence education or safer sexting? *Cyberpsychology* **2014**, *8*, 9. [CrossRef]
13. Renfrow, D.G.; Rollo, E.A. Sexting on campus: Minimizing perceived risks and neutralizing behaviors. *Deviant Behav.* **2014**, *35*, 903–920. [CrossRef]
14. Salter, M.; Crofts, T. Responding to revenge porn: Challenges to online legal impunity. In *New Views on Pornography: Sexuality, Politics, and the Law*; Comella, L., Tarrant, S., Eds.; Praeger Publishers: Santa Barbara, CA, USA, 2015; pp. 233–256.
15. Stroud, S.R. The Dark Side of the Online Self: A Pragmatist Critique of the Growing Plague of Revenge Porn. *J. Mass Media Ethics* **2014**, *29*, 168–183. [CrossRef]
16. Temple, J.R.; Le, V.D.; van den Berg, P.; Ling, Y.; Paul, J.A.; Temple, B.W. Brief report: Teen sexting and psychosocial health. *J. Adolesc.* **2014**, *37*, 33–36. [CrossRef]
17. Dir, A.L.; Coskunpinar, A.; Steiner, J.L.; Cyders, M.A. Understanding Differences in Sexting Behaviors Across Gender, Relationship Status, and Sexual Identity, and the Role of Expectancies in Sexting. *Cyberpsychol. Behav. Soc. Netw.* **2013**, *16*, 568–574. [CrossRef]
18. Champion, A.R.; Pedersen, C.L. Investigating differences between sexters and non-sexters on attitudes, subjective norms, and risky sexual behaviours. *Can. J. Hum. Sex.* **2015**, *24*, 205–214. [CrossRef]
19. Rentschler, C. #Safetytipsforladies: Feminist Twitter Takedowns of Victim Blaming. *Fem. Media Stud.* **2015**, *15*, 353–356.
20. Henry, N.; Powell, A. Beyond the "sext": Technology-facilitated sexual violence and harassment against adult women. *Aust. N. Z. J. Criminol.* **2015**, *48*, 104–118. [CrossRef]
21. Hall, R. "It can happen to you": Rape prevention in the age of risk management. *Hypatia* **2004**, *19*, 1–18.
22. Rentschler, C.A. Rape culture and the feminist politics of social media. *Girlhood Stud.* **2014**, *7*, 65–82. [CrossRef]
23. Fraser, C. From "Ladies First" to "Asking for It": Benevolent Sexism in the Maintenance of Rape Culture. *Calif. Law Rev.* **2015**, *103*, 141–204.
24. Brownmiller, S. *Against our will: Women and rape*; Simon and Schuster: New York, NY, USA, 1975.
25. Burt, M.R. Cultural myths and supports for rape. *J. Pers. Soc. Psychol.* **1980**, *38*, 217–230. [CrossRef] [PubMed]
26. Vance, K.; Sutter, M.; Perrin, P.B.; Heesacker, M. The Media's Sexual Objectification of Women, Rape Myth Acceptance, and Interpersonal Violence. *J. Aggress. Maltreat. Trauma* **2015**, *24*, 569–587. [CrossRef]

27. Lonsway, K.A.; Fitzgerald, L.F. Rape myths: In review. *Psychol. Women Q.* **1994**, *18*, 133–164. [CrossRef]
28. Szymanski, D.M.; Moffitt, L.B.; Carr, E.R. Sexual Objectification of Women: Advances to Theory and Research. *Couns. Psychol.* **2011**, *39*, 6–38. [CrossRef]
29. Fredrickson, B.L.; Roberts, T.-A. Objectification theory. *Psychol. Women Q.* **1997**, *21*, 173–206. [CrossRef]
30. Moradi, B.; Huang, Y.-P. Objectification theory and psychology of women: A decade of advances and future directions. *Psychol. Women Q.* **2008**, *32*, 377–398. [CrossRef]
31. Bartky, S.L. *Femininity and Domination: Studies in the Phenomenology of Oppression*; Psychology Press: New York, NY, USA, 1990.
32. Gervais, S.J.; Holland, A.M.; Dodd, M.D. My Eyes Are Up Here: The Nature of the Objectifying Gaze Toward Women. *Sex Roles* **2013**, *69*, 557–570. [CrossRef]
33. Bohner, G. *Vergewaltigungsmythen [Rape myths]*; Verlag Empirische Pädagogik: Landau, Germany, 1998.
34. Eyssel, F.; Bohner, G. Schema Effects of Rape Myth Acceptance on Judgments of Guilt and Blame in Rape Cases: The Role of Perceived Entitlement to Judge. *J. Interpers. Violence* **2011**, *26*, 1579–1605. [CrossRef] [PubMed]
35. Süssenbach, P.; Bohner, G.; Eyssel, F. Schematic influences of rape myth acceptance on visual information processing: An eye tracking approach. *J. Exp. Soc. Psychol.* **2012**, *48*, 660–668. [CrossRef]
36. Süssenbach, P.; Eyssel, F.; Rees, J.; Bohner, G. Looking for Blame Rape Myth Acceptance and Attention to Victim and Perpetrator. *J. Interpers. Violence* **2017**, *32*, 2323–2344. [CrossRef]
37. Rollero, C.; Tartaglia, S. The effects of objectification on stereotypical perception and attractiveness of women and men. *Psihologija* **2016**, *49*, 231–243. [CrossRef]
38. Perkins, A.B.; Becker, J.V.; Tehee, M.; Mackelprang, E. Sexting Behaviors Among College Students: Cause for Concern? *Int. J. Sex. Health* **2014**, *26*, 79–92. [CrossRef]
39. Noll, S.M.; Fredrickson, B.L. A mediational model linking self-objectification, body shame, and disordered eating. *Psychol. Women Q.* **1998**, *22*, 623–636. [CrossRef]
40. Strelan, P.; Hargreaves, D. Women Who Objectify Other Women: The Vicious Circle of Objectification? *Sex Roles* **2005**, *52*, 707–712. [CrossRef]
41. Gerger, H.; Kley, H.; Bohner, G.; Siebler, F. The acceptance of modern myths about sexual aggression scale: Development and validation in German and English. *Aggress. Behav.* **2007**, *33*, 422–440. [CrossRef]
42. Kleinbaum, D.G.; Klein, M. *Logistic Regression*; Springer: New York, NY, USA, 2010.
43. Draper, N.R.A. Is Your Teen at Risk? Discourses of adolescent sexting in United States television news. *J. Child. Media* **2012**, *6*, 221–236. [CrossRef]
44. Ringrose, J.; Harvey, L.; Gill, R.; Livingstone, S. Teen girls, sexual double standards and "sexting": Gendered value in digital image exchange. *Fem. Theory* **2013**, *14*, 305–323. [CrossRef]
45. Henry, N.; Powell, A. Technology-Facilitated Sexual Violence: A Literature Review of Empirical Research. *Trauma Violence Abuse* **2018**, *19*, 195–208. [CrossRef]
46. Bates, S. Revenge Porn and Mental Health. A Qualitative Analysis of the Mental Health Effects of Revenge Porn on Female Survivors. *Fem. Criminol.* **2017**, *12*, 22–42. [CrossRef]
47. Gill, R. Media, Empowerment and the "Sexualization of Culture" Debates. *Sex Roles* **2012**, *66*, 736–745. [CrossRef]
48. Englander, E. Coerced Sexting and Revenge Porn Among Teens. *Bullying Teen Aggress. Soc. Media* **2015**, *1*, 19–21.
49. Rohlinger, D.A. Eroticizing men: Cultural influences on advertising and male objectification. *Sex Roles* **2002**, *46*, 61–74. [CrossRef]
50. Ward, L.M. Media and Sexualization: State of Empirical Research, 1995–2015. *J. Sex Res.* **2016**, *53*, 560–577. [CrossRef]
51. Davidson, M.M.; Gervais, S.J.; Canivez, G.L.; Cole, B.P. A psychometric examination of the Interpersonal Sexual Objectification Scale among college men. *J. Couns. Psychol.* **2013**, *60*, 239–250. [CrossRef]
52. Engeln-Maddox, R.; Miller, S.A.; Doyle, D.M. Tests of Objectification Theory in Gay, Lesbian, and Heterosexual Community Samples: Mixed Evidence for Proposed Pathways. *Sex Roles* **2011**, *65*, 518–532. [CrossRef]
53. Bernard, P.; Loughnan, S.; Marchal, C.; Godart, A.; Klein, O. The Exonerating Effect of Sexual Objectification: Sexual Objectification Decreases Rapist Blame in a Stranger Rape Context. *Sex Roles* **2015**, *72*, 499–508. [CrossRef]

54. Gervais, S.J.; Bernard, P.; Klein, O.; Allen, J. Toward a Unified Theory of Objectification and Dehumanization. In *Objectification and (De)Humanization: 60th Nebraska Symposium on Motivation*; Gervais, S.J., Ed.; Springer: New York, NY, USA, 2013; pp. 1–23.
55. Heflick, N.A.; Goldenberg, J.L.; Cooper, D.P.; Puvia, E. From women to objects: Appearance focus, target gender, and perceptions of warmth, morality and competence. *J. Exp. Soc. Psychol.* **2011**, *47*, 572–581. [CrossRef]
56. Puvia, E.; Vaes, J. Being a Body: Women's Appearance Related Self-Views and their Dehumanization of Sexually Objectified Female Targets. *Sex Roles* **2013**, *68*, 484–495. [CrossRef]
57. Hall, C.; Hogue, T.; Guo, K. Differential Gaze Behavior towards Sexually Preferred and Non-Preferred Human Figures. *J. Sex Res.* **2011**, *48*, 461–469. [CrossRef] [PubMed]
58. Hewig, J.; Trippe, R.H.; Hecht, H.; Straube, T.; Miltner, W.H.R. Gender Differences for Specific Body Regions When Looking at Men and Women. *J. Nonverbal Behav.* **2008**, *32*, 67–78. [CrossRef]
59. Lykins, A.D.; Meana, M.; Strauss, G.P. Sex Differences in Visual Attention to Erotic and Non-Erotic Stimuli. *Arch. Sex. Behav.* **2008**, *37*, 219–228. [CrossRef] [PubMed]
60. Nummenmaa, L.; Hietanen, J.K.; Santtila, P.; Hyona, J. Gender and Visibility of Sexual Cues Influence Eye Movements While Viewing Faces and Bodies. *Arch. Sex. Behav.* **2012**, *41*, 1439–1451. [CrossRef] [PubMed]
61. Bolmont, M.; Cacioppo, J.T.; Cacioppo, S. Love Is in the Gaze: An Eye tracking Study of Love and Sexual Desire. *Psychol. Sci.* **2014**, *25*, 1748–1756. [CrossRef]
62. Bohner, G.; Eyssel, F.; Pina, A.; Siebler, F.; Viki, G.T. Rape myth acceptance: Cognitive, affective and behavioural effects of beliefs that blame the victim and exonerate the perpetrator. In *Rape: Challenging contemporary thinking*; Horvath, M., Brown, J.M., Eds.; Willan Publishing: Cullompton, UK, 2009; pp. 17–45.
63. Swim, J.K.; Aikin, K.J.; Hall, W.S.; Hunter, B.A. Sexism and racism: Old-fashioned and modern prejudices. *J. Pers. Soc. Psychol.* **1995**, *68*, 199–214. [CrossRef]
64. Salter, M. Justice and revenge in online counter-publics: Emerging responses to sexual violence in the age of social media. *Crime Media Cult.* **2013**, *9*, 225–242. [CrossRef]
65. Blais, C.; Jack, R.E.; Scheepers, C.; Fiset, D.; Caldara, R. Culture Shapes How We Look at Faces. *PLoS ONE* **2008**, *3*, e3022. [CrossRef] [PubMed]
66. Loughnan, S.; Fernandez-Campos, S.; Vaes, J.; Anjum, G.; Aziz, M.; Harada, C.; Holland, E.; Singh, I.; Purvia, E.; Tsuchiya, K. Exploring the role of culture in sexual objectification: A seven nations study. *Revue Internationale de Psychologie Sociale* **2015**, *28*, 125–152.
67. Buchanan, N.T.; Ormerod, A.J. Racialized sexual harassment in the lives of African American women. *Women Ther.* **2002**, *25*, 107–124. [CrossRef]
68. Ho, I.K.; Dinh, K.T.; Bellefontaine, S.A.; Irving, A.L. Sexual Harassment and Posttraumatic Stress Symptoms among Asian and White Women. *J. Aggress. Maltreat. Trauma* **2012**, *21*, 95–113. [CrossRef]
69. Lee, M.; Crofts, T. Gender, pressure, coercion and pleasure: Untangling motivations for sexting between young people. *Br. J. Criminol.* **2015**, *55*, 454–473. [CrossRef]
70. Capodilupo, C.M.; Nadal, K.L.; Corman, L.; Hamit, S.; Lyons, O.B.; Weinberg, A. The manifestation of gender microaggressions. In *Microaggressions and Marginality: Manifestation, Dynamics, and Impact*; Wing Sue, D., Ed.; John Wiley & Sons: Somerset, NJ, USA, 2010; pp. 193–216.
71. Papp, L.J.; Erchull, M.J. Objectification and System Justification Impact Rape Avoidance Behaviors. *Sex Roles* **2017**, *76*, 110–120. [CrossRef]
72. Tolman, D.L. Female Adolescents, Sexual Empowerment and Desire: A Missing Discourse of Gender Inequity. *Sex Roles* **2012**, *66*, 746–757. [CrossRef]
73. Egan, R.D. *Becoming sexual: A critical appraisal of the sexualization of girls*; Polity Press: Cambridge, UK, 2013.
74. Daniels, E.A.; Zurbriggen, E.L. The price of sexy: Viewers' perceptions of a sexualized versus nonsexualized Facebook profile photograph. *Psychol. Pop. Media Cult.* **2016**, *5*, 2–14. [CrossRef]
75. Manago, A.M.; Graham, M.B.; Greenfield, P.M.; Salimkhan, G. Self-presentation and gender on MySpace. *J. Appl. Dev. Psychol.* **2008**, *29*, 446–458. [CrossRef]
76. Seidman, G.; Miller, O.S. Effects of Gender and Physical Attractiveness on Visual Attention to Facebook Profiles. *Cyberpsychol. Behav. Soc. Netw* **2013**, *16*, 20–24. [CrossRef] [PubMed]
77. Hall, C.L.; Hogue, T.; Guo, K. Sexual Cognition Guides Viewing Strategies to Human Figures. *J. Sex Res.* **2014**, *51*, 184–196. [CrossRef] [PubMed]

78. Chalfen, R. Commentary Sexting as Adolescent Social Communication. *J. Child. Media* **2010**, *4*, 350–354. [CrossRef]
79. Hasinoff, A.A. Sexting as media production: Rethinking social media and sexuality. *New. Media Soc.* **2013**, *15*, 449–465. [CrossRef]
80. Lerum, K.; Dworkin, S.L. "Bad Girls Rule": An Interdisciplinary Feminist Commentary on the Report of the APA Task Force on the Sexualization of Girls. *J. Sex Res.* **2009**, *46*, 250–263. [CrossRef] [PubMed]

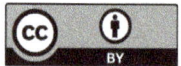

© 2019 by the authors. Licensee MDPI, Basel, Switzerland. This article is an open access article distributed under the terms and conditions of the Creative Commons Attribution (CC BY) license (http://creativecommons.org/licenses/by/4.0/).

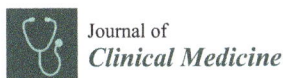

Article

Sexual Satisfaction and Mental Health in Prison Inmates

Rodrigo J. Carcedo [1], Daniel Perlman [2], Noelia Fernández-Rouco [3,*], Fernando Pérez [1] and Diego Hervalejo [1]

[1] Department of Developmental and Educational Psychology, University of Salamanca, Salamanca 37005, Spain; rcarcedo@usal.es (R.J.C.); ferp95@usal.es (F.P.); diegoherva@usal.es (D.H.)
[2] Department of Human Development and Family Studies, University of North Carolina at Greensboro, Greensboro, NC 27402, USA; d_perlma@uncg.edu
[3] Department of Education, University of Cantabria, Santander 39005, Spain
* Correspondence: fernandezrn@unican.es; Tel.: +34-942-201-179

Received: 30 April 2019; Accepted: 14 May 2019; Published: 17 May 2019

Abstract: The main goal of this study was to investigate the association between sexual satisfaction and mental health, and the combined effect of two previously found, statistically significant moderators: partner status and sexual abstinence. In-person interviews were conducted with 223 participants (49.327% males and 50.673% females). The effect of sexual satisfaction on mental health and the interactions of sexual satisfaction × partner status, sexual satisfaction × sexual abstinence, and sexual satisfaction × partner status × sexual abstinence were examined using simple moderation and moderated moderation tests after controlling for a set of sociodemographic, penitentiary, and interpersonal variables. Results revealed a direct relationship between sexual satisfaction and mental health only for the sexually abstinent group. Partner status was not significant as a moderator. It seems that the lack of sexual relationships is more powerful as a moderator than the lack of a romantic relationship. Additionally, the sexually abstinent group showed lower levels of sexual satisfaction in those with a partner outside or inside prison, and lower mental health independently of the current romantic status, than sexually active inmates. These findings point to the importance of sexual satisfaction to mental health in sexual situations of extreme disadvantage.

Keywords: sexual satisfaction; sexual abstinence; partner status; mental health; prison inmates

1. Introduction

More than 10 million people are living in jails and prisons worldwide [1], and considerably larger numbers of ex-prisoners are living in society [2]. A high prevalence of mental health problems is present in prison populations [3]. There is also increasing epidemiological evidence that prisoners are more likely to suffer from mental health problems than the average population [4–7].

In the most representative Spanish study that included 28.8% of the inmate populations in five different prisons, the lifetime prevalence rate of mental disorders was 84.4%. The prevalence of any mental disorder in the last month before the time of interview was 41.2% [8]. These results were confirmed more recently by a study with a smaller sample size ($n = 184$), obtained from three prototypical Spanish prisons [9]. A total percentage of 90.2% inmates had suffered a mental disorder during their lives. Also, 55.2% were suffering a mental disorder at the time. Finally, in this study, the inmate population was 5.3 times more likely to have a mental health problem than the general population.

These mental health problems are risk factors for a range of adverse outcomes in prison and on release including self-harm [10], suicide [11–16], and violence inside prison [17], and reoffending in released prisoners [2,18,19].

In sum, most prevalence studies have been conducted in developed countries and consistently show that a very high proportion of prisoners suffer from poor mental health [3,20]. Despite the high level of need, these disorders are frequently underdiagnosed and poorly treated [20]. In addition, a growing literature documents the detrimental consequences of incarceration for mental health [21–24]. For example, early scholars believed being imprisoned is associated with having higher rates of mental health disorders than inmates would have had if they had remained in the community [25]. Massoglia found evidence of persisting elevated mental health issues in previously incarcerated individuals [26]. Furthermore, incarceration is negatively associated with finances [27], family ties [28], and physical health [29] as well as a greater risk for sexual victimization [20].

All this makes the mental health status of current and former prison inmates an important public health issue [3]. Following the World Health Organization's definition, this study will consider mental health as not merely the absence of illness but "a state of well-being in which every individual realizes his or her own potential, can cope with the normal stresses of life, can work productively and fruitfully, and is able to make a contribution to her or his community" [30]. Thus, this concept includes mental illness but also understands mental health as a positive dimension of well-being [31].

One of the possible causes of prison inmates being an at-risk population for poor mental health is that they encounter difficulties in having a satisfactory sex life [32–35]. Linville found that approximately 75 percent of a sample of 100 male inmates in a minimum-security prison reported emotional problems due to sexual deprivation [36]. As a result of the sexual deprivation inmates experience, they may seek relief in alternative, less satisfactory and/or riskier ways [37]. Different studies have demonstrated a high rate of masturbation [38–40], and the presence of consensual homosexual behavior as alternative forms of sexual behaviors [41,42]. Such behaviors are sometimes coercive [43–45], and can lead to the transmission of sexual diseases such as HIV [46]. Conjugal visitations have been suggested as one possible solution. Consistent with this view, states that permit conjugal visits have lower instances of reported rape and other sexual offenses in their prisons [47]. Nonetheless, the low frequency of visits, the lack of good conditions [48], and their being restricted to married or committed partners limits the efficacy of conjugal visits.

All these experiences are evaluated by prison inmates determining their level of sexual satisfaction. Sexual satisfaction has been defined as "an affective response arising from one's subjective evaluation of the positive and negative dimensions associated with one's sexual relationship" [49] (p. 258). It is regarded as a fundamental dimension of the quality of sexual activity. Research on sexual satisfaction in prison inmates has generally shown very low levels of sexual satisfaction except for those with a romantic partner inside the same prison and those who did not remain abstinent [48,50,51]. Taken altogether, sexual needs are not well satisfied in prison.

Arguably, sexual satisfaction can be considered an essential component of general well-being and mental health. Empirically, higher sexual satisfaction is associated higher mental health and lower depression [52–54]. The recognition of the need to be loved, appreciated and cared for, and of the desire for intimate relationships that provide emotional sustenance and empathy, have been considered important aspects for maintaining mental health in prisons [30].

1.1. The Sexual Satisfaction and Mental Health Relationship Moderated by Partner Status and Sexual Abstinence

Research on the relationship between sexual satisfaction and mental health in prison inmates is in a fledgling state. Researchers have largely overlooked the part sexual satisfaction can play in inmates' mental health and well-being. Research involving these variables conducted with other populations is more extensive.

1.1.1. Research Conducted Outside Prisons

The consequences of a satisfying sex life are important areas of research that are gaining increasing attention in the psychological and medical literature, suggesting that sexuality maintains its importance even in the context of serious health concerns [55]. In this way, higher sexual satisfaction is associated with low levels of sexual anxiety [56,57], low psychopathological symptoms [57,58], and good mental health [59,60].

Furthermore, fostering patients' quality of life and mental health are key aims of health care in which subjective factors are commonly seen as central [61]. One subjective factor that has received very little attention is patients' sexual satisfaction, although Mallis et al.'s results showed that sexual satisfaction and quality of life are "strongly connected" (p. 447) [62]. Other research has found sexual dissatisfaction is higher in patients with depression than in those without depressive symptoms [63].

Turning to relationship status and its role in the association between sexual satisfaction and mental health, in both non-clinical and clinical samples, partnered compared to single individuals have tended to report higher sexual satisfaction and sexual activity [52,64,65]. Having a partner does not necessarily mean that couples live together or that they have an active sex life, but it increases the likelihood that partners do have consistent sexual contact. Furthermore, tight-knit social structures such as being in a close relationship often, but not always, lead to better mental health outcomes [66]. Consistent with the beneficial view of tight structures, Holt-Lunstad, Birmingham, and Jones [67] and others (e.g., [68]) have found that being married is associated with better mental and physical health. Analyses such as this typically lump everyone together and do not examine other predictors of mental within subgroups.

Although the moderating effect of partner status between sexual satisfaction and mental health was not specifically investigated in the aforementioned studies of partner status, there is important evidence that the negative aspects of romantic life (e.g., loneliness and dissatisfaction, two aspects related to the fact of not having a partner or not having a satisfactory relationship for meeting one's emotional needs) predict personal well-being more strongly than the positive aspects (e.g., marital satisfaction) [69]. Complementing the negative is stronger than the positive, other non-prison studies have found a strong relationship between sexual satisfaction and general well-being including mental health for those who had been sexually deprived due to the presence of sexual dysfunctions [70,71], physical disabilities [72], amputations [73], and having had germ-cell tumor therapy [74].

Other interpersonal variables, a category in which sexuality belongs [75], have a differential effect on mental health depending on partner status. For example, friendship quality only correlated significantly with depression among a group of college students without a romantic partner whereas no association was found in the group in a current romantic relationship [76].

Furthermore, Taleporos and McCabe compared the strength of this relationship for a group of people with and without sexual difficulty (physical disability vs. no physical disability) [72]. In this case, for both genders, the relationships between sexual satisfaction and indicators of mental health such as depression and self-esteem were stronger for people with physical disabilities than for able-bodied people. In other words, sexual satisfaction was a stronger predictor for the mental health of the group in a less favorable and more restrained condition. This situation might be comparable with the situation of sexually abstinent prison inmates who have shown much lower levels of sexual satisfaction than sexually active ones. In this comparison it is the sexually abstinent inmates who are in a more restrained and difficult situation.

Complementing Taleporos and McCabe's results, Laumann et al. found that in the cluster of countries where average levels of sexual satisfaction were low (male-centered regimes; in a worse situation with a less freedom of choice) there was a stronger relationship between sexual well-being and happiness, which may be considered as an indirect indicator of positive mental health status, than in the cluster of countries where average levels of sexual satisfaction were higher (gender-equal sexual regime; in a better and free situation) [77]. If results in this vein generalize, one would then expect the association between sexual satisfaction and mental health to be stronger among sexually abstinent inmates. Also, based on prisoners' previously mentioned negative feelings toward abstinence and the available data, we would expect the sexually abstinent inmates to have low sexual satisfaction.

1.1.2. Research Conducted in Prison Contexts

Sexual satisfaction, mental health and other well-being-related measures have been found to be significantly correlated in studies conducted in prison settings [48,50,51,78]. The findings revealed that higher levels of sexual satisfaction were associated with higher levels of mental health and other well-being related measures.

Typically, in these studies the association between sexual satisfaction and mental health has been examined without considering the participants' relationship status. The meaning of sexual experiences may vary depending on individuals' romantic situation, especially among prison inmates who have stringent restrictions imposed on their sexual activities. In fact, research has shown that prison inmates without a partner or with a partner outside the prison had lower levels of sexual satisfaction and mental health than those inmates with a partner inside the same prison [48]. In a later study, a moderating effect of partner status on the relationship between sexual satisfaction and mental health was found. Lower sexual satisfaction was associated with lower mental health only for those without a partner [50]. These latter findings illustrate a pattern suggested in non-prison studies that the association between sexual satisfaction and mental health is intensified for those in a less desirable romantic status.

In arguing that a lack of sexual satisfaction can negatively impact prison inmates' mental health, most authors [33–35,79] were referring mainly to inmates who had not had heterosexual relationships during their incarceration. Thus, these investigators were defacto ignoring inmates who were engaging in sanctioned sexual activities with their partners. Sexual satisfaction reflects a self-evaluation of one's current sexual life; sexual abstinence refers to a complete lack of sexual relationships during a period of time. In reporting their sexual satisfaction, abstinent inmates were reporting on their satisfaction with not having sanctioned partnered sex whereas partnered inmates were reporting on the partnered sexual activities they were permitted to have. As has been found, an inmate may have been sexually abstinent during the last 6 months, yet show reasonable high sexual satisfaction [32]. By contrast, an individual may have been sexually active and show low sexual satisfaction. Thus in a noteworthy way, the referent for their judgments of sexual satisfaction is different for abstinent inmates than it is for partnered inmates.

This opens the possibility that the relationship between inmates' sexual satisfaction and mental health may be different for sexual abstainers than for sexually active individuals. An earlier prison study found such a moderating effect [51]: sexual satisfaction was significantly associated with psychological health only for the group of inmates who had not had sexual relationships during the last 6 months, in other words, sexual abstainers.

In sum, previous research findings showed lower levels of sexual satisfaction and mental health in sexually abstinent inmates [32,51]. More importantly, an association between low sexual satisfaction and low mental health was only found for those who did not have a partner in the same prison (versus without a partner) [50] and those who remained sexual abstainers (versus non-abstainers) [32,51]. However, these two interaction effects have not been tested together to study (a) whether both are significant, (b) whether the proportion of variance for which they account is similar or different, and (c) whether there is a higher order interaction formed by sexual satisfaction, partner status, and sexual abstinence.

This study will focus on the new knowledge gained by including both abstinence and partner status. This current investigation also refines a previous study [50] because it includes three different partner statuses (no partner, partner outside of prison, and partner inside the same prison) instead of two (partner vs. no partner). Clearly there is a need of differentiating inmates with a partner inside or outside because these situations delineate different experiences.

In addition, this study benefits from a larger sample size and the addition of a set of control variables that have previously been demonstrated to have significant effects on mental health. Namely, poorer mental health has been exhibited by inmates who are younger, Caucasian [80], and married [80,81]; who have longer sentences and a longer expected time prior to their release [82]; who report poor general health [83]; who show higher levels of social and emotional loneliness [32,50,51,78]; and who, based on non-prison studies [84–86], masturbate more frequently. All these variables will be entered in the models as covariates.

1.1.3. Research Questions

Flowing from the summary of the aforementioned evidence found, two research questions emerge, a first and central question and an ancillary second one: (a) Will partner status and sexual activity level play a moderator role in the relationship between sexual satisfaction and mental health, after controlling for sociodemographic (sex, age, and nationality), penitentiary (total time in prison and estimated time to parole), and personal, social, and sexual well-being aspects (self-rated health, social, family, and romantic loneliness, and frequency of masturbation)? (see Figure 1) and (b) Will partner status and sexual abstinence be associated with inmates' sexual satisfaction and mental health, after controlling for sociodemographic (sex, age, and nationality), penitentiary (total time in prison and estimated time to parole), and personal, social, and sexual well-being aspects (self-rated health; social, family, and romantic loneliness; and frequency of masturbation)?

2. Experimental Section

2.1. Participants

Participants for this study were entirely inmates from the medium-security Topas penitentiary, located in Salamanca (Spain). This prison houses men and women in the same prison but in different modules. The prison administration decided from which men's and women's modules the investigators could recruit participants. After stratifying by gender, 80% of the participants were randomly selected, whereas 20% were selected under a "snowball" sampling scheme [36]. Participants were excluded from this study if they (a) had been in prison for less than 6 months, the time considered necessary to become adapted to prison life and develop new relationships inside the facility; (b) did not speak Spanish or English; (c) had been diagnosed with a serious mental disorder; or (d) were not in an optimal condition to be interviewed (e.g., under the influence of drugs or expressing high levels of anxiety or distrust toward the interviewer). Only twelve potential participants declined being interviewed. All of the participants found the interview to be a positive experience.

Due to the difficulties collecting information from this specific population, we retained for analyses in the present report participants in two of Carcedo et al.'s previous studies [50,51] that had 119 and 173 participants, respectively. For this study, a sample of 223 inmates from 20 to 62 years old (M = 35.172, SD = 7.823) was used. We selected the increase in sample size to ensure reasonable power for testing the interaction effects of interest in the current analyses. This increase resulted in successfully having at least 10 participants per subgroup formed by crossing partner status (inside, outside, no partner) and sexual abstinence categories (abstinent vs. non-abstinent). Although males and females in prison are not equal in number, we selected a roughly equal number of male (n = 110) and female (n = 113) participants in order to explore the possible effect of sex on the results and, consequently, the results' interpretation and discussion. Nationality was encoded in two levels: Spanish nationality (n = 103) and foreign, unspecified origin country (n = 120). Regarding the two moderators in this study, 76 inmates had no partner (34.080%), 61 had a partner outside the prison (27.354%), and 86 had a partner inside the prison (38.565%); also, 122 inmates reported having had sex in the last six months (54.709%) and 101 kept sexually abstinent (45.291%).

In comparison with inmates with a current romantic partner outside the prison, those in a relationship inside the same prison presented a higher frequency of in-person contact (t (145) = −12.413, $p > 0.001$; outside: M = 3.311, SD = 1.679; inside: M = 5.698, SD = 0.510; variable coding: 1 "never", 2 "more than 6 months", 3 "3–6 months", 4 "each 1–2 months", 5 "each 7–15 days", and 6 "every day or almost every day", and satisfaction with the current relationship (t (145) = −2.746, $p < 0.001$; outside: M = 3.510, SD = 1.678; inside: M = 4.358, SD = 1.326; variable coding: 1 "totally unsatisfied" and 5 "totally satisfied") and lower duration of the union in months (t (145) = 3.588, $p < 0.001$; outside: M = 102.459, SD = 100.593; inside: M = 49.831, SD = 77.172).

All sexually active inmates reported they had engaged in heterosexual behavior at least once in the last six months. Regarding frequency, 63.934% of sexually active inmates had had sexual relationships at least once every 15 days, 24.590% every 2 months, and 11.475% every 6 months. Most of these sexual relationships occurred in conjugal visit rooms (76.471%), but also in other locations inside the prison (shared areas such as the sociocultural module, prison laundry, kitchen, gym, etc. (19.328%) and family visit rooms (1.681%)) and during furloughs outside the prison (2.521%). Inmates reported that their sexual relationships had included vaginal coitus at least once in the last 6 months. It is also important to mention that three sexually active participants also reported to have had some homosexual contact in prison. Finally, no sexually active inmate was convicted of sex crimes.

Preliminary analyses did not find any significant effect of sex, in the presence of partner status and sexual activity level, on sexual satisfaction and mental health nor a moderating effect between these two variables. Therefore, both sexes were analyzed together and sex was only included as a control variable in all the analyses.

2.2. Design and Procedure

This study used a short-term longitudinal design. Two interview sessions were carried out with a difference of a week between them. The main associated variable and control variables were extracted from the first interview and the outcome (mental health) was taken from the second one. Each participant was interviewed in a private room located in his or her prison module, separated from the rest of the inmates. The interviews were kept short (approximately 30 min without counting the time dedicated to create a good relationship) to ensure that participants did not get tired and to avoid "interrogation effects".

All the interviews were conducted by the same interviewer to foster consistency. Before starting the interview, the interviewer spent a significant amount of time building a trustful relationship with every inmate (usually about 20–30 min, but depending on the speed of establishing rapport, in some cases it took up to 2 h). Afterwards, participants were invited to participate and were informed about the possibility of leaving the study whenever they wished to do so. Participants were informed about the confidentiality and anonymity of the study and all the participants signed consent forms. We consider that respecting all of these conditions is extremely important in collecting good-quality data from this population. Ignoring these conditions can easily increase distrust among the prison inmates. Finally, it is important to state that this study respected the norms of the Declaration of Helsinki's ethical principles for medical research involving human subjects.

2.3. Measures

2.3.1. Sexual Satisfaction

The sexual satisfaction subscale of the Multidimensional Sexual Self-Concept Questionnaire (MSSCQ) [87] was used to measure the main variable of this study. A total of five items were scored on a five-point Likert-type scale that ranged from 1 (not at all characteristic of me) to 5 (very characteristic of me). Cronbach's alpha for this scale was 0.960.

2.3.2. Moderating Variables: Sexual Activity Level and Partner Status

This variable was recorded as 0 for the inmates who had experienced sexual relationships in the past 6 months (non-abstinent), and 1 for the inmates who had not (abstinent). Sexual relationships were understood as any sexual behavior with another person including vaginal or anal intercourse, oral sex, and mutual masturbation and genital caresses, excluding kisses, hugs, and non-genital caress. Partner status was coded to have three categorical levels: no partner (0), partner outside (1), and partner inside the prison (2). Partner status was defined as a relationship deemed, in the inmate's mind, as one that both partners considered serious.

2.3.3. Outcome Variable: Mental Health

This construct was measured with the short Spanish version of the Psychological health subscale included in the World Health Quality of Life scale (WHOQOL-BREF) [88]. Six items were scored on a five-point Likert-type scale that ranged, with different labels, from 1 (not at all; very dissatisfied; never) to 5 (extremely-completely; very satisfied; always). Cronbach's alpha was 0.709. Sample items include "To what extent do you feel your life to be meaningful?" and "How often do you have negative feelings such as blue mood, despair, anxiety, depression?" This scale was selected for multiple reasons: It is brief; it conceptualizes mental health not only as the absence of illness but also the presence of positive aspects of mental health; and its concurrent validity as indicated by its high correlation ($r = 0.70$) with the widely used SF-36 (36-Item Short-Form Health Survey) mental health subscale [89].

2.3.4. Control Variables: Sociodemographic, Penitentiary, and Personal, Social, and Sexual Well-Being Variables

Considering sociodemographic variables, sex was codified as 0 for male and 1 for female inmates, age was asked directly to each inmate and confirmed against inmate penitentiary records for accuracy, and nationality was dichotomized into Spaniards (0) versus foreigners (1). Regarding penitentiary variables, total time in prison refers to the total time spent in prison for previous and current offenses. This information was collected by reviewing inmates' penitentiary records, and it was recorded in months. Estimated time to parole was captured by asking the inmates how much time they expected to be in prison from that moment, based on the information they possessed. This variable was also computed in months.

With respect to personal, social, and sexual well-being variables, self-rated health was measured by asking the participants "in general, would you say your health is: excellent (4); very good (3); good (2); fair (1); or poor (0)?" [90]. The short version of the Social and Emotional Loneliness Scale for Adults (SELSA-S) [91] was used to measure both types of loneliness. SELSA-S consists of three subscales labeled (a) social loneliness, (b) family-emotional loneliness, and (c) romantic-emotional loneliness. Participants rated 15 items (five per scale) on a seven-point Likert-type scale that ranged from 1 (strongly disagree) to 7 (strongly agree). Cronbach's alphas were 0.829, 0.898, and 0.840 for social, family-emotional, and romantic-emotional loneliness, respectively. Finally, masturbation frequency was codified into six levels based on the frequency inmates reported having masturbated during the last 6 months: (1) never, (2) less than once a month, (3) once or twice a month, (4) once or twice a week, (5) once a day, (6) twice a day or more.

Each scale or subscale score was obtained by adding the item scores and dividing them by the number of items answered. Higher scores represented higher levels in that dimension for all the variables included in this study.

2.4. Statistical Analysis

A 3 × 2, partner status (no partner, partner outside the prison, and partner inside) by sexual activity (abstinent vs. non-abstinent inmates) ANCOVA was used to first analyze the differences in sexual satisfaction and then performed again with mental health as the outcome variable. Each analysis controlled for sociodemographic, penitentiary, personal, social, and sexual well-being variables. If the partner status by sexual activity interaction between factors was statistically significant, Bonferroni post-hoc tests for multiple comparisons were conducted. Statistical significance was defined as $p < 0.05$.

The Breuch–Pagan test was conducted to test heteroscedasticity between sexual satisfaction and mental health. The macro heteroscedasticity test for SPSS [92] was utilized for this purpose. To study the relationships of sexual satisfaction with mental health and the moderating effects of partner status and sexual activity level, the PROCESS 3.2. macro for SPSS [93] was utilized. PROCESS's models number one and two for two-way interactions (also called simple moderation), and three for the three-way interaction (also named moderated moderation) were used. Additionally, 95% confidence intervals were calculated based on 5000 bootstrap samples. The HC3 heteroscedasticity-consistent standard error estimator was applied [94] due to the violation of homoscedasticity. All the statistical analyses were conducted using the IBM SPSS 23 package (IBM Corp., Armonk, NY, USA).

3. Results

Descriptive information for the variables considered in this study are included in Table 1. With sexual satisfaction as the outcome variable, the 3 × 2 partner status by sexual activity level ANCOVA yielded significant effects for sexual activity level ($F_{(1, 207)} = 47.115$, $p < 0.001$, $\eta^2_p = 0.185$) and the partner status × sexual activity level interaction ($F_{(2, 207)} = 14.638$, $p < 0.001$, $\eta^2_p = 0.124$). Bonferroni post-hoc comparisons revealed lower levels of sexual satisfaction in sexually abstinent inmates in comparison with non-abstinent for those who had a partner outside ($p < 0.001$; abstinent: $M = 0.838$, $SE = 0.237$; non-abstinent: $M = 2.979$, $SE = 0.178$) or inside the same prison ($p < 0.001$; abstinent: $M = 1.094$, $SE = 0.302$; non-abstinent: $M = 3.006$, $SE = 0.155$). However, no differences in sexual satisfaction between abstinent and non-abstinent inmates were found for those who were not involved in a romantic relationship ($p > 0.05$; abstinent: $M = 2.462$, $SE = 0.197$; non-abstinent: $M = 2.312$, $SE = 0.354$).

In the 3 × 2 ANCOVA with mental health as the outcome measure, sexual activity level yielded a significant effect ($F_{(1, 207)} = 10.182$, $p < 0.01$, $\eta^2_p = 0.047$). Those who were sexually abstinent ($M = 3.260$, $SE = 0.081$) presented lower levels of mental health in comparison with non-abstinent inmates ($M = 3.633$, $SE = 0.080$). The effect due to partner status was non-significant.

Regarding associations with mental health, the Breuch–Pagan test yielded a significant result for heteroscedasticity ($LM = 3.883$, $p < 0.05$). Thus the HC3 heteroscedasticity-consistent standard error estimator was used [42] to run the regression model. The three-way interaction of sexual satisfaction × partner status × sexual activity level was not significant ($\Delta R^2 = 0.001$, $F_{(2, 201)} = 0.174$, $p > 0.05$). By contrast, the two-way sexual satisfaction × sexual activity level interaction was statistically significant ($\Delta R^2 = 0.016$, $F_{(2, 205)} = 8.298$, $p < 0.01$), whereas the sexual satisfaction × partner status interaction was not ($\Delta R^2 = 0.007$, $F_{(1, 205)} = 1.590$, $p > 0.05$). In the former case, the conditional effects of sexual satisfaction at the values of the moderators showed lower levels of mental health only for those who were abstinent during the last six months. This result was found significant across the three levels of partner status (see Table 2 and Figure 1) and for the whole sample (sexual abstinent group: $B = 0.176$, $SE = 0.089$, $t = 1.990$, $p < 0.05$, 95% CI = (−0.346, 0.129)). No significant effect was observed for sexually active individuals.

Table 1. Correlations, means, and standard deviations of the variables considered in this study.

	Mean	SD	%(1)	1	2	3	4	5	6	7	8	9	10	11a	11b	11c	12	13	14
1. Sex (0 = male; 1 = female)			50.673		0.032	−0.033	−0.348 ***	0.102	−0.019	−0.259 ***	−0.070	−0.257 ***	−0.485 ***	−0.199 **	0.002	0.192 **	−0.364 ***	0.264 ***	0.048
2. Age	35.172	7.822				−0.108	0.156 *	0.006	−0.164 *	0.098	−0.027	−0.074	−0.146 *	0.006	0.074	−0.074	0.054	0.072	−0.014
3. Nationality (0 = Spanish; 1 = foreigner)			53.812				−0.269 ***	0.016	0.014	0.089	0.029	0.057	0.046	0.021	0.044	−0.061	0.120	−0.059	0.163 *
4. Total time in prison	54.337	48.623						−0.020	−0.010	0.178 **	0.165 *	0.139 *	0.265 ***	−0.162 *	−0.204 **	0.029	0.176 **	−0.125	−0.041
5. Time to parole	19.878	21.763							−0.088	0.029	0.025	0.001	−0.062	−0.081	0.082	0.004	−0.018	0.055	−0.141 *
6. Self-rated health	3.466	1.280								−0.165 **	−0.086	−0.148 *	0.053	−0.085	−0.106	0.180 **	−0.050	0.096	0.300 ***
7. Social loneliness	3.479	1.790									0.317 ***	0.274 ***	0.160 *	0.233 ***	−0.042	−0.189 **	0.265 ***	−0.211 **	−0.371 ***
8. Family loneliness	2.175	1.690										0.086	0.132 *	0.118	−0.098	−0.026	0.101	0.017	−0.090
9. Romantic loneliness	4.034	2.111											0.104	0.826 ***	−0.245 ***	−0.579 ***	0.547 ***	−0.563 ***	−0.198 **
10. Masturbation frequency	2.740	1.403												0.147 *	−0.181 **	0.022	0.143 *	−0.122	0.063
11a. No partner (0 = other; 1 = no partner)			34.081												−0.441 ***	−0.570 ***	0.600 ***	−0.449 ***	−0.164 *
11b. Partner inside (0 = other; 1 = partner inside)			38.565													−0.486 ***	−0.094	0.010	−0.024
11c. Partner outside (0 = other; 1 = partner outside)			27.354														−0.499 ***	0.428 ***	0.181 **
12. Sexual activity level (0 = active; 1 = abstinent)			45.291															−0.611 ***	−0.252 ***
13. Sexual satisfaction	2.483	3.449																	0.309 ***
14. Mental health	1.467	0.724																	

* $p < 0.05$; ** $p < 0.01$; *** $p < 0.001$. %(1): Percentage of group with label "1" (females, foreigner, partner status, and abstinent) for dichotomous variables.

Table 2. Multiple regression analysis on mental health and conditional effects of sexual satisfaction at values of the moderators (partner status and sexual activity level).

	Mental Health			
	B	SE	t	95% CI
Sociodemographic and penitentiary variables				
Sex	−0.043	0.117	−0.366	(−0.273, 0.188)
Age	0.008	0.006	1.252	(−0.005, 0.021)
Nationality	0.359	0.092	3.899 ***	(0.178, 0.541)
Total time in prison	0.001	0.001	0.996	(−0.001, 0.003)
Time to parole	−0.004	0.002	−2.092 *	(−0.008, 0.001)
Personal, social, and sexual well-being variables				
Self-rated health	0.133	0.036	3.685 ***	(0.062, 0.204)
Social loneliness	−0.13	0.028	−4.592 ***	(−0.186, −0.074)
Family loneliness	−0.002	0.027	−0.072	(−0.056, 0.052)
Romantic loneliness	0.030	0.05	0.597	(−0.069, 0.129)
Masturbation frequency	0.058	0.038	1.515	(−0.017, 0.133)
Conditional effects				
Partner outside	−0.271	0.324	−0.835	(−0.910, 0.369)
Partner inside	−0.180	0.317	−0.566	(−0.805, 0.445)
Sexual activity level	−0.628	0.224	−2.800 **	(−1069, −0.186)
Sexual satisfaction	−0.108	0.121	−0.899	(−0.346, 0.129)
Two-way interaction model				
Sexual satisfaction × Partner status (outside)	0.221	0.124	1.781	(−0.024, 0.467)
Sexual satisfaction × Partner status (inside)	0.175	0.116	1.500	(−0.055, 0.404)
Sexual satisfaction × Sexual activity level	0.285	0.099	2.881 **	(0.090, 0.479)
R^2	0.355 ***			
Sexual satisfaction at values of the moderators				
Non-sexual abstinent—No partner	−0.108	0.121	−0.899	(−0.346, 0.129)
Non-sexual abstinent—Partner outside	0.113	0.063	1.791	(−0.011, 0.237)
Non-sexual abstinent—Partner inside	0.066	0.057	1.157	(−0.047, 0.179)
Sexual abstinent—No partner	0.176	0.089	1.990 *	(0.002, 0.351)
Sexual abstinent—Partner outside	0.398	0.104	3.835 ***	(0.193, 0.602)
Sexual abstinent—Partner inside	0.351	0.098	3.577 ***	(0.157, 0.544)

* $p < 0.05$; ** $p < 0.01$; *** $p < 0.001$. B, Unstandardized coefficient; SE, Standard Error.

As clearly can be seen in Figure 1, the interaction effect of sexual satisfaction × sexual activity presents a similar pattern for the groups of inmates without a partner, and in a current relationship outside or inside the prison. It is important to highlight that overall a decrease in sexual satisfaction of the sexually abstinent group is associated with a reduction of mental health levels, and the contrary, an increase in sexual satisfaction is related to an improvement in mental health.

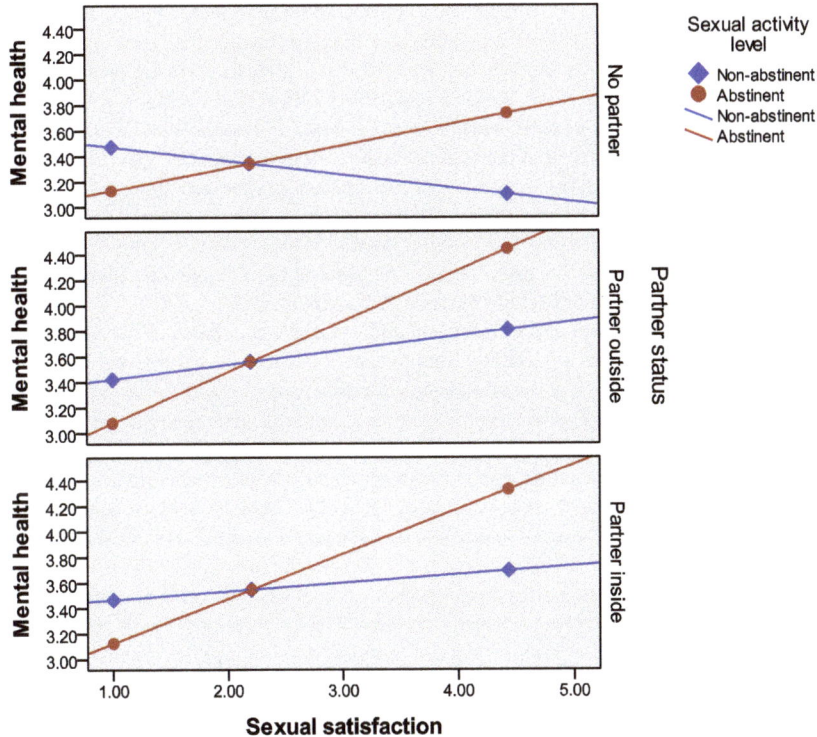

Figure 1. Sexual satisfaction × sexual activity level interaction associated with mental health for three different partner status groups.

4. Discussion

A direct relationship between sexual satisfaction and mental health was only found for the sexually abstinent group in this study. Partner status did not appear as a significant moderator. However, among those with a partner outside or inside prison, the sexually abstinent group showed lower levels of sexual satisfaction and mental health than sexually active inmates.

Again, sexual satisfaction was found to be significantly associated with mental health, as in other prison studies [36,50,51,78] and non-prison studies [52–54,56–60,63]. In this study, however, the sexual satisfaction, mental health association was only obtained for those who had remained sexually abstinent for at least the last six months. Previous research testing just one moderator has found that higher levels of sexual satisfaction were associated with higher levels of mental health only for prison inmates without a partner [50] and inmates who were sexually abstinent [51]. The current study examined the impact of both moderators, partner status and sexual activity level, together on the sexual satisfaction, mental health association. The results of this analysis showed that only the sexual satisfaction × sexual activity interaction was statistically significant. Neither the sexual satisfaction × partner status interaction nor the three-way interaction was significant. Thus a key implication of this study is that the lack of sexual relationships is more powerful as a moderator than the lack of a romantic relationship.

An important question here is why the lack of sexual relationships emerged in the regression analysis as significantly associated with mental health, whereas partner status did not. We speculate that sexual needs may be more important or basic than the emotional needs associated with romantic relationships. Sexuality, and more specifically sexual desire, comprises cognitive, emotional, and physiological processes and is consubstantial to the fact of being humans. Sexual desire may be a stimulus that sparks the inmates' sensitivity to their lack of sexual satisfaction. Lack of sexual contact in prison has even been named by inmates as "sexual torture" [32]. By contrast, wishing to be in a romantic relationship in a prison where the pool of eligible partners may not be especially attractive, may produce either lower levels of reactance and/or lower levels of dissatisfaction with not having a partner. In addition, intimacy and emotional needs can be solved by other ties, like close friends [75]. This suggests that future research could profitably focus on the role of sexual desire levels as a means of dealing effectively with inmates' sexual deprivation and/or the role that non-romantic, personal relationships contribute to improving their mental health. Hence, the damaging impact of being exposed to circumstances perceived as negative could be lessened by promoting positive interpersonal experiences and healthy interactions within inmates' daily experiences.

Prison settings are an unconventional, yet potentially diagnostic, context in which to study the sexual satisfaction, mental health association. Similar contexts would be worth considering in other public health studies. The meaning of sexual satisfaction may be completely different for those who are sexually inactive or suffering from serious restrictions vis-a-vis sexual activities than for those who are sexually active. The current results have possible implications for other populations whose freedom to choose has been reduced or eliminated due to constraining situations or who are involved in more negative or difficult circumstances. As noted previously, strong associations between sexual satisfaction and mental health or other well-being related measures have been found in other populations afflicted by different medical conditions [70–74] or living in a more sexually restrained culture [77].

This study also found significantly lower levels of sexual satisfaction in the abstinent group. This result is consistent with previous research in prison [32,51]. Furthermore, there were parallel significant differences in sexual satisfaction between abstinent and sexually active inmates in both the groups with a partner outside and inside the prison (not all inmates with a partner were sexually active), but not for those without a partner. Having a partner and not having access to sexual relationships can generate even more reactance and/or create a worse position than not having a partner and sexual relationships. Additionally, sexually abstinent inmates showed low mental health. Presumably the abstinent inmates were in a worse situation and experiencing greater reactance to the loss of freedom with respect to their sexual lives than the sexually active inmates. All these results are consistent with previous research developed within prison contexts, highlighting inmates' difficulties in meeting their sexual needs [32–35,51] and, as a consequence of this, presenting mental and emotional health problems [36].

Findings stemming from the two research questions of this study point to the crucial role sexual abstinence can have for mental health in some circumstances. Low sexual satisfaction (only for inmates with a partner outside or inside the prison) correlated with poorer mental health and a significant relationship between sexual satisfaction and mental health was observed in sexual abstainers. The abstinent group may be increasing their desire for sexual relationships due to their sexual deprivation [95]. Individuals wish to operate with a freedom to choose behaviors to satisfy their needs and if their freedom is reduced, threatened, or eliminated, individuals will become "motivationally aroused" to regain this freedom (see reactance theory [96,97]). Also, as seen in our results, this group is afflicted by sexual dissatisfaction, possibly the result of a large gap between their desires and their reality. Negative information and events (e.g., being abandoned by partners, losing friends, etc.) per se have been shown to have more impact on individuals' judgments and well-being than positive ones (e.g., gaining friends, partners, etc.) (see "the bad is stronger than good approach" [98]), especially in stigmatizing contexts [99]. This association has also been found in romantic relationships in non-prison studies [69].

The reactance and the bad is stronger than good explanations complement one another but do differ. The reactance interpretation sees motivation as a triggering factor in the linkage between sexual abstinence and mental health. The "bad is better than good" interpretation places primary emphasis on evaluation per se as crucial in the sexual abstinence-mental health association. Future research might profitably examine whether the processes implied by one of these explanations is more applicable than the processes implied by the other and test this current study's findings in other populations where individuals are afflicted by sexual deprivation or restriction due to different medical conditions or social factors.

In sum, this current investigation has found (a) lower levels of both sexual satisfaction and mental health in the sexually abstinent group, and (b) a stronger sexual satisfaction and mental health association in that group. Our perspective is that sexual satisfaction has been strongly correlated with mental health for the abstinent inmates likely because they are in a sexually worse or more deprived situation, and a similar, strong sexual satisfaction-mental health correlation should be observable in other comparably compromised situations or populations.

Our findings have important implications. First, inmates, especially those who are not sexually active, may benefit from prison policies that ease access to romantic and, especially, sexual relationships. We would note that inmates scoring higher on mental health have lower levels of misconduct [100] and lower recidivism rate after release [101]. Promoting positive mental health in prison inmates during incarceration and therefore increasing the likelihood of a successful reentry into society is a central concern with important consequences for public health, security, and the economy. According to this, clinical interventions to increase sexual access could be introduced to enhance inmates' sexual satisfaction. This in turn should be associated with an increase in their mental health. Such changes, however, should take into account the risk profile of inmates because it may be an important variable influencing the choice of interventions.

Assuming inmates will not be able to engage in sexual activities with a partner, other policies and interventions may also be helpful. A shift in cognitions and/or attitudes might influence inmates' evaluation of their sexual satisfaction. Cognitive restructuring techniques might be useful in this regard. Also, helping inmates to focus on other activities, especially ones that they pursue passionately, may relieve part of the distress associated with abstinence. In his dual theory of passion, Vallerand has shown that what he calls harmonious engagement in activities leads to psychological well-being [102]. Finally, increasing privacy in prison cells could facilitate masturbation as another way to obtain some sexual pleasure. Future research should address possible differences in sexual satisfaction between inmates who do, or do not, share their cells with other inmates. Also, it would be worthwhile to compare inmates living alone in a cell but in different prisons where inmates have more or less privacy (e.g., cameras in the rooms, prison officers entering in the cell without asking in advance, etc.).

We also believe that clinicians working with other populations who see their sexual freedom threatened (e.g., physical disabilities, older adults in nursing homes, etc.) can benefit from considering the implications of this study. Populations at risk of mental health problems should also be questioned about the presence or absence of sexual activity in their lives as a means of improving diagnosis and a more accurate intervention plan. Including sexual satisfaction in any diagnosis of mental health and its subsequent intervention seems sensible to consider, especially for those who have difficulties in meeting their sexual needs. Working on external impediments or barriers to having access to sexual relationships should be addressed too. Finally, clinical strategies aimed at reducing patients' reactance and negative evaluations of their sexual deprivation coupled with helping patients discover and perform new highly motivating activities may help patients overcome part of the distress associated with their actual sexual situation.

Apropos of the limitations of this work, this study is correlational so causation is difficult to infer although we used a short-term longitudinal design. Also, a few participants affirmed engaging in homosexual behavior. Despite our stressing the confidentiality and anonymity of the study, homosexual contacts might have been underreported by the inmates. The Spanish context is conservative in character, where heteronormativity (the cultural assumption that heterosexuality is the only valid social norm) is tied deeply to culture [103]. These values are definitely prone to be found in prison inmates too [104]. In this context it is not easy to acknowledge engaging in homosexual behaviors. However, all the participants pointed out they felt very comfortable during the interview and disclosed information that they considered sensitive and important.

5. Conclusions

In sum, correctional systems often adopt deprivation as a solution to inmates' sexual desires during incarceration. This study offers evidence regarding the importance of sexual satisfaction for their mental health, especially for abstinent inmates. A clear implication of this work is to urge prison administrators to find different solutions for inmates' sexuality that helps them to deal with their sexual desires. But not only that, this study adds new evidence to highlight the importance of considering sexual satisfaction as a predictor of mental health especially in those populations whose freedom to engage in partnered sexual activity has been threatened. From a public health perspective, the association between sexual satisfaction and mental health can vary depending on an individual's sexual activity level, as has been found in this study. Clinicians and health professional should take into consideration this possibility as part of their patients' evaluation and intervention.

Author Contributions: Conceptualization, R.J.C., D.P. and N.F.-R.; Methodology, R.C., D.P., F.P., and N.F.-R.; Software, R.J.C. and F.P.; Validation, R.J.C., F.P. and N.F.-R.; Formal analysis, R.J.C., F.P., and N.F.-R.; Investigation, R.J.C. and D.H.; Resources, R.J.C. and D.H.; Data curation, R.J.C. F.P., N.F.-R., and D.H.; Writing—original draft preparation, R.J.C., D.P., F.P., N.F.-R., and D.H.; Writing—review and editing, R.J.C., D.P., F.P., N.F.-R., and D.H.; Visualization, R.J.C., F.P., N.F.-R., and D.H.; Supervision, R.J.C.; Project administration, R.J.C.; Funding acquisition, R.J.C.

Funding: This research was funded by the regional education authority of Castile and Leon (Junta de Castilla y León, ref. SA007B08).

Conflicts of Interest: The authors declare no conflict of interest.

References

1. Walmsley, R. *World Prison Population List*; International Center for Prison Studies: London, UK, 2013.
2. Chang, Z.; Larsson, H.; Lichtenstein, P.; Fazel, S. Psychiatric disorders and violent reoffending: A national cohort study of convicted prisoners in Sweden. *Lancet Psychiatry* **2015**, *2*, 891–900. [CrossRef]
3. Schildbach, C.; Schildbach, S. Yield and efficiency of mental disorder screening at intake to prison: A comparison of DIA-X short-and long-screening-protocols in compensation prisoners. *Front. Psychiatry* **2018**, *9*, 538. [CrossRef]
4. Alevizopoulos, G.; Igoumenou, A. Psychiatric disorders and criminal history in male prisoners in Greece. *Int. J. Law Psychiatry* **2016**, *47*, 171–175. [CrossRef]
5. Daquin, J.C.; Daigle, L.E. Mental disorder and victimisation in prison: Examining the role of mental health treatment. *Crim. Behav. Ment. Health* **2018**, *28*, 141–151. [CrossRef]
6. Fazel, S.; Danesh, J. Serious mental disorder in 23000 prisoners: A systematic review of 62 surveys. *Lancet* **2002**, *359*, 545–550. [CrossRef]
7. White, L.M.; Lau, K.S.L.; Aalsma, M.C. Detained adolescents: Mental health needs, treatment use, and recidivism. *J. Am. Acad. Psychiatry Law* **2016**, *44*, 200–212. [PubMed]
8. Vicens, E.; Tort, V.; Dueñas, R.M.; Muro, A.; Pérez-Arnau, F.; Arroyo, J.M.; Acín, E.; de Vicente, A.; Guerrero, R.; Lluch, J.; et al. The prevalence of mental disorders in Spanish prisons. *Crim. Behav. Ment. Health* **2011**, *21*, 321–332. [CrossRef] [PubMed]
9. Zabala-Baños, M.C.; Segura, A.; Maestre-Miquel, C.; Martínez-Lorca, M.; Rodríguez-Martín, B.; Romero, D.; Rodríguez, M. Prevalencia de trastorno mental y factores de riesgo asociados en tres prisiones de España [Mental disorder prevalence and associated risk factors in three prisons of Spain]. *Rev. Esp. Sanid. Penit.* **2016**, *18*, 13–23. [CrossRef] [PubMed]
10. Hawton, K.; Linsell, L.; Adeniji, T.; Sariaslan, A.; Fazel, S. Self-harm in prisons in England and Wales: An epidemiological study of prevalence, risk factors, clustering, and subsequent suicide. *Lancet* **2014**, *383*, 1147–1154. [CrossRef]
11. Fazel, S.; Cartwright, J.; Norman-Nott, A.; Hawton, K. Suicide in prisoners: A systematic review of risk factors. *J. Clin. Psychiatry* **2008**, *69*, 1721–1731. [CrossRef]

12. Fazel, S.; Grann, M.; Kling, B.; Hawton, K. Prison suicide in 12 countries: An ecological study of 861 suicides during 2003–2007. *Soc. Psychiatry Psychiatr. Epidemiol.* **2011**, *46*, 191–195. [CrossRef]
13. Haglund, A.; Tidemalm, D.; Jokinen, J.; Långström, N.; Liechtenstein, P.; Fazel, S.; Runeson, B. Suicide after release from prison-a population-based cohort study from Sweden. *J. Clin. Psychiatry* **2014**, *75*, 1047. [CrossRef]
14. Pratt, D.; Piper, M.; Appleby, L.; Webb, R.; Shaw, J. Suicide in recently released prisoners: A population-based cohort study. *Lancet* **2006**, *368*, 119–123. [CrossRef]
15. Rivlin, A.; Hawton, K.; Marzano, L.; Fazel, S. Psychiatric disorders in male prisoners who made near-lethal suicide attempts: Case–control study. *Br. J. Psychiatry* **2010**, *197*, 313–319. [CrossRef]
16. Verona, E.; Hicks, B.M.; Patrick, C.J. Psychopathy and suicidality in female offenders: Mediating influences of personality and abuse. *J. Consult. Clin. Psychol.* **2005**, *73*, 1065. [CrossRef] [PubMed]
17. Gonçalves, L.C.; Gonçalves, R.A.; Martins, C.; Dirkzwager, A.J. Predicting infractions and health care utilization in prison: A meta-analysis. *Crim. Justice Behav.* **2014**, *41*, 921–942. [CrossRef]
18. Baillargeon, J.; Binswanger, I.A.; Penn, J.V.; Williams, B.A.; Murray, O.J. Psychiatric disorders and repeat incarcerations: The revolving prison door. *Am. J. Psychiatry* **2009**, *166*, 103–109. [CrossRef]
19. Shaffer, H.J.; Nelson, S.E.; LaPlante, D.A.; LaBrie, R.A.; Albanese, M.; Caro, G. The epidemiology of psychiatric disorders among repeat DUI offenders accepting a treatment-sentencing option. *J. Consult. Clin. Psychol.* **2007**, *75*, 795. [CrossRef]
20. Fazel, S.; Hayes, A.J.; Bartellas, K.; Clerici, M.; Trestman, R. Mental health of prisoners: Prevalence, adverse outcomes, and interventions. *Lancet Psychiatry* **2016**, *3*, 871–881. [CrossRef]
21. Kaeble, D.; Glaze, L.; Tsoutis, A.; Minton, T. *Correctional Populations in the United States*; NCJ 249513; U.S. Department of Justice: Washington, DC, USA, September 2015.
22. Porter, L.C.; DeMarco, L.M. Beyond the dichotomy: Incarceration dosage and mental health. *Criminology* **2019**, *57*, 136–156. [CrossRef]
23. Toch, H. *Living in Prison: The Ecology of Survival*; Free Press: New York, NY, USA, 1977.
24. Zamble, E.; Porporino, F.J. *Coping, Behavior, and Adaptation in Prison Inmates*; Springer-Verlag Publishing: New York, NY, USA, 1988.
25. Sykes, G.M. *The Society of Captives: A Study of a Maximum Security Prison*; Princeton University Press: Princeton, NJ, USA, 2007; Original work published 1958.
26. Massoglia, M. Incarceration as exposure: The prison, infectious disease, and other stress-related illnesses. *J. Health Soc. Behav.* **2008**, *49*, 56–71. [CrossRef]
27. Western, B. *Punishment and Inequality in America*; Russell Sage Foundation: New York, NY, USA, 2006.
28. Lopoo, L.M.; Western, B. Incarceration and the formation and stability of marital unions. *J. Marriage Fam.* **2005**, *67*, 721–734. [CrossRef]
29. Allen, S.A.; Wakeman, S.E.; Cohen, R.L.; Rich, J.D. Physicians in US prisons in the era of mass incarceration. *Int. J. Prison Health* **2010**, *6*, 100.
30. Durcan, G.; Zwemstra, J.C. Mental health in prison. In *Prisons and Health*; Enggist, S., Møller, L., Galea, G., Udesen, U., Eds.; WHO Regional Office for Europe: Copenhagen, Denmark, 2014; pp. 87–95.
31. King, M.; Nazareth, I.; Levy, G.; Walker, C.; Morris, R.; Weich, S.; Bellón-Saameño, J.A.; Moreno, B.; Svab, I.; Rotar, D.; et al. Prevalence of common mental disorders in general practice attendees across Europe. *Br. J. Psychiatry* **2008**, *192*, 362–367. [CrossRef]
32. Carcedo, R.J. *Necesidades Sociales, Emocionales y Sexuales: Estudio en un Centro Penitenciario [Social, Emotional, and Sexual Needs: Study in a Penitentiary]*; Servicio de Publicaciones de la Universidad de Salamanca: Salamanca, Spain, 2005.
33. Levenson, L. Sexual attitudes of males in a protected environment. *J. Am. Soc. Psychosom. Dent. Med.* **1983**, *30*, 135–136.
34. Maeve, M.K. The social construction of love and sexuality in a women's prison. *ANS Adv. Nurs. Sci.* **1999**, *21*, 46–65. [CrossRef] [PubMed]
35. Neuman, E. *El Problema Sexual en las Cárceles [The Sexual Problem in Prisons]*; Editorial Universidad: Buenos Aires, Argentina, 1982.
36. Linville, S.L. *Assessing Sexual Attitudes and Behaviors of Incarcerated Males in a Minimum Security Institution*; West Virginia University: Morgantown, WV, USA, 1981.

37. Worley, R.M.; Worley, V. Inmate public autoerotism uncovered: Exploring the dynamics of masturbatory behavior within correctional facilities. *Deviant Behav.* **2013**, *34*, 11–24. [CrossRef]
38. Hensley, C.; Tewksbury, R.; Koscheski, M. Masturbation uncovered: Autoeroticism in a female prison. *Prison J.* **2001**, *81*, 491–501. [CrossRef]
39. Hensley, C.; Tewksbury, R.; Wright, J. Exploring the dynamics of masturbation and consensual same-sex activity within a male maximum security prison. *J. Men's Stud.* **2001**, *10*, 59–71. [CrossRef]
40. Marcum, C.D. Examining prison sex culture. In *Sex in Prison: Myths and Realities*; Marcum, C.D., Castle, T.L., Eds.; Lynne Rienner: London, UK, 2014; pp. 1–12.
41. Fleisher, M.S.; Krienert, J.L. *The Myth of Prison Rape: Sexual Culture in American Prisons*; Rowman and Littlefield: New York, NY, USA, 2009.
42. Levan, K. Consensual sex. In *Sex in Prison: Myths and Realities*; Marcum, C.D., Castle, T.L., Eds.; Lynne Rienner: London, UK, 2014; pp. 13–24.
43. Beck, A.J.; Harrison, P. *Sexual Victimization in Prisons and Jails Reported by Inmates, 2008–2009 (NCJ No. 231169)*; US Department of Justice, Office of Justice Programs: Washington, DC, USA, 2010.
44. Caravaca-Sánchez, F.; Wolff, N. Prevalence and Predictors of Sexual Victimization Among Incarcerated Men and Women in Spanish Prisons. *Crim. Justice Behav.* **2016**, *43*, 977–991. [CrossRef]
45. Tewksbury, R.; Connor, D.P. Sexual victimization. In *Sex in Prison: Myths and Realities*; Marcum, C.D., Castle, T.L., Eds.; Lynne Rienner: London, UK, 2014; pp. 25–51.
46. Potter, R.H.; Rosky, J. Health issues. In *Sex in Prison: Myths and Realities*; Marcum, C.D., Castle, T.L., Eds.; Lynne Rienner: London, UK, 2014; pp. 25–51.
47. D'Alessio, S.J.; Flexon, J.; Stolzenberg, L. The effect of conjugal visitation on sexual violence in prison. *Am. J. Crim. Justice* **2013**, *38*, 13–26. [CrossRef]
48. Carcedo, R.J.; Perlman, D.; Orgaz, M.B.; López, F.; Fernández-Rouco, N.; Faldowski, R.A. Heterosexual romantic relationships inside of prison: Partner status as predictor of loneliness, sexual satisfaction, and quality of life. *Int. J. Offender Ther. Comp. Criminol.* **2011**, *55*, 898–924. [CrossRef]
49. Byers, E.S.; Demmons, S.; Lawrance, K. Sexual satisfaction within dating relationships: A test of the interpersonal exchange model of sexual satisfaction. *J. Soc. Pers. Relatsh.* **1998**, *15*, 257–267. [CrossRef]
50. Carcedo, R.J.; Perlman, D.; López, F.; Orgaz, M.B. Heterosexual romantic relationships, interpersonal needs, and quality of life in prison. *Span. J. Psychol.* **2012**, *15*, 187–198. [CrossRef]
51. Carcedo, R.J.; Perlman, D.; López, F.; Orgaz, M.B.; Fernández-Rouco, N. The relationship between sexual satisfaction and psychological health of prison inmates. *Prison J.* **2015**, *95*, 43–65. [CrossRef]
52. Sánchez-Fuentes, M.M.; Santos-Iglesias, P.; Sierra, J.C. A systematic review of sexual satisfaction. *Int. J. Clin. Health Psychol.* **2014**, *14*, 67–75. [CrossRef]
53. Shindel, A.W.; Eisenberg, M.L.; Breyer, B.N.; Sharlip, I.D.; Smith, J.F. Sexual function and depressive symptoms among female North American medical students. *J. Sex. Med.* **2011**, *8*, 391–399. [CrossRef] [PubMed]
54. Davison, S.L.; Bell, R.J.; LaChina, M.; Holden, S.L.; Davis, S.R. The relationship between self-reported sexual satisfaction and general well-being in women. *J. Sex. Med.* **2009**, *6*, 2690–2697. [CrossRef] [PubMed]
55. Stephenson, K.R.; Meston, C.M. The conditional importance of sex: Exploring the association between sexual well-being and life satisfaction. *J. Sex Marital Ther.* **2015**, *41*, 25–38. [CrossRef]
56. Cohen, J.N.; Byers, E.S. Beyond lesbian bed death: Enhancing our understanding of the sexuality of sexual-minority women in relationships. *J. Sex Res.* **2014**, *51*, 893–903. [CrossRef] [PubMed]
57. De Ryck, I.; Van Laeken, D.; Nöstlinger, C.; Platteau, T.; Colebunders, R. Sexual satisfaction among men living with HIV in Europe. *AIDS Behav.* **2012**, *16*, 225–230. [CrossRef] [PubMed]
58. Sánchez-Fuentes, M.; Sierra, J.C. Sexual satisfaction in a heterosexual and homosexual Spanish sample: The role of socio-demographic characteristics, health indicators, and relational factors. *Sex. Relatsh. Ther.* **2015**, *30*, 226–242. [CrossRef]
59. Holmberg, D.; Blair, K.L.; Phillips, M. Women's sexual satisfaction as a predictor of well-being in same-sex versus mixed-sex relationships. *J. Sex Res.* **2010**, *47*, 1–11. [CrossRef]
60. Totenhagen, C.J.; Butler, E.A.; Ridley, C.A. Daily stress, closeness, and satisfaction in gay and lesbian couples. *Pers. Relatsh.* **2012**, *19*, 219–233. [CrossRef]

61. Priebe, S.; Reininghaus, U.; McCabe, R.; Burns, T.; Eklund, M.; Hansson, L.; Junghan, U.; Kallert, T.; van Nieuwenhuizen, C.; Ruggeri, M.; et al. Factors influencing subjective quality of life in patients with schizophrenia and other mental disorders: A pooled analysis. *Schizophr. Res.* **2010**, *121*, 251–258. [CrossRef] [PubMed]
62. Mallis, D.; Moisidis, K.; Kirana, P.S.; Papaharitou, S.; Simos, G.; Hatzichristou, D. Psychology: Moderate and severe erectile dysfunction equally affects life satisfaction. *J. Sex. Med.* **2006**, *3*, 442–449. [CrossRef]
63. Field, N.; Mercer, C.H.; Sonnenberg, P.; Tanton, C.; Clifton, S.; Mitchell, K.R.; Erens, B.; Macdowall, W.; Wu, F.; Datta, J. Associations between health and sexual lifestyles in Britain: Findings from the third National Survey of Sexual Attitudes and Lifestyles (Natsal-3). *Lancet* **2013**, *382*, 1830–1844. [CrossRef]
64. Laxhman, N.; Greenberg, L.; Priebe, S. Satisfaction with sex life among patients with schizophrenia. *Schizophr. Res.* **2017**, *190*, 63–67. [CrossRef]
65. Træen, B.; Štulhofer, A.; Janssen, E.; Carvalheira, A.A.; Hald, G.M.; Lange, T.; Graham, C. Sexual activity and sexual satisfaction among older adults in four European countries. *Arch. Sex. Behav.* **2019**, *48*, 815–829. [CrossRef]
66. Kawachi, I.; Berkman, L.F. Social ties and mental health. *J. Urban Health* **2001**, *78*, 458–467. [CrossRef] [PubMed]
67. Holt-Lunstad, J.; Birmingham, W.; Jones, B.Q. Is there something unique about marriage? The relative impact of marital status, relationship quality, and network social support on ambulatory blood pressure and mental health. *Ann. Behav. Med.* **2008**, *35*, 239–244. [CrossRef]
68. Waite, L.; Gallagher, M. *The Case for Marriage: Why Married People Are Happier, Healthier and Better Off Financially*; Broadway Books: New York, NY, USA, 2002.
69. Proulx, C.M.; Helms, H.M.; Buehler, C. Marital quality and personal well-being: A meta-analysis. *J. Marriage Fam.* **2007**, *69*, 576–593. [CrossRef]
70. Lau, J.T.F.; Wang, Q.; Cheng, Y.; Yang, X. Prevalence and risk factors of sexual dysfunction among younger married men in a rural area in China. *Urology* **2005**, *66*, 616–622. [CrossRef]
71. Ventegodt, S. Sex and quality of life in Denmark. *Arch. Sex. Behav.* **1998**, *27*, 295–307. [CrossRef]
72. Taleporos, G.; McCabe, M.P. The impact of sexual esteem, body esteem, and sexual satisfaction on psychological well-being in people with physical disability. *Sex. Disabil.* **2002**, *20*, 177–183. [CrossRef]
73. Walters, A.S.; Williamson, G.M. Sexual satisfaction predicts quality of life: A study of adult amputees. *Sex. Disabil.* **1998**, *16*, 103–115. [CrossRef]
74. Fegg, M.J.; Gerl, A.; Vollmer, T.C.; Gruber, U.; Jost, C.; Meiler, S.; Hiddemann, W. Subjective quality of life and sexual functioning after germ-cell tumour therapy. *Br. J. Cancer* **2003**, *89*, 2202–2206. [CrossRef]
75. López, F. *Necesidades en la Infancia y en la Adolescencia. Respuesta Familiar, Escolar y Social [Needs in Childhood and Adolescence. Family, School and Social Response]*; Pirámide: Madrid, Spain, 2008.
76. Demir, M.; Tyrell, F. Friendship and well-being among young adults with/out a romantic partner. In Proceedings of the International Association of Relationship Research Conference, Providence, RI, USA, 17–20 July 2008.
77. Laumann, E.O.; Paik, A.; Glasser, D.B.; Kang, J.H.; Wang, T.; Levinson, B.; Moreira, E.D., Jr.; Nicolosi, A.; Gingell, C. A cross-national study of subjective sexual well-being among older women and men: Findings from the Global Study of Sexual Attitudes and Behaviors. *Arch. Sex. Behav.* **2006**, *35*, 143–159. [CrossRef]
78. Carcedo, R.J.; Perlman, D.; López, F.; Orgaz, M.B.; Toth, K.; Fernández-Rouco, N. Men and women in the same prison: Interpersonal needs and psychological health of prison inmates. *Int. J. Offender Ther. Comp. Criminol.* **2008**, *52*, 641–657. [CrossRef]
79. Sánchez, M.G. *La Abstinencia Sexual Forzosa de las Reclusas en los Establecimientos Carcelarios de Venezuela [Forced Sexual Abstinence of Female Prison Inmates in Venezuela]*; Composición Comput: Coro, Venezuela, 1995.
80. Lindquist, C.H. Social integration and mental well-being among jail inmates. *Sociol. Forum.* **2000**, *15*, 431–455. [CrossRef]
81. Lindquist, C.H.; Lindquist, C.A. Gender differences in distress: Mental health consequences of environmental stress among jail inmates. *Behav. Sci. Law* **1997**, *15*, 503–523. [CrossRef]
82. James, D.J.; Glaze, L.E. *Bureau of Justice Statistics Special Report: Mental Health Problems of Prison and Jail Inmates*; US Department of Justice: Washington, DC, USA, 2006.
83. McDonald, B.; Kulkarni, M.; Andkhoie, M.; Kendall, J.; Gall, S.; Chelladurai, S.; Yaghoubi, M.; McClean, S.; Szafron, M.; Farag, M. Determinants of self-reported mental health and utilization of mental health services in Canada. *Int. J. Ment. Health* **2017**, *46*, 299–311. [CrossRef]

84. Brody, S. The relative health benefits of different sexual activities. *J. Sex. Med.* **2010**, *7*, 1336–1361. [CrossRef]
85. Costa, R.M. Masturbation is related to psychopathology and prostate dysfunction: Comment on Quinsey. *Arch. Sex. Behav.* **2012**, *41*, 539–540. [CrossRef]
86. Das, A. Masturbation in the United States. *J. Sex. Marital Ther.* **2007**, *33*, 301–317. [CrossRef]
87. Snell, W.E. The Multidimensional Sexual Self-Concept Questionnaire. In *Handbook of Sexuality Related Measures*; Davis, C.M., Yarber, W.L., Bauserman, R., Schreer, G., Davis, S.L., Eds.; Sage: Riverside County, CA, USA, 1995; pp. 521–527.
88. Lucas, R. *Versión Española del WHOQOL [Spanish Version of WHOQOL]*; Ergón: Madrid, Spain, 1998.
89. Skevington, S.M.; McCrate, F.M. Expecting a good quality of life in health: Assessing people with diverse diseases and conditions using the WHOQOL-BREF. *Health Expect.* **2012**, *15*, 49–62. [CrossRef] [PubMed]
90. Jylhä, M. What is self-rated health and why does it predict mortality? Towards a unified conceptual model. *Soc. Sci. Med.* **2009**, *69*, 307–316. [CrossRef]
91. Ditommaso, E.; Brannen, C.; Best, L.A. Measurement and validity characteristics of the short version of the social and emotional loneliness scale for adults. *Educ. Psychol. Meas.* **2004**, *64*, 99–119. [CrossRef]
92. Daryanto, A. Heteroskedasticity Test for SPSS (2nd Version). 2018. Available online: https://sites.google.com/site/ahmaddaryanto/scripts/Heterogeneity-test (accessed on 28 January 2018).
93. Hayes, A.F.; Little, T.D. *Introduction to Mediation, Moderation, and Conditional Process Analysis: A Regression-Based Approach*, 2nd ed.; Guilford Press: New York, NY, USA, 2018.
94. Davidson, R.; MacKinnon, J. *Estimation and Inference in Econometrics*; Oxford University Press: Oxford, UK, 1993.
95. Bushman, B.J.; Bonacci, A.M.; Van Dijk, M.; Baumeister, R.F. Narcissism, sexual refusal, and aggression: Testing a narcissistic reactance model of sexual coercion. *J. Pers. Soc. Psych.* **2003**, *84*, 1027. [CrossRef]
96. Brehm, J.W. *A Theory of Psychological Reactance*; Academic Press: New York, NY, USA, 1966.
97. Brehm, S.S.; Brehm, J.W. *Psychological Reactance: A Theory of Freedom and Control*; Academic Press: New York, NY, USA, 1981.
98. Baumeister, R.F.; Bratslavsky, E.; Finkenauer, C.; Vohs, K.D. Bad is stronger than good. *Rev. Gen. Psychol.* **2001**, *5*, 323–370. [CrossRef]
99. Paolini, S.; McIntyre, K. Bad is stronger than good for stigmatized, but not admired outgroups: Meta-analytical tests of intergroup valence asymmetry in individual-to-group generalization experiments. *Pers. Soc. Psych. Rev.* **2019**, *23*, 3–47. [CrossRef] [PubMed]
100. Wright, E.M.; Salisbury, E.J.; Van Voorhis, P. Predicting the prison misconducts of women offenders: The importance of gender-responsive needs. *J. Contemp. Crim. Justice* **2007**, *23*, 310–340. [CrossRef]
101. Gendreau, P.; Little, T.; Goggin, C. A meta-analysis of the predictors of adult offender recidivism: What works! *Criminology* **1996**, *34*, 575–608. [CrossRef]
102. Vallerand, R.J. From motivation to passion: In search of the motivational processes involved in a meaningful life. *Can. Psychol.* **2012**, *53*, 42–52. [CrossRef]
103. Fernández-Rouco, N.; Carcedo, R.J.; Yeadon-Lee, T. Transgender Identities, Pressures and Social Policy: A Study Carried Out in Spain. *J. Homosex.* **2018**, 1–19. [CrossRef] [PubMed]
104. Hefner, M.K. Queering Prison Masculinity: Exploring the Organization of Gender and Sexuality within Men's Prison. *Men Masc.* **2018**, *21*, 230–253. [CrossRef]

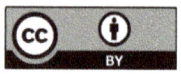

© 2019 by the authors. Licensee MDPI, Basel, Switzerland. This article is an open access article distributed under the terms and conditions of the Creative Commons Attribution (CC BY) license (http://creativecommons.org/licenses/by/4.0/).

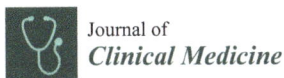

Article

Sexual Distress in Patients with Hidradenitis Suppurativa: A Cross-Sectional Study

Carlos Cuenca-Barrales [1], Ricardo Ruiz-Villaverde [1] and Alejandro Molina-Leyva [2,3,4,*]

[1] Dermatology, Hospital Universitario San Cecilio, Avenida de la Investigación s/n, 18016 Granada, Spain; carloscuenca1991@gmail.com (C.C.-B.); ismenios@hotmail.com (R.R.-V.)
[2] Dermatology, Hidradenitis Suppurativa Clinic, Hospital Universitario Virgen de las Nieves, Avenida de las Fuerzas Armadas 2, 18014 Granada, Spain
[3] European Hidradenitis Suppurativa Foundation (EHSF), 06847 Dessau-Roßlau, Germany
[4] Instituto de Investigación Biosanitaria Granada, 18016 Granada, Spain
* Correspondence: alejandromolinaleyva@gmail.com; Tel.: +34-686731837

Received: 7 April 2019; Accepted: 16 April 2019; Published: 18 April 2019

Abstract: Hidradenitis suppurativa (HS) is a chronic auto-inflammatory skin disease with a great impact in quality of life. However, there is little research about the impact of HS on sex life. The aims of this study are to describe the frequency of sexual distress (SD) in patients with HS and to explore potentially associated epidemiological and clinical factors. We conducted a cross-sectional study by means of a crowd-sourced online questionnaire hosted by the Spanish hidradenitis suppurativa patients' association (ASENDHI). Sexual distress (SD) was evaluated with a Numeric Rating Scale (NRS) for HS impact on sex life. A total of 393 participants answered the questionnaire. The mean NRS for HS impact on sex life was 7.24 (2.77) in women and 6.39 (3.44) in men ($p < 0.05$). Variables significantly associated ($p < 0.05$) with SD in the multiple linear regression model were sex, with a higher risk in females, the presence of active lesions in the groin and genitals and NRS for pain and unpleasant odor; being in a stable relationship was an important protector factor. Regarding these results, it seems that SD in HS patients is due, at least in part, to disease symptoms and active lesions in specific locations, emphasizing the importance of disease control with a proper treatment according to management guidelines. Women and single patients are more likely to suffer from sexual distress.

Keywords: sexuality; mental health; mental disorder; sexual dysfunction; hidradenitis suppurativa

1. Introduction

Hidradenitis suppurativa (HS) is a chronic auto-inflammatory skin disease characterized by recurrent nodules, abscesses and fistulae and which involves hair follicles, predominantly in intertriginous areas [1]. These lesions cause pain, unpleasant odor, itching and suppuration. When the disease progresses to advanced stages, there may be a permanent negative effect on body image due to scarring.

According to recent studies, the reduction in HS patients' quality of life is one of the most significant among dermatological patients [2,3] and similar to other non-dermatological illnesses such as chronic obstructive pulmonary disease, diabetes mellitus, cardiovascular disease and cancer [4]. Some research indicates that pain or pruritus may negatively affect quality of life [5,6].

Sexuality is a basic need and one which cannot be separated from other aspects of human life, being extremely important for maintaining good mental health [7]. Several studies show a direct relationship between sexual function and quality of life [8,9]. Sexual functionality can be impaired by chronic diseases because of factors related to the disease itself, its treatments, or alterations in body image [10]. Due to the chronic relapsing course of HS and the disease's characteristics, HS may affect patients' sexuality. Numerous publications have associated HS with depression, anxiety, low self-esteem, loneliness, stigmatization, suicide risk, or impact on working life [2,3,11–16]. However, there is little research about the impact of HS on sex life.

The aims of this study are to describe the frequency of sexual distress (SD) in patients with HS and to explore potentially associated epidemiological and clinical factors.

2. Experimental Section

2.1. Patients and Design

We conducted a cross-sectional study by means of a crowd-sourced online questionnaire. Participants were recruited from 1 March to 1 April 2018. The Spanish hidradenitis suppurativa patients' association (ASENDHI) hosted the questionnaire and invited people with HS to participate in the study [17].

The selection criterion was self-referred diagnosis of HS. Participants were aware of the questionnaire's anonymity and the use of their data for research purposes. The study was approved on May 2017 by the ethics committee of Hospital Universitario San Cecilio and is in accordance with the World Health Organization Declaration of Helsinki.

2.2. Questionnaire

The questionnaire was developed with Google® Forms suite. Socio-demographic data, biometric parameters, use of medication for other comorbidities and several characteristics of the disease, such as age of onset, time under medical attention and affected areas were collected. Disease severity was assessed by patients' self-reported Hurley stage, since patients with HS are capable of self-assessing their Hurley stage with a good correlation with physician assessment [18].

Disease activity was assessed by Patients' Global Assessment (PtGA), including five categories (inactive, very low, low, mild and severe) [19], and intensity of symptoms by Numeric Rating Scales (NRS) [20]. These scales show the subjective impact of the disease on patients, with equal or greater importance than objective scales.

SD was evaluated with a NRS for HS impact on sex life, in which participants were asked to measure from 0 to 10 how much the disease affects their sex life. This scale reflects the subjective suffering and distress caused by the disease to patients' sex lives. Its concordance with the Female Sexual Function Index-6 (FSFI-6) and the International Index of Erectile Function-5 (IIEF-5), two validated questionnaires that explore female sexual dysfunction and erectile dysfunction respectively, was also assessed.

2.3. Statistical Analysis

Statistical analyses were performed using JMP version 9.0.1 (SAS institute, Inc., Cary, NC, USA). When there were missing data in any of the variables of interest, patients were excluded from the study. When missing data were found in other variables, they were imputed. To explore the characteristics of the sample, descriptive statistics were used. Continuous variables were expressed as means and standard deviations. Qualitative variables were expressed as absolute and relative frequencies.

The main outcome of interest was SD, measured by the NRS for HS impact on sex life. To explore possibly associated factors, simple linear regression was used for continuous variables, Student's t-test for dichotomous variables, and one-way analysis of variance for nominal variables with two or more categories (Levene's test was used to assess the equality of variances, standardized residual plots to check independence and Normality was assumed because of the sample size). Significantly associated variables ($p < 0.05$) or those showing trends towards statistical significance ($p < 0.20$) were included in a multiple linear regression model to assess the factors associated with SD. Statistical significance was considered if p values were less than 0.05.

The correlation of NRS for HS impact on sex life with FSFI-6 and IIEF-5 was checked with simple linear regression. Student's t-test was used to assess differences between NRS for HS impact in sex life means in participants with and without sexual or erectile dysfunction according to the FSFI-6 or IIEF-5 scores, respectively. The cut-off point for sexual dysfunction using the NRS for HS impact on sex life was assessed by ROC curve analysis.

3. Results

3.1. Baseline

Three hundred and ninety three participants answered the questionnaire. Seven of them filled out the questionnaire incompletely, so the final sample consisted of 386 participants (319 (82.6%) from Spain, 57 (14.8%) from abroad, and 10 (2.6%) did not provide their country of residence). The ratio of women to men was 3.8:1 (306 (79.27%) women and 80 (20.73%) men). Their socio-demographic characteristics and comorbidities are shown in Table 1; current smoking was higher among men, body mass index was 1.5 greater in women, and the prevalence of diabetes mellitus type II and antidepressant consumption was higher among women, but these differences did not reach statistical significance. HS baseline characteristics are shown in Table 2. Age of onset was earlier in women (19.09 ± 7.1 vs. 23.57 ± 9.45, $p < 0.0001$), with a medium diagnosis delay of 11.23 ± 9.55 in women and 8.86 ± 9.13 in men. The groin was the location most affected in women, either by active lesions (65.7%) or scars (57.2%). In men, groin was the location more frequently affected by active lesions (53.8%), and axilla by scars (47.5%). Genitals were affected by active lesions in 111 (36.3%) of women and in 31 (38.8%) of men, and by scars in 82 (26.8%) of women and in 28 (35%) of men. The presence of active lesions in the perianal region (35 (43.8%) vs. 50 (16.3%), $p < 0.0001$) and on the buttocks (35 (43.8%) vs. 95 (31%), $p <0.05$) were higher among men, while the breast region was more frequently affected in women (90 (29.4%) vs. 2 (2.5%), $p < 0.0001$).

Table 1. Socio-demographic characteristics and comorbidities.

	Men ($n = 80$)	Women ($n = 306$)	All ($n = 386$)
Age	39.21 ± 11.15	37.44 ± 8.69	37.81 ± 9.26
BMI	28.12 ± 5.03	29.67 ± 7.05	29.35 ± 6.71
Current smoker			
No	28 (35%)	135 (44.1%)	163 (42.2%)
Yes	52 (65%)	171 (55.9%)	223 (57.8%)
Comorbidities			
HBP	4 (5%)	21 (6.9%)	25 (6.5%)
DM2	2 (2.5%)	20 (6.5%)	22 (5.7%)
Dyslipidemia	3 (3.8%)	9 (2.9%)	12 (3.1%)
Antidepressant use	4 (5%)	31 (10.1%)	35 (9.1%)
Benzodiazepine use	4 (5%)	18 (5.9%)	22 (5.7%)
Stable relationship	54 (67.5%)	236 (77.1%)	290 (75.1%)

Continuous variables are expressed as means ± standard deviation and qualitative variables as absolute (relative) frequencies. BMI: body mass index. HBP: high blood pressure. DM2: diabetes mellitus type 2.

Table 2. Hidradenitis suppurativa (HS) patients' baseline characteristics.

	Men ($n = 80$)	Women ($n = 306$)	All ($n = 386$)
Time of evolution	15.64 ± 10.53	18.33 ± 9.3	17.77 ± 9.62
Time under medical attention	6.79 ± 7.21	7.1 ± 7.29	7.03 ± 7.27
Number of active regions	2.73 ± 1.79	2.5 ± 1.57	2.55 ± 1.62
Number of regions with scars	2.34 ± 2.29	2.31 ± 2.06	2.31 ± 2.1

Table 2. Cont.

	Men ($n = 80$)	Women ($n = 306$)	All ($n = 386$)
Hurley state			
I	13 (16.3%)	55 (18%)	68 (17.6%)
II	25 (31.3%)	149 (48.7%)	174 (45.1%)
III	42 (52.5%)	102 (33.3%)	144 (37.3%)
PtGA	3.73 ± 1.04	3.65 ± 1.11	3.66 ± 1.09
NRS pain	6.64 ± 2.81	6.52 ± 2.98	6.54 ± 2.95
NRS pruritus	6.24 ± 2.67	6.48 ± 3.03	6.43 ± 2.96
NRS unpleasant odor	6.11 ± 3.05	5.47 ± 3.45	5.6 ± 3.38
NRS suppuration	6.84 ± 3.04	6.39 ± 3.21	6.48 ± 3.18

Continuous variables are expressed as means ± standard deviation and qualitative variables as absolute (relative) frequencies. PtGA: Patient's Global Assessment; values range from 1 (inactive disease) to 5 (severe disease). NRS: Numeric Rating Scale; values range from 0 (no symptoms) to 10 (maximum intensity of symptoms).

3.2. Sexual Distress and Related Factors in Patients with Hidradenitis Suppurativa

The mean NRS for HS impact on sex life was 7.24 (2.77) in women and 6.39 (3.44) in men ($p < 0.05$). Results from univariate analysis of factors possibly related to NRS for HS impact on sex life are shown in Table 3.

Table 3. Univariate analysis of factors associated with sexual distress in patients with HS.

KERRYPNX	Univariate Analysis	p-Value
Sex		
Female	$\bar{x} = 7.24\ (0.17)$	0.021 *
Male	$\bar{x} = 6.39\ (0.33)$	
Age	$\beta = -0.01\ (0.02)$	0.738
Current smoker		
Yes	$\bar{x} = 7.35\ (0.2)$	0.023 *
No	$\bar{x} = 6.66\ (0.23)$	
Antidepressant use		
Yes	$\bar{x} = 7.37\ (0.5)$	0.51
No	$\bar{x} = 7.03\ (0.16)$	
Benzodiazepine use		
Yes	$\bar{x} = 6.82\ (0.63)$	0.692
No	$\bar{x} = 7.07\ (0.15)$	
Age of onset	$\beta = -0.01\ (0.02)$	0.667
Time under medical attention	$\beta = 0.04\ (0.02)$	0.042 *
Active lesions in axilla		
Yes	$\bar{x} = 7.16\ (0.22)$	0.532
No	$\bar{x} = 6.97\ (0.21)$	
Scars in axilla		
Yes	$\bar{x} = 7.15\ (0.22)$	0.607
No	$\bar{x} = 6.99\ (0.2)$	
Active lesions in groin		
Yes	$\bar{x} = 7.63\ (0.18)$	<0.0001 *
No	$\bar{x} = 6.09\ (0.24)$	
Scars in groin		
Yes	$\bar{x} = 7.25\ (0.2)$	0.169
No	$\bar{x} = 6.84\ (0.22)$	
Active lesions on genitals		
Yes	$\bar{x} = 7.99\ (0.24)$	<0.0001 *
No	$\bar{x} = 6.16\ (0.18)$	

Table 3. Cont.

KERRYPNX	Univariate Analysis	p-Value
Scars on genitals		
Yes	x̄ = 7.6 (0.28)	0.022 *
No	x̄ = 6.84 (0.18)	
Active lesions on buttocks		
Yes	x̄ = 7.45 (0.26)	0.065
No	x̄ = 6.86 (0.18)	
Scars on buttocks		
Yes	x̄ = 6.94 (0.26)	0.566
No	x̄ = 7.12 (0.18)	
Active lesions on breast		
Yes	x̄ = 7.65 (0.3)	0.026 *
No	x̄ = 6.87 (0.17)	
Scars on breast		
Yes	x̄ = 7.33 (0.31)	0.327
No	x̄ = 6.98 (0.17)	
Active lesions on abdomen		
Yes	x̄ = 7.6 (0.46)	0.219
No	x̄ = 7 (0.16)	
Scars on abdomen		
Yes	x̄ = 7.18 (0.44)	0.77
No	x̄ = 7.04 (0.16)	
Active lesions in perianal region		
Yes	x̄ = 7.47 (0.32)	0.144
No	x̄ = 6.94 (0.17)	
Scars in perianal region		
Yes	x̄ = 7.46 (0.33)	0.168
No	x̄ = 6.95 (0.17)	
Active lesions on neck		
Yes	x̄ = 7.2 (0.59)	0.805
No	x̄ = 7.05 (0.16)	
Scars on neck		
Yes	x̄ = 7.22 (0.61)	0.791
No	x̄ = 7.05 (0.15)	
Number of regions with active lesions	β = 0.48 (0.09)	<0.0001 *
Number of regions with scars	β = 0.1 (0.07)	0.182
Hurley stage		
I	x̄ = 6.21 (0.35)	
II	x̄ = 7.02 (0.22)	0.01 *
III	x̄ = 7.51 (0.24)	
Treatment with oral antibiotics		
Yes	x̄ = 7.48 (0.28)	0.074
No	x̄ = 6.89 (0.18)	
Treatment with oral contraceptives		
Yes	x̄ = 7.13 (0.38)	0.833
No	x̄ = 7.05 (0.16)	
Treatment with adalimumab		
Yes	x̄ = 7.82 (0.38)	0.03 *
No	x̄ = 6.92 (0.16)	
PtGA	β = 0.87 (0.13)	<0.0001 *
NRS for pain	β = 0.32 (0.05)	<0.0001 *
NRS for pruritus	β = 0.27 (0.05)	<0.0001 *
NRS for unpleasant odor	β = 0.25 (0.04)	<0.0001 *
NRS for suppuration	β = 0.25 (0.05)	<0.0001 *
Stable relationship		
Yes	x̄ = 6.88 (0.17)	0.032 *
No	x̄ = 7.62 (0.3)	

p-values of variables significantly associated are marked with * PtGA: Patient's Global Assessment; values range from 1 (inactive disease) to 5 (severe disease). NRS: Numeric Rating Scale; values range from 0 (no symptoms) to 10 (maximum intensity of symptoms).

Variables that were significantly associated or showed trends towards statistical significance ($p < 0.20$) were included in the multiple linear regression model, whose results are shown in Table 4. Variables significantly associated with SD were sex, with a higher risk in females, the presence of active lesions in the groin and genitals and NRS for pain and unpleasant odor; being in a stable relationship was an important protector factor for SD. Current smoking, PtGA, time under medical attention and treatment with adalimumab showed trends toward statistical significance.

Table 4. Multivariate analysis of factors associated with sexual distress in patients with HS.

	Multivariate Analysis	p-Value
Sex (female)	$\beta = 0.57$ (0.19)	0.003 *
Current smoker	$\beta = 0.27$ (0.14)	0.059
Time under medical attention	$\beta = 0.03$ (0.02)	0.088
Active lesions in groin	$\beta = 0.44$ (0.18)	0.015 *
Scars in groin	$\beta = 0.15$ (0.19)	0.449
Active lesions on genitals	$\beta = 0.4$ (0.19)	0.033 *
Scars on genitals	$\beta = 0.05$ (0.21)	0.812
Active lesions on buttocks	$\beta = 0.19$ (0.18)	0.296
Active lesions on breast	$\beta = 0.09$ (0.21)	0.666
Active lesions in perianal region	$\beta = 0.15$ (0.21)	0.463
Scars in perianal region	$\beta = 0.23$ (0.21)	0.28
Number of regions with active lesions	$\beta = 0.15$ (0.19)	0.44
Number of regions with scars	$\beta = 0.14$ (0.12)	0.24
Hurley stage III vs. I III vs. II	$\beta = 0.07$ (0.26) $\beta = 0.03$ (0.19)	0.804 0.866
Treatment with oral antibiotics	$\beta = 0.02$ (0.16)	0.9
Treatment with adalimumab	$\beta = 0.38$ (0.2)	0.054
PtGA	$\beta = 0.3$ (0.19)	0.115
NRS for pain	$\beta = 0.15$ (0.08)	0.049 *
NRS for pruritus	$\beta = 0.03$ (0.06)	0.615
NRS for unpleasant odor	$\beta = 0.13$ (0.06)	0.035 *
NRS for suppuration	$\beta = 0.05$ (0.07)	0.489
Stable relationship	$\beta = -0.56$ (0.16)	<0.001 *

p values of variables significantly associated are marked with * PtGA: Patient's Global Assessment; values range from 1 (inactive disease) to 5 (severe disease). NRS: Numeric Rating Scale; values range from 0 (no symptoms) to 10 (maximum intensity of symptoms).

3.3. Correlation between NRS for HS Impact on Sex Life and FSFI-6/IIEF-5 Scores

Scores from NRS for HS impact on sex life and FSFI-6 showed a negative correlation ($\beta = -0.15 \pm 0.02$, $r^2 = 0.16$, $p < 0.0001$), indicating a good concordance between both questionnaires. Scores from NRS for HS impact on sex life and IIEF-5 also showed a negative correlation ($\beta = -0.21 \pm 0.05$, $r^2 = 0.15$, $p < 0.001$). The mean score on the NRS for HS impact on sex life was 8.27 ± 0.21 in women with sexual dysfunction, and 6.16 ± 0.21 in women without sexual dysfunction ($p < 0.0001$). In men, the mean score on the NRS for HS impact on sex life was 7.31 ± 0.47 in those with erectile dysfunction, and 5 ± 0.58 in those without erectile dysfunction ($p < 0.01$).

In women, a score of 8 or more on the NRS for HS impact on sex life was indicative of sexual dysfunction according to FSFI-6 scores, with a sensitivity of 73% and a specificity of 64% (Figure 1). In men, a score of 9 or more on the NRS for HS impact on sex life was indicative of erectile dysfunction according to IIEF-5 scores, with a sensitivity of 52% and a specificity of 81% (Figure 2).

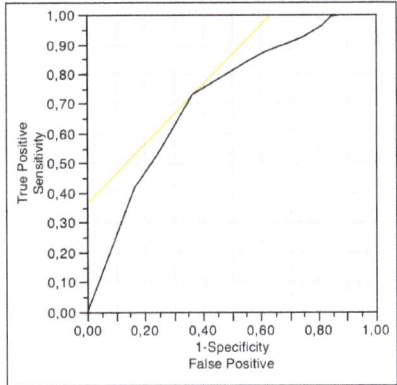

Figure 1. ROC curve analysis for comparison between scores of NRS of HS impact on sex life and FSFI-6.

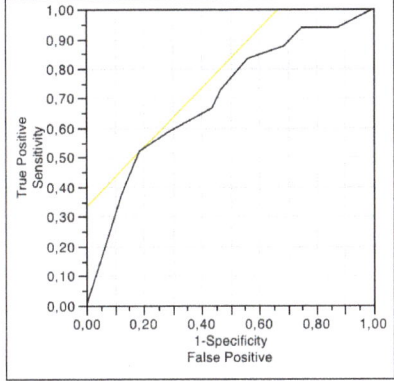

Figure 2. ROC curve analysis for comparison between scores of NRS of HS impact on sex life and IIEF-5.

4. Discussion

To our best knowledge, this is the largest cross-sectional study about the impact of HS on sexuality. Socio-demographic and disease characteristics did not differ from those previously reported in the literature, and were representative of the general HS population [21–28].

The mean NRS score for HS impact on sex life was significantly higher in women, which tallies with previous research that indicates higher sexual distress in women than in men with HS [29] or psoriasis [30]. These differences have been associated with cultural aspects and differences in emotional and neuroendocrine responses to disfigurement, and with the earlier onset of HS in women (4.5 years earlier in our sample) [29]. A higher prevalence of lesions at the lower abdomen has also been posed as a reason for this higher distress in women [29], but in our sample we only observed more involvement below the abdomen in the groin.

Although in psoriasis the involvement of the anogenital area has been related to sexual dysfunction [31–33], in HS anogenital involvement has been related to a reduction in quality of life [2,34], but there are no locations related to sexual dysfunction or to sexual distress [29,34]. In our investigation, we found an association between active lesions in the groin and genitals and SD, so a properly medical/surgical intervention at this level could turn into a better sexual life. In previous research about sexual health in patients with HS, samples were taken from hospital departments [29,34] and from a patient's association [34], and there were no important differences in patients' baseline characteristics, with the exception of a more prevalent Hurley III stage in our sample. Therefore, these findings were probably made possible due to the larger size of our sample.

Moreover, subjective symptoms caused sexual distress. The intensity of pain and unpleasant odor were related with higher scores on NRS for HS impact on sex life. This association may be due to factors directly related to the nature of the sexual act and/or to psychological factors that could be related to disease activity [2], highlighting the importance of symptom management to improve sexual health in patients with HS. Other factors such as antidepressant or benzodiazepine use were not statistically associated with SD, suggesting that SD is directly related to organic symptoms.

The absence of a stable relationship was not associated with sexual dysfunction in previous research [29,34]. Nevertheless, we observed that the presence of a stable partner was importantly related to lower SD. Since having a partner is associated with less self-consciousness and less orgasm difficulty in both men and women [35], probably feelings of shame, distrust, shyness and rejection influence SD, which could be lessened by the trust built in a relationship.

There were other factors that showed trends toward statistical significance in the multiple linear regression model: (1) PtGA, pointing to the importance of disease activity in sexual distress and the need to control the inflammatory load; (2) current smoking, because it is related to greater disease activity, since it favors follicular occlusion, a proinflammatory state with activation of neutrophils and Th17 lymphocytes, induces biofilm formation and suppresses notch signaling, among other effects [36]; moreover, smoking cessation is associated with clinical improvement [37]; (3) time under medical care, since it reflects time of disease evolution, with cumulative life course impairment [38]; and (4) Treatment with adalimumab, probably because in our sample it is a better predictor of severity than Hurley, since the patients treated with adalimumab are the most severe.

Finally, we found a good correlation between the scores on NRS for HS impact on sex life and those of FSFI-6 and IIEF-5, which indicates an association between the subjective and objective involvement of the sexual sphere in participants. However, despite this concordance, the ROC curve analyses revealed that the NRS for HS impact on sex life was not a good tool to assess sexual dysfunction in women or erectile dysfunction in men, because the cut-off points reach neither an acceptable sensitivity nor specificity. It is important to the clinician to distinguish between sexual distress and sexual dysfunction, because the first reveals the suffering of the subject, whereas the second may mean a worse sexual experience for both members of the stable/sporadic relationship. Therefore, clinicians should assess both aspects when patients' sexuality is addressed.

There are some methodological weaknesses in our study: (1) A possible selection bias, since it only represents patients in contact with support groups and Internet access. The elderly, who may use the Internet less frequently, or those with low sociocultural status or fear of new technologies, could be under-represented [39]. Moreover, people already concerned about sexual problems may have been more likely to answer the questionnaire. Nonetheless, the baseline characteristics of our sample did not differ from those previously reported in the literature, either in hospital-based or population-based studies. Given the scarcity of information about HS and sexuality we consider that this study is a good introduction to the problem, and could lay the foundation for future research. (2) A possible classification bias, because it was an online questionnaire and HS diagnosis could not be confirmed; HS characteristics were also self-referred. Nevertheless, an informed population can properly identify HS, because of its apparent and distinctive clinical manifestations. Since a patients' association hosted the questionnaire, it is expected that the participants did suffer from the disease.

5. Conclusions

This is the largest cross-sectional study about HS and sexuality. We have observed important sexual distress in patients with HS. Factors related to SD were female sex, the presence of active lesions in the groin and genital areas, and the intensity of pain and unpleasant odor. Being in a stable relationship has been an important protector factor against SD. Regarding these results, it seems that SD in HS patients is due, at least in part, to disease symptoms and active lesions in specific locations, emphasizing the importance of proper control of the disease based on management guidelines to improve their sexual health. Women and single patients are more likely to suffer from sexual distress, so special medical care should be given to them.

Author Contributions: Conceptualization, C.C.-B. and A.M.-L.; methodology, C.C.-B. and A.M.-L.; software, A.M.-L.; validation, C.C.-B., R.R.-V. and A.M.-L.; formal analysis, C.C.-B.; investigation, C.C.-B. and A.M.-L.; resources, A.M.-L.; data curation, C.C.-B.; writing—original draft preparation, C.C.-B.; writing—review and editing, R.R.-V. and A.M.-L.; visualization, C.C.-B., R.R.-V. and A.M.-L.; supervision, R.R.-V. and A.M.-L.; project administration, A.M.-L.

Acknowledgments: We would like to thank José Juan Jiménez Moleón for his contribution to the development of this study; Charlotte Bower, for improving the English of this manuscript; the Spanish hidradenitis suppurativa patients' association (ASENDHI) for their help and valuable collaboration to develop the study, as well as for hosting the questionnaire; and all the patients who have participated in this survey. The results of this study are part of Carlos Cuenca-Barrales' PhD.

Conflicts of Interest: The authors declare no conflict of interest.

References

1. Jemec, G.B. Clinical practice. Hidradenitis suppurativa. *N. Engl. J. Med.* **2012**, *366*, 158–164. [CrossRef] [PubMed]
2. Matusiak, L.; Bieniek, A.; Szepietowski, J.C. Psychophysical aspects of hidradenitis suppurativa. *Acta Derm. Venereol.* **2010**, *90*, 264–268. [CrossRef]
3. Onderdijk, A.J.; van der Zee, H.H.; Esmann, S.; Lophaven, S.; Dufour, D.N.; Jemec, G.B.; Boer, J. Depression in patients with hidradenitis suppurativa. *J. Eur. Acad. Dermatol. Venereol.* **2013**, *27*, 473–478. [CrossRef] [PubMed]
4. Balieva, F.; Kupfer, J.; Lien, L.; Gieler, U.; Finlay, A.Y.; Tomas-Aragones, L.; Poot, F.; Misery, L.; Sampogna, F.; van Middendorp, H.; et al. The burden of common skin diseases assessed with the EQ5D: A European multicentre study in 13 countries. *Br. J. Dermatol.* **2017**, *176*, 1170–1178. [CrossRef] [PubMed]
5. Matusiak, L.; Szczech, J.; Kaaz, K.; Lelonek, E.; Szepietowski, J.C. Clinical Characteristics of Pruritus and Pain in Patients with Hidradenitis Suppurativa. *Acta Derm. Venereol.* **2018**, *98*, 191–194. [CrossRef]
6. Vossen, A.; Schoenmakers, A.; van Straalen, K.R.; Prens, E.P.; van der Zee, H.H. Assessing Pruritus in Hidradenitis Suppurativa: A Cross-Sectional Study. *Am. J. Clin. Dermatol.* **2017**, *18*, 687–695. [CrossRef]
7. Molina-Leyva, A.; Almodovar-Real, A.; Carrascosa, J.C.; Molina-Leyva, I.; Naranjo-Sintes, R.; Jimenez-Moleon, J.J. Distribution pattern of psoriasis, anxiety and depression as possible causes of sexual dysfunction in patients with moderate to severe psoriasis. *Anais Bras. Dermatol.* **2015**, *90*, 338–345. [CrossRef]
8. Nazarpour, S.; Simbar, M.; Ramezani Tehrani, F.; Alavi Majd, H. Quality of life and sexual function in postmenopausal women. *J. Women Aging* **2018**, *30*, 299–309. [CrossRef]
9. Nappi, R.E.; Cucinella, L.; Martella, S.; Rossi, M.; Tiranini, L.; Martini, E. Female sexual dysfunction (FSD): Prevalence and impact on quality of life (QoL). *Maturitas* **2016**, *94*, 87–91. [CrossRef]
10. Nusbaum, M.R.; Hamilton, C.; Lenahan, P. Chronic illness and sexual functioning. *Am. Fam. Physician* **2003**, *67*, 347–354.
11. Kouris, A.; Platsidaki, E.; Christodoulou, C.; Efstathiou, V.; Dessinioti, C.; Tzanetakou, V.; Korkoliakou, P.; Zisimou, C.; Antoniou, C.; Kontochristopoulos, G. Quality of Life and Psychosocial Implications in Patients with Hidradenitis Suppurativa. *Dermatology* **2016**, *232*, 687–691. [CrossRef] [PubMed]
12. Kurek, A.; Johanne Peters, E.M.; Sabat, R.; Sterry, W.; Schneider-Burrus, S. Depression is a frequent co-morbidity in patients with acne inversa. *JDDG* **2013**, *11*, 743–749. [CrossRef] [PubMed]
13. Shavit, E.; Dreiher, J.; Freud, T.; Halevy, S.; Vinker, S.; Cohen, A.D. Psychiatric comorbidities in 3207 patients with hidradenitis suppurativa. *J. Eur. Acad. Dermatol. Venereol.* **2015**, *29*, 371–376. [CrossRef] [PubMed]

14. Thorlacius, L.; Cohen, A.D.; Gislason, G.H.; Jemec, G.B.E.; Egeberg, A. Increased Suicide Risk in Patients with Hidradenitis Suppurativa. *J. Investig. Dermatol.* **2018**, *138*, 52–57. [CrossRef] [PubMed]
15. Theut Riis, P.; Thorlacius, L.; Knudsen List, E.; Jemec, G.B.E. A pilot study of unemployment in patients with hidradenitis suppurativa in Denmark. *Br. J. Dermatol.* **2017**, *176*, 1083–1085. [CrossRef] [PubMed]
16. Matusiak, L.; Bieniek, A.; Szepietowski, J.C. Hidradenitis suppurativa markedly decreases quality of life and professional activity. *J. Am. Acad. Dermatol.* **2010**, *62*, 706–708. [CrossRef] [PubMed]
17. ASENDHI [Internet]. Madrid: ASENDHI. 2008. Available online: http://asendhi.org/ (accessed on 28 September 2018).
18. Deckers, I.E.; Mihajlovic, D.; Prens, E.P.; Boer, J. Hidradenitis suppurativa: A pilot study to determine the capability of patients to self-assess their Hurley stage. *Br. J. Dermatol.* **2015**, *172*, 1418–1419. [CrossRef]
19. Lubrano, E.; Perrotta, F.M.; Parsons, W.J.; Marchesoni, A. Patient's Global Assessment as an Outcome Measure for Psoriatic Arthritis in Clinical Practice: A Surrogate for Measuring Low Disease Activity? *J. Rheumatol.* **2015**, *42*, 2332–2338. [CrossRef]
20. Zouboulis, C.C.; Desai, N.; Emtestam, L.; Hunger, R.E.; Ioannides, D.; Juhasz, I.; Lapins, J.; Matusiak, L.; Prens, E.P.; Revuz, J.; et al. European S1 guideline for the treatment of hidradenitis suppurativa/acne inversa. *J. Eur. Acad. Dermatol. Venereol.* **2015**, *29*, 619–644. [CrossRef]
21. Vinding, G.R.; Miller, I.M.; Zarchi, K.; Ibler, K.S.; Ellervik, C.; Jemec, G.B. The prevalence of inverse recurrent suppuration: A population-based study of possible hidradenitis suppurativa. *Br. J. Dermatol.* **2014**, *170*, 884–889. [CrossRef]
22. Revuz, J.E.; Canoui-Poitrine, F.; Wolkenstein, P.; Viallette, C.; Gabison, G.; Pouget, F.; Poli, F.; Faye, O.; Roujeau, J.C.; Bonnelye, G.; et al. Prevalence and factors associated with hidradenitis suppurativa: Results from two case-control studies. *J. Am. Acad. Dermatol.* **2008**, *59*, 596–601. [CrossRef] [PubMed]
23. Ingram, J.R.; Jenkins-Jones, S.; Knipe, D.W.; Morgan, C.L.I.; Cannings-John, R.; Piguet, V. Population-based Clinical Practice Research Datalink study using algorithm modelling to identify the true burden of hidradenitis suppurativa. *Br. J. Dermatol.* **2018**, *178*, 917–924. [CrossRef] [PubMed]
24. Vazquez, B.G.; Alikhan, A.; Weaver, A.L.; Wetter, D.A.; Davis, M.D. Incidence of hidradenitis suppurativa and associated factors: A population-based study of Olmsted County, Minnesota. *J. Investig. Dermatol.* **2013**, *133*, 97–103. [CrossRef] [PubMed]
25. Bettoli, V.; Naldi, L.; Cazzaniga, S.; Zauli, S.; Atzori, L.; Borghi, A.; Capezzera, R.; Caproni, M.; Cardinali, C.; De Vita, V.; et al. Overweight, diabetes and disease duration influence clinical severity in hidradenitis suppurativa-acne inversa: Evidence from the national Italian registry. *Br. J. Dermatol.* **2016**, *174*, 195–197. [CrossRef] [PubMed]
26. Deckers, I.E.; Janse, I.C.; van der Zee, H.H.; Nijsten, T.; Boer, J.; Horvath, B.; Prens, E.P. Hidradenitis suppurativa (HS) is associated with low socioeconomic status (SES): A cross-sectional reference study. *J. Am. Acad. Dermatol.* **2016**, *75*, 755–759.e1. [CrossRef]
27. Deckers, I.E.; van der Zee, H.H.; Boer, J.; Prens, E.P. Correlation of early-onset hidradenitis suppurativa with stronger genetic susceptibility and more widespread involvement. *J. Am. Acad. Dermatol.* **2015**, *72*, 485–488. [CrossRef]
28. Schrader, A.M.; Deckers, I.E.; van der Zee, H.H.; Boer, J.; Prens, E.P. Hidradenitis suppurativa: A retrospective study of 846 Dutch patients to identify factors associated with disease severity. *J. Am. Acad. Dermatol.* **2014**, *71*, 460–467. [CrossRef]
29. Kurek, A.; Peters, E.M.; Chanwangpong, A.; Sabat, R.; Sterry, W.; Schneider-Burrus, S. Profound disturbances of sexual health in patients with acne inversa. *J. Am. Acad. Dermatol.* **2012**, *67*, 422–428. [CrossRef] [PubMed]
30. Molina-Leyva, A.; Jimenez-Moleon, J.J.; Naranjo-Sintes, R.; Ruiz-Carrascosa, J.C. Sexual dysfunction in psoriasis: A systematic review. *J. Eur. Acad. Dermatol. Venereol.* **2015**, *29*, 649–655. [CrossRef]
31. Wu, T.; Duan, X.; Chen, S.; Chen, X.; Yu, R.; Yu, X. Association Between Psoriasis and Erectile Dysfunction: A Meta-Analysis. *J. Sex. Med.* **2018**, *15*, 839–847. [CrossRef]
32. Maaty, A.S.; Gomaa, A.H.; Mohammed, G.F.; Youssef, I.M.; Eyada, M.M. Assessment of female sexual function in patients with psoriasis. *J. Sex. Med.* **2013**, *10*, 1545–1548. [CrossRef]
33. Molina-Leyva, A.; Almodovar-Real, A.; Ruiz-Carrascosa, J.C.; Naranjo-Sintes, R.; Serrano-Ortega, S.; Jimenez-Moleon, J.J. Distribution pattern of psoriasis affects sexual function in moderate to severe psoriasis: A prospective case series study. *J. Sex. Med.* **2014**, *11*, 2882–2889. [CrossRef] [PubMed]

34. Janse, I.C.; Deckers, I.E.; van der Maten, A.D.; Evers, A.W.M.; Boer, J.; van der Zee, H.H.; Prens, E.P.; Horváth, B. Sexual health and quality of life are impaired in hidradenitis suppurativa: A multicentre cross-sectional study. *Br. J. Dermatol.* **2017**, *176*, 1042–1047. [CrossRef]
35. Sanchez, D.T.; Kiefer, A.K. Body concerns in and out of the bedroom: Implications for sexual pleasure and problems. *Arch. Sex. Behav.* **2007**, *36*, 808–820. [CrossRef]
36. Prens, E.; Deckers, I. Pathophysiology of hidradenitis suppurativa: An update. *J. Am. Acad. Dermatol.* **2015**, *73* (Suppl. 1), S8–S11. [CrossRef] [PubMed]
37. Micheletti, R. Tobacco smoking and hidradenitis suppurativa: Associated disease and an important modifiable risk factor. *Br. J. Dermatol.* **2018**, *178*, 587–588. [CrossRef] [PubMed]
38. Ibler, K.S.; Jemec, G.B. Cumulative life course impairment in other chronic or recurrent dermatologic diseases. *Curr. Probl. Dermatol.* **2013**, *44*, 130–136. [CrossRef] [PubMed]
39. Molina-Leyva, A.; Caparros-Del Moral, I.; Gomez-Avivar, P.; Alcalde-Alonso, M.; Jimenez-Moleon, J.J. Psychosocial Impairment as a Possible Cause of Sexual Dysfunction among Young Men with Mild Androgenetic Alopecia: A Cross-sectional Crowdsourcing Web-based Study. *Acta Dermatovenerol. Croat.* **2016**, *24*, 42–48. [PubMed]

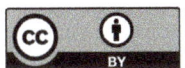

© 2019 by the authors. Licensee MDPI, Basel, Switzerland. This article is an open access article distributed under the terms and conditions of the Creative Commons Attribution (CC BY) license (http://creativecommons.org/licenses/by/4.0/).

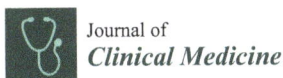

Article

Predictors of Sexual Dysfunction in Veterans with Post-Traumatic Stress Disorder

Marina Letica-Crepulja [1,2,*], Aleksandra Stevanović [1,2,3], Marina Protuđer [4], Božidar Popović [5], Darija Salopek-Žiha [5] and Snježana Vondraček [5]

1. Department of Psychiatry and Psychological Medicine, Faculty of Medicine, University of Rijeka, 51000 Rijeka, Croatia; aleksandras@medri.uniri.hr
2. Department of Psychiatry, Clinical Hospital Center Rijeka, Referral Center of the Ministry of Health of the Republic of Croatia, 51000 Rijeka, Croatia
3. Department of Basic Medical Sciences, Faculty of Health Studies, University of rijeka, 51000 Rijeka, Croatia
4. County General Hospital Varaždin, 42000 Varaždin, Croatia; marina2ri@yahoo.com
5. County General Hospital Našice, 31500 Našice, Croatia; salutogeneza1@gmail.com (B.P.); mentordsz@gmail.com (D.S.-Ž.); bolnica@obnasice.hr (S.V.)
* Correspondence: marinalc@medri.uniri.hr; Tel.: +385-51-658-321

Received: 18 February 2019; Accepted: 27 March 2019; Published: 29 March 2019

Abstract: Background: The problems in sexual functioning among patients with post-traumatic stress disorder (PTSD) are often overlooked, although scientific research confirms high rates of sexual dysfunctions (SD) particularly among veterans with PTSD. The main objective of this study was to systematically identify predictors of SD among veterans with PTSD. Methods: Three hundred veterans with PTSD were included in the cross-sectional study. The subjects were assessed by the Mini-International Neuropsychiatric Interview (MINI) and self-report questionnaires: PCL-5, i.e., PTSD Checklist for Diagnostic and Statistical Manual of Mental Disorders, Fifth Edition (DSM-5) with Criterion A, International Index of Erectile Function (IIEF), Premature Ejaculation Diagnostic Tool (PEDT), and Relationship Assessment Scale (RAS). Several hierarchical multiple regressions were performed to test for the best prediction models for outcome variables of different types of SD. Results: 65% of participants received a provisional diagnosis of SD. All tested prediction models showed a good model fit. The significant individual predictors were cluster D (Trauma-Related Negative Alterations in Cognition and Mood) symptoms (for all types of SD) and in a relationship status/relationship satisfaction (all, except for premature ejaculation (PE)). Conclusions: The most salient implication of this study is the importance of sexual health assessment in veterans with PTSD. Therapeutic interventions should be focused on D symptoms and intended to improve relationship functioning with the aim to lessen the rates of SD. Psychotropic treatment with fewer adverse sexual effects is of utmost importance if pharmacotherapy is applied. Appropriate prevention, screening, and treatment of medical conditions could improve sexual functioning in veterans with PTSD.

Keywords: post-traumatic stress disorder; sexual dysfunction; veterans; predictors

1. Introduction

The problems in sexual functioning among patients with post-traumatic stress disorder (PTSD) are often overlooked clinically and receive little attention in research. However, an increasing body of scientific research regarding sexual dysfunctions (SD) among veterans who were exposed to military trauma confirms much higher rates of problems in sexual functioning among veterans with PTSD than in those without PTSD or in adults without exposure to military trauma [1–5]. The rates of SD differ across the studies, mainly because of methodological differences. Systematic reviews reported a prevalence of SD between 8.4% and 88.6% among male veterans with PTSD [3,5]. Persons with PTSD, compared with similarly exposed survivors without it, have an increased risk of SD implying that PTSD, rather than trauma exposure per se, is the more proximal antecedent to sexual problems [3,6–10]. Studies revealed correlation of PTSD with a variety of impairments in the specific domains of sexuality (desire, arousal, orgasm, resolution) [1–7]. On the other hand, the specific PTSD symptoms or PTSD symptom clusters may influence the prevalence of SD unevenly. The emotional numbing and avoidance cluster, for example, appeared to be intimately tied to impairment in sexual functioning and higher level of sexual anxiety [2,11,12].

1.1. Predictors of Sexual Dysfunction in Veterans with PTSD

Only a few studies and systematic reviews have addressed the possible predictors that have an impact on sexual functioning in the population of veterans with or without PTSD. Considering the relationship between overall PTSD symptom severity and SD, studies revealed conflicting results [5]. Particular PTSD clusters and symptoms have been studied, and it was hypothesized that autonomic arousal, anger/hostility [13], emotional numbing/avoidance symptoms [2,11,12], and chronic autonomic arousal and intrusive symptoms [3,14,15] were mostly associated with sexual problems among veterans with PTSD. Recent studies indicate that emotional numbing may impede intimacy and attachment, thus serving as a potential mechanism through which symptoms of PTSD may drive problems and predict SD in these patients. According to the Diagnostic and Statistical Manual of Mental Disorders, Fifth Edition (DSM-5) [16], numbing symptoms (low positive emotions and negative emotional state) were included in the new D symptom cluster (Trauma-Related Negative Alterations in Cognition and Mood). These and other symptoms from this cluster, such as diminished interest or participation in significant activities, a feeling of detachment or estrangement from others, and guilt and shame, may impede sexual functioning in veterans with PTSD. SD is more common among veterans who are male, older, separated, divorced, or widowed, have lower annual income, mental health diagnoses—particularly PTSD—hypertension, and are prescribed psychiatric medications [1,4,17]. Returning combat veterans with SD have a reduced quality of life, decreased sexual intimacy, and increased health-care utilization [18]. PTSD is associated with impairments in romantic relationship satisfaction [19,20]. Recent research revealed that marital dissatisfaction is the factor that mediates the relationship between the number of PTSD symptoms and sexual dissatisfaction [21]. Considering the specific types of SD, age appeared to be the only significant predictor of erectile dysfunction; age, race, depression, and social support predicted self-reported sexual arousal problems; and race, combat exposure, social support, and avoidance/numbing symptoms of PTSD predicted self-reported sexual desire problems in male combat veterans seeking outpatient treatment for PTSD [2].

1.2. Predictors of Sexual Dysfunction in the General Population

Generally speaking, the predictors, risk, or etiological factors of SD can be separated in two groups: "organic" (such as diabetes, peripheral vascular disease or venous leaks, injury of the spinal cord, etc.) and "non-organic" (such as anxiety, depression, cultural taboos, ignorance, relationship problems, poor communication skills, etc.). However, there is substantial evidence indicating a multifactorial etiology of sexual function and dysfunction, meaning that the sexual response can be described as a complex interaction of psychological, interpersonal, social, cultural, physiological, and gender-influenced processes [22,23]. SD is strongly associated with certain health conditions and diseases, psychiatric disorders, medication or substance use, lack of knowledge, psychological or behavioral factors, relationship and cultural factors processes [23].

1.3. Study Background

More than 20 years after the Homeland War in Croatia (1991–1995), veterans still suffer from numerous health problems. Patients and/or health professionals may be reluctant to mention and discuss sexual symptoms [24], and a huge proportion of SD remains undiagnosed. Despite that, clinical observations and rising awareness have encouraged the recognition and assessment of SD in this patient group, and case reports [25] and research articles [26,27] regarding SD in veterans with PTSD in Croatia have been published.

The main objective of this research is to systematically identify predictors of SD among veterans with PTSD. The main hypothesis of the study is that SD are predicted by overall PTSD symptom severity and by severity of D symptom cluster (Trauma-Related Negative Alterations in Cognition and Mood).

2. Experimental Section

2.1. Participants and Procedure

Participants were male war veterans ($N = 300$) recruited from a pool of patients referred to the Regional Center for Psychotrauma (RCP) and Department of Psychiatry within the Clinical Hospital Center (CHC) Rijeka, the Referral Center for PTSD of the Ministry for Health of the Republic of Croatia ($N = 250$), and the Daily Hospital for PTSD and Department of Psychiatry within the General Hospital (GH) Našice for treatment. Most of the veterans participated in operations on different and almost all battlefields. Thirteen of those whom we approached refused to participate, while two patients did not complete the questionnaires.

Eligibility was determined by meeting diagnostic criteria for war-related PTSD as defined in DSM-5 [16]. Three patients were not eligible for the study as they did not meet the criteria for PTSD diagnosis. We continued recruiting patients until the number of 300 participants was reached. There were no differences in sociodemographic characteristics between those who refused to participate, those who did not complete the questionnaires, and those who were not eligible for the study.

The inclusion criteria for the study were: participation in the Homeland War as a soldier, experiencing at least one war-related traumatic event defined in the DSM-5 criteria for PTSD (personal experience of combat or exposure to a war zone), male gender, and age below 65. The exclusion criteria for the study were: active psychosis, moderate or high suicide risk measured by the Mini-International Neuropsychiatric Interview (MINI) for DSM-IV [28], and deformities, injury, or mutilation of the genital organs. None of the participants met the exclusion criteria.

Research consisted of two parts, i.e., a clinical interview and self-report questionnaires. The interviews were conducted by five psychiatrists and two psychologists from the two study sites. Sociodemographic data were collected through a questionnaire created for study purposes. The interviews and filling in of the questionnaires were usually completed in one or two sessions. The study was approved by the Ethics Committees of the Faculty of Medicine, University of Rijeka, CHC Rijeka, and GH Našice. Written informed consent was obtained from all participants after detailed information about the study was provided to them.

The study sample included a total of 300 male veterans. At the time of participation in the study, the majority of participants were in ambulatory treatment (66.8%), while other participants were involved in day-hospital treatment (19.3%) or club for PTSD (7.5%), or were hospitalized (6.4%). Table 1 provides further information on sample demographics.

Table 1. Sociodemographic characteristic and differences according to the presence of sexual dysfunction.

	All $n = 300$	Sexual Dysfunction NO $n = 98$	Sexual Dysfunction YES $n = 181$	Statistics	Probability
	M(sd) or N(%)	M(sd) or N(%)	M(sd) or N(%)		
Age (years)	52.4 (5.82)	52.4 (5.15)	52.1 (5.74)	$t = 0.470$	0.639
Marital Status (yes)					
Married	197 (65.7%)	68 (57.4%)	116 (63%)	$\chi^2 = 0.795$	0.373
Cohabitation	18 (6%)	5 (31.2%)	11 (68.8%)	$\chi^2 = 0.112$	0.738
Divorced	33 (11%)	9 (29%)	22 (71%)	$\chi^2 = 0.568$	0.451
Widower	2 (0.7%)	–	–		
Not married	37 (12.3%)	9 (27.3%)	24 (72.7%)	$\chi^2 = 1.013$	0.314
Other	12 (4%)	7 (58.3%)	5 (41.7%)	$\chi^2 = 2.964$	0.085
In a relationship (yes)	259 (86.3%)	94 (38.8%)	148 (61.2%)	$\chi^2 = 11.067$	0.001
Financial Status (yes)					
Low income	96 (32.7%)	25 (27.5%)	66 (72.5%)	$\chi^2 = 3.471$	0.062
Medium income	186 (63.3%)	71 (39.7%)	75 (60.3%)	$\chi^2 = 4.516$	0.034
High income	12 (4.1%)	2 (22.2%)	7 (77.8%)	$\chi^2 = 0.679$	0.410
Education (yes)					
Elementary	39 (13.1%)	14 (40%)	21 (60%)	$\chi^2 = 0.417$	0.518
Secondary	231 (77.5%)	77 (34.8%)	144 (65.2%)	$\chi^2 = 0.038$	0.846
Higher	26 (8.7%)	7 (30.4%)	16 (69.6%)	$\chi^2 = 0.242$	0.697
In the Last Month [1] (yes)					
Alcohol	33 (89%)	6 (20.7%)	23 (79.3%)	$\chi^2 = 2.960$	0.085
Cigarettes	50 (16.7%)	21 (42.9%)	28 (57.1%)	$\chi^2 = 2.837$	0.092
Marijuana	4 (1.3%)	–	–		
War deployment (months)	29.6 (19.2)	29.6 (19.34)	30 (19.51)	$t = -0.163$	0.871
Cluster B symptoms	15 (3.25)	15.1 (2.92)	14.9 (3.32)	$t = 0.534$	0.594
Cluster C symptoms	6.2 (1.47)	6.1 (1.48)	6.3 (1.46)	$t = -1.047$	0.296
Cluster D symptoms	18.7 (5.15)	17.2 (4.81)	19.4 (5,06)	$t = -3.612$	<0.001
Cluster E symptoms	17.7 (3.9)	16.9 (4.27)	18 (3.64)	$t = -2.422$	0.016
Total PTSD symptoms	57.5 (10.92)	55.2 (10.46)	58.6 (10.71)	$t = -2.559$	0.011
Relationship satisfaction	25.9 (6.37) [1]	28.1 (5.15) [2]	24.8 (6.01) [3]	$t = 4.298$	<0.001

[1] $n = 256$, range 7–35; [2] $n = 148$; [3] $n = 98$.

2.2. Measures

2.2.1. PTSD Checklist for DSM-5 (PCL-5) with Criterion A

The PCL-5 with Criterion A [29] is a self-report measure was revised to match the adapted DSM-5 criteria for PTSD. The interpretation of the PCL-5 should be made by a clinician. A PTSD diagnosis can be made provisionally considering items rated 2 = moderately or higher as a symptom endorsed according to the DSM-5 diagnostic rule (at least one B, one C, two D, and two E symptoms present). DSM-5 symptom cluster severity scores can be obtained by summing the scores for the items within a given cluster, i.e., cluster B (items 1–5), cluster C (items 6–7), cluster D (items 8–14), and cluster E (items 15–20). A total symptom severity score (range 0–80) can be obtained by summing the scores for each of the 20 items. Preliminary validation work was sufficient to make a cut-point score of 33, which was chosen for the purpose of this study [29]. Previous validation studies showed good psychometric properties for evaluating PTSD [30–33]. Cronbach's alpha in our study for clusters of symptoms ranged from 0.67 to 0.85, and to 0.89 for total PCL-5. The Criterion A measure was included in the assesment according the criteria of DSM-5 [16].

2.2.2. The International Index of Erectile Function (IIEF)

IIEF [34] is a widely used, multi-dimensional self-report instrument for the evaluation of male sexual function over the last four weeks [34]. It consists of 15 questions grouped into five domains that assess erectile function (Q1,2,3,4,5,15), intercourse satisfaction (Q6,7,8), orgasmic function (Q9,10), sexual desire (Q11,12), and overall satisfaction (Q13,14). Each item is rated from 1 (very low; almost never or never; extremely difficult) to 5 (very high; almost always or always; not difficult). Scores for domains are calculated as the sum of the answers, with lower scores indicating worse functioning. The score for erectile function can be calculated and used to classify the severity of dysfunction as severe, moderate, mild, or no dysfunction. For other domains, a higher score indicates better function. The IIEF meets psychometric criteria for test reliability and validity, has a high degree of sensitivity and specificity, and correlates well with other measures of treatment outcome [34–37]. Cronbach's alpha was 0.96 for erectile function, 0.91 for orgasmic function, 0.89 for sexual desire, and 0.91 for intercourse satisfaction and overall satisfaction.

2.2.3. Premature Ejaculation Diagnostic Tool (PEDT)

PEDT [38,39] is a self-report instrument for the evaluation of the presence and severity of premature ejaculation. Each PEDT item is rated from 0 (not difficult at all; almost never or never; not at all) to 4 (extremely difficult; almost always or always, extremely), with a higher score indicating more difficulties with premature ejaculation. Previous validation studies have shown satisfactory feasibility, reliability, and validity of the PEDT [38,39]. Cronbach's alpha for PEDT scale in our study was 0.87.

2.2.4. Male Sexual Dysfunction Criteria

The DSM-5 [16] classification recognizes four male sexual dysfunctions: delayed ejaculation (DE), erectile disorder (ED), male hypoactive sexual desire (HSD), and premature (early) ejaculation. To be diagnosed with SD, the symptoms must be present for at least six months, cause significant distress, and not be caused exclusively by a non-sexual mental disorder, significant relationship distress, medical illness, or medication. Also, these diagnoses are applicable to men who engage in non-vaginal sexual activity, but unfortunately, the specific duration criteria remain unknown [16]. For the purposes of this study, the following criteria were applied for a provisional diagnosis:

- DE—items Q9 or Q10 on IIEF rated 2 or less.
- ED—sum of scores on IIEF items Q1-Q5 and Q15 was 16 or less.
- HSD—items Q11 or Q12 on IIEF rated 2 or less.
- PE—item 2 on PEDT (*Do you ejaculate before you want to?*) rated 3 (Over half the time—>75%) or 4 (Always or Almost always—100%).

2.2.5. Relationship Assessment Scale (RAS)

The RAS [40,41] is a seven-item measure of global relationship satisfaction. Responses are on a five-point Likert scale, and either the total or the average score can be used in the interpretation. Average scores range from 1 to 5; total scores range from 7 to 35 (used in this study). Higher scores indicate greater relationship satisfaction. The reliability and validity of the English RAS have been established [41]. Cronbach's alpha in our study was 0.87.

2.2.6. Mini-International Neuropsychiatric Interview (MINI)

Comorbid psychiatric disorders were diagnosed using the Croatian version of MINI for DSM-IV [28]. It is a brief and valid structured clinical interview meeting the need for a short but accurate structured psychiatric interview for multicenter clinical trials and epidemiology studies, to be used as a first step in outcome tracking in nonresearch clinical settings. This interview enables researchers to assess the 17 most common psychiatric disorders in DSM-IV.

2.2.7. Anatomical Therapeutic Chemical (ATC) Classification System

Self-reported data about drug consumption are classified in accordance with the ATC classification [42]. In brief, the ATC system classifies therapeutic drugs. The purpose of the system is to serve as a tool for drug utilization research in order to improve the quality of drug use. In the ATC classification system, the drugs are divided into different groups according to the organ or system on which they act and their chemical, pharmacological, and therapeutic properties. Drugs are classified into five different groups.

2.3. Data Analysis

2.3.1. Data Analysis Plan

The aim of the study was to assess the predictive models of several sexual dysfunctions in male veterans with PTSD. Average score of erectile function, orgasmic function, sexual desire, intercourse satisfaction, overall satisfaction (all measured by IIEF), and premature ejaculation (measured by PEDT) were the outcome variables. Prediction variables were characteristics identified as relevant for sexual dysfunction in previous studies. Two sets of hierarchical regression analyses were executed for each of the sexual functions (one without and one with relationship satisfaction) in order to assess the best models for the overall sample of veterans with PTSD and for the subset of veterans in relationship. In order to control for covariances, predictor variables were entered in the following steps/models: (1) sociodemographic variables, (2) comorbid disorders (psychiatric and others), (3) medication used (psychotropic and other drugs), (4) variables related to PTSD (deployment duration and PTSD symptoms), and (5) relationship satisfaction (subset sample of veterans in relationship). The exclusion criterion for dichotomous predictors was set to 10 or less events per variable [43]. The inclusion criterion for a prediction variable was a significant association with the outcome variable.

2.3.2. Statistical Analysis

Statistical analysis was performed with Statistica software, version 12 (Dell Inc. Inc., Tulsa, OK, USA). Data are presented as N (%) or M (sd). Chi-square tests for categorical variables and independent sample t-tests for continuous variables were used to compare veterans with or without provisional diagnosis of sexual dysfunction. Pearson and Spearman correlation coefficients were calculated between sexual functions and the variables of interest. Several hierarchical multiple regressions were performed to test for the best prediction models for the outcome variables of erectile function, orgasmic function, sexual desire, intercourse satisfaction, overall satisfaction, and premature ejaculation. All models were controlled for basic assumptions. Two issues with multicollinearity were encountered, i.e., between cluster D and cluster E symptoms with overall PTSD symptoms, and between in-a-relationship status and relationship satisfaction in the subset sample. Overall PTSD symptoms were excluded from both sets of samples, and the in-a-relationship status variable from the subset sample. Missing values were controlled for listwise. Probability significance was set to $p \leq 0.05$.

3. Results

3.1. Sociodemographic Data

Sociodemographic data for the overall sample are presented in Table 1.

3.2. Trauma Exposure and PTSD

The average duration of active participation in the Homeland war was 30 (19.516) months, ranging from 1 month to 70 months.

Twenty-three percent of participants had sought psychiatric help in the period from 1991 to 1995, while the war was ongoing. The average intensity for overall PTSD symptoms was 57.5 (10.92) within the range of 33 to 80. The average intensity of B symptoms was 15 (3.25), of C symptoms 6.2 (1.47), of D symptoms 18.7 (5.15), and of E symptoms 17.7 (3.90).

3.3. Prevalence of SD and Association with Sociodemographic Data and PTSD

The average score for erectile function was 16 (9.71), which relates to moderate dysfunction. The average score for orgasmic function was 5.8 (3.31) (theoretical maximum = 8), for sexual desire 5.8 (2.47) (theoretical maximum = 8), for intercourse satisfaction 6.51 (4.71) (theoretical maximum = 12), and for overall satisfaction 6.3 (2.44) (theoretical maximum = 8). The average score for PEDT was 7.43 (5.14) within the range of 0 to 20.

According to provisional criteria for male sexual dysfunction (described in methodology), the following rates were found: DE 124 (44%, n = 282), ED 134 (46.2%, n = 290), HSD 128 (44.6%, n = 287), and PE 59 (21.3%, n = 277). Overall, on the basis of self-reported data, 98 (35.1%) of veterans with PTSD did not meet, while 181 (64.9%) participants met provisional criteria for at least one male SD in the last month. Out of possible four SD, one SD had 49 (17.6%) participants, two SDs had 36 participants (12.9%) participants, three SD had 80 participants (28.7%), and four SD had 16 participants (5.7%).

As presented in Table 1, participants in a relationship and participants with medium income were less likely to have a provisional diagnosis of SD. Participants who met the provisional diagnosis of SD were significantly less satisfied with their relationship compared to participants without SD. Veterans with SD had significantly greater severity of cluster D, cluster E, and overall symptoms of PTSD. They did not differ for duration of deployment or for cluster B and cluster C symptoms.

Prevalence of comorbid disorders and drug use and association with SD are presented in Supplementary Materials: Material S1.

3.4. Prediction Models of Sexual Dysfunctions among War Veterans with PTSD

Predictor variables for each model (i.e., sexual function) were selected on the basis of the following criteria: variables with events greater than 10 and significant correlation with the outcome variable (Table S2). However, some variables were included regardless, such as age and all clusters of PTSD symptoms. Also, analysis showed great correlation coefficients between overall PTSD symptoms intensity and cluster D and E symptom intensity (variance inflation factor (VIF) > 8). Because of the multicollinearity issues, overall PTSD symptoms were not included in the models. The variable "in a relationship" had high multicollinearity with relationship satisfaction (VIF > 8), and, therefore, only relationship satisfaction was included in the models for the subset of veterans in a relationship. The final steps for all tested models are presented in Supplementary material (Tables S3 and S4). An overview of individual significant predictors for each sexual function is given in Tables 2 and 3.

Table 2. Overview of individual significant predictors in the final step of hierarchical regression analysis for the overall sample.

	Erectile Function		Orgasmic Function		Sexual Desire		Inter-Course Satisfaction		Overall Satisfaction		Premature Ejaculation	
	B	β	B	β	B	β	B	β	B	β	B	β
In a relationship	7.69	**0.28 ****	1.98	**0.21 ***	0.93	**0.13 ***	3.94	**0.30 ****	1.17	**0.15 ***	1.99	0.13
Alcohol use dis. [1]					−1.62	**−0.13 ***			−1.47	**−0.12 ***		
Diabetes mellitus											1.71	**0.12 ***
Hypertension, esse. [2]	−3.99	**−0.20 ****	−0.98	**−0.15 ***			−1.49	**−0.15 ****	−0.71	**−0.14 ***		
Antidepressant	−1.3	−0.06	−1.12	**−0.15 ****	−0.71	**−0.14 ***			−0.36	−0.07		
Cluster D symptoms	−0.46	**−0.24 ****	−0.15	**−0.23 ****	−0.14	**−0.29 ****	−0.23	**−0.25 ****	−0.11	**−0.23 ****	0.21	**0.21 ***

* $p \leq 0.05$; ** $p \leq 0.01$; [1] Alcohol use disorders; [2] Hypertension, essential; significant values are in bold.

Table 3. Overview of individual significant predictors in the final step of hierarchical regression analysis for the subset sample of veterans in a relationship.

	Erectile Function		Orgasmic Function		Sexual Desire		Inter-Course Satisfaction		Overall Satisfaction		Premature Ejaculation	
	B	β	B	β	B	β	B	β	B	β	B	β
Diabetes mellitus											1.91	0.14 *
Hypertension, esse. [1]	−3.08	−0.17 **	−0.78	−0.12 *			−0.84	−0.09	−0.48	−0.10		
Hyperplasia prost. [2]	−2.88	−0.05	−169	−0.08			−2.19	−0.08	−1.99	−0.13 *		
Antidepressant	−1.17	−0.06	−0.96	−0.15 *	−0.73	−0.15 *			−0.47	−0.11 *		
Cluster D symptoms	−0.38	−0.21 **	−0.15	−0.24 **	−0.14	−0.30 **	−0.11	−0.23 **	−0.09	−0.19 **	0.23	0.23 **
Relationship satisf. [3]	0.43	0.29 **	0.14	0.28 **	0.06	0.16 **	0.27	0.39 **	0.16	0.44 **	0.05	0.07

* $p \leq 0.05$; ** $p \leq 0.01$; [1] Hypertension, essential; [2] Hyperplasia of prostate; [3] Relationship satisfaction; significant values are in bold.

3.4.1. Erectile Function

The initial model tested for erectile function included age, low income, medium income, not married, married, "in a relationship" status (Model 1: $R^2 = 0.134$, $F = 7.060$, $p < 0.001$). In the second step ongoing major depressive episode (MDE), panic disorder lifetime, essential hypertension, and hyperplasia of prostate (Model 2: $R^2 = 0.181$, $F = 5.816$, $p < 0.001$) were included; in the third step, use of antidepressants, hypnotics, and sedatives (Model 3: $R^2 = 0.184$, $F = 5.514$, $p < 0.001$) was added; in the fourth step, war deployment in months and cluster B, C, D, and E symptoms were added (model 4: $R^2 = 0.257$, $F = 5.651$, $p < 0.001$). Significant predictors did not change through the models. The final model explained 25.7% of the variance of erectile function. Variables with significant independent contribution were being in a relationship, having essential hypertension, and severity of D cluster symptoms (Table 2).

In the subset of participants in a relationship, Model 1, containing age, low income, medium income, not married, and married, was not significant, since the variable relationship status was removed. Model 2 accounted for 9.3% ($F = 2.200$, $p = 0.019$), Model 3 for 9.98% ($F = 2.097$, $p = 0.22$), and Model 4 for 20.1% ($F = 3.273$, $p < 0.001$) of the variance of erectile function. The final model with relationship satisfaction added explained 27.9% of the variance of erectile function ($F = 5.457$, $p < 0.001$). Significant individual predictors were having essential hypertension, severity of cluster D symptoms, and relationship satisfaction. (Table 3).

3.4.2. Orgasmic Function

The initial model tested for orgasmic function included age, higher education, low income, medium income, married, and "in a relationship" status (Model 1: $R^2 = 0.100$, $F = 4.619$, $p < 0.001$). In the second step, ongoing MDE, panic disorder lifetime, essential hypertension, hyperplasia of prostate, and disorders of lipoprotein metabolism were added (Model 2: $R^2 = 0.165$, $F = 4.397$, $p < 0.001$); in the third step, use of antidepressants, hypnotics, and sedatives (Model 3: $R^2 = 0.189$, $F = 4.751$, $p < 0.001$) was included; in the fourth step, cluster B, C, D, and E symptoms (Model 4: $R^2 = 0.248$, $F = 4.628$, $p < 0.001$) were added. Higher education level was a significant individual contributor until psychotropic medication was introduced in the third step. The final model explained 24.8% of the variance of orgasmic function. Significant independent predictors were being in a relationship, use of antidepressants, having hypertension, and severity of cluster D symptoms (Table 2).

In the subset of participants who were in a relationship, Model 1 was not significant and accounted for 5.4% variance of orgasmic function. Model 2 ($R^2 = 0.121$, $F = 2.601$, $p = 0.004$), Model 3 ($R^2 = 0.152$, $F = 3.098$, $p < 0.001$), and Model 4 ($R^2 = 0.244$, $F = 3.839$, $p < 0.001$) were all significant. The final model explained 29.5% of the variance of orgasmic function ($F = 4.679$, $p < 0.001$). Significant individual predictors were: use of antidepressants, presence of essential hypertension, severity of cluster D symptoms, and relationship satisfaction (Table 3). There was no significant change in the significance of individual predictors through the models.

3.4.3. Sexual Desire

The initial model for sexual desire included age, low and medium income, and "in a relationship" status (Model 1: $R^2 = 0.055$, $F = 4.131$, $p = 0.003$). In the second model, alcohol use disorder (AUD) was added (Model 2: $R^2 = 0.074$, $F = 4.521$, $p = 0.001$); in the third model, antidepressant use was included (Model 3: $R^2 = 0.095$, $F = 4.901$, $p < 0.001$); in the fourth model, cluster B, C, D, and E symptoms (Model 4: $R^2 = 0.166$, $F = 5.482$, $p < 0.001$) were added. All the models were significant, and there was no change in the significance of individual predictors. The final model explained 16.6% of the variance of sexual desire in the entire sample. Predictors with independent contribution were being in a relationship, presence of an AUD, use of antidepressant, and severity of cluster D symptoms (Table 2).

In the subset sample of veterans in a relationship, the sociodemographic variables entered did not significantly contribute to the variance of sexual desire (Model 1: $R^2 = 0.035$, $F = 2.219$, $p = 0.068$) Addition of AUD in step two (Model 2: $R^2 = 0.054$, $F = 2.789$, $p = 0.018$), antidepressant in step three (Model 3: $R^2 = 0.081$, $F = 3.536$, $p = 0.002$), and clusters of PTSD symptoms in step four (Model 4: $R^2 = 0.172$, $F = 4.930$, $p < 0.001$) significantly increased the variance of sexual desire. The final model which included relationship satisfaction explained 19.6% of sexual desire in veterans in a relationship ($F = 5.227$, $p < 0.001$). As in the total sample, predictors with significant independent contribution were use of an antidepressant and severity of cluster D symptoms, but not AUD. A significant contributor was also relationship satisfaction (Table 3). The significant predictors did not change through the models.

3.4.4. Intercourse Satisfaction (IS)

The initial model for the intercourse satisfaction consisted of age, low income, medium income, not married, divorced, married and relationship status (Model 1: $R^2 = 0.139$, $F = 6.748$, $p < 0.001$). In the second model, ongoing MDE, other anxiety disorders, essential hypertension, and hyperplasia of prostate were added (Model 2: $R^2 = 0.168$, $F = 5.287$, $p < 0.001$); in the third (final) model, war deployment in months, cluster B, C, D, and E symptoms (Model 3: $R^2 = 0.251$, $F = 5.714$, $p < 0.001$) were included. There was no change in individual predictors through the models, and the final model explained 25.1% of intercourse satisfaction in veterans with PTSD. The identified significant predictors were being in a relationship, presence of essential hypertension, and severity of cluster D symptoms (Table 2).

In the subset sample of veterans who were in a relationship, the final model accounted for 31.6% of intercourse satisfaction ($F = 7.382$, $p < 0.001$). All tested models were significant (Model 1: $R^2 = 0.067$, $F = 2.982$, $p = 0.008$; Model 2: $R^2 = 0.102$, $F = 2.788$, $p = 0.003$; Model 3: $R^2 = 0.188$, $F = 3.987$, $p < 0.001$). The significance of predictors did not change through the models. In contrast to the overall sample, essential hypertension was not a significant predictor of IS among veterans in a relationship. Severity of D cluster symptoms and relationship satisfaction were independent significant contributors (Table 3).

3.4.5. Overall Satisfaction

In the first model for overall satisfaction, the following variables were entered: age, low income, medium income, and "in a relationship" status (Model 1: $R^2 = 0.061$, $F = 4.474$, $p = 0.002$). In the next step, comorbid diseases, ongoing MDE, panic disorder lifetime, other anxiety disorders, AUD, essential hypertension, and hyperplasia of prostate were entered (Model 2: $R^2 = 0.140$, $F = 4.371$ $p < 0.001$); in the third step, use of antidepressants (Model 3: $R^2 = 0.145$, $F = 4.125$, $p < 0.001$) was included; in the fourth step, clusters B, C, D, and E symptoms (Model 4: $R^2 = 0.210$, $F = 4.652$, $p < 0.001$) were added. Recurrent panic disorder was a significant predictor until PTSD symptoms were entered in the last step. The final model explained 21% of the variance of overall satisfaction in veterans with PTSD. Significant individual predictors of overall satisfaction were being in a relationship, presence of an AUD, presence of essential hypertension, and severity of cluster D symptoms (Table 2).

All the models tested for overall satisfaction among veterans with PTSD who were in a relationship were significant (Model 1: $R^2 = 0.038$, $F = 3.188$, $p = 0.024$; Model 2: $R^2 = 0.117$, $F = 3.457$, $p < 0.001$; Model 3: $R^2 = 0.136$, $F = 3.717$, $p < 0.001$; Model 4: $R^2 = 0.215$, $F = 4.570$, $p < 0.001$). The "other anxiety disorders" variable was a significant predictor until PTSD symptoms were entered in the fourth step. The final model in the subset sample explained 38.4% of the variance of overall satisfaction ($F = 9.651$, $p < 0.001$). Significant individual predictors were: presence of hyperplasia of prostate, use of an antidepressants, severity of cluster D symptoms, and relationship satisfaction (Table 3). It is important to note that relationship satisfaction by itself ($\beta = 0.435$) explained most of the variance of overall sexual satisfaction.

3.4.6. Premature Ejaculation

In the first model of premature ejaculation in the overall sample, the following sociodemographic variables were entered: age, not married, married, and "in a relationship" status (Model 1: $R^2 = 0.054$, $F = 3.779$, $p < 0.01$). In Model 2, diabetes mellitus (DM) was added ($R^2 = 0.067$, $F = 3.795$, $p < 0.01$), and cluster B, C, D, and E symptoms were added in Model 3. Significant individual predictors were DM and severity of cluster D symptoms (Table 2).

Similar findings were reported in the subset sample of veterans in a relationship, as the final model contributed to 10.7% of the variance of premature ejaculation ($F = 3.019$, $p < 0.001$) with the independent significant contributors DM and cluster D symptoms (Table 3). Model 1, containing sociodemographic variables ($R^2 = 0.016$, $F = 1.257$, $p = 0.290$), and Model 2 ($R^2 = 0.035$, $F = 2.079$, $p = 0.054$), containing comorbid diseases, did not contribute significantly to the variance of premature ejaculation. Model 3, which included clusters of PTDS symptoms, was significant ($R^2 = 0.104$, $F = 3.277$, $p < 0.001$). Relationship satisfaction added in the final model did not alter significantly the variance explained.

4. Discussion

To the best of our knowledge, the present study is the first to suggest patterns of association of PTSD with different types of SD and to determine the predictors of this relationship. The results of the study support the main hypothesis that SD in veterans with PTSD are predicted by the severity of the D cluster of PTSD symptoms. The second part of the hypothesis that states SD are predicted by overall PTSD symptom severity is partially supported. We found that veterans with SD had significantly higher PTSD symptom scores than veterans without SD. Furthermore, overall PTSD symptom severity was significantly correlated with all types of SD (DE, ED, HSD, and PE) as well as intercourse satisfaction (IS) and overall satisfaction (OS). Analysis revealed significant multicollinearity of this predictor with D symptoms of PTSD, which implies that the association of PTSD symptom severity with SD is mediated and mostly depends on the quantity and severity of trauma-related negative alterations in cognition and mood. Previous studies found high rates of SD among male veterans with PTSD [1–5]. The results of our study are consistent with the scarce but increasing body of research that indicates that the severity of PTSD measured by overall scores on PTSD scales is not a significant predictor of SD in veterans with PTSD [2,5,11,12].

Beside the prevalence and correlation of SD with PTSD, it is important to understand the background of this relationship. A high score of D symptoms (Trauma-Related Negative Alterations in Cognition and Mood) appears to be the most prevalent predictor of SD among veterans with PTSD, emerging as a significant predictor of all types of SD (DE, ED, HSD, PE) as well as of IS and OS. D cluster includes three new symptoms according to the DSM-5 classification: negative expectations of self, others, or the world (replacing the sense of foreshortened future), persistent distorted blame of self or other for trauma, and pervasive negative emotional state. The presence of these symptoms and/or other symptoms from the D cluster, such as diminished interest or participation in significant activities, a feeling of detachment or estrangement from others, or a persistent inability to experience positive emotions, precludes a person's capacity to engage adequately in sexual behavior(s). As a result, D symptoms predict lower levels of satisfaction in sexual life. The current DSM-5 classification embraces the four-factor model, as it provides a better representation of PTSD's latent structure than the tripartite model of DSM-IV [43–46], which has received extensive criticism [47]. Our findings in veterans are consistent with prior research demonstrating that avoidance/numbing symptoms of PTSD are strongly linked to self-reported problems in sexual functioning. Nunnink and colleagues found that self-reported symptoms of emotional numbing predicted a greater likelihood of endorsing sexual problems [11]. The results of another study that investigated predictors of ED and self-reported sexual problems among 150 male combat veterans seeking outpatient treatment for PTSD revealed, beside various demographic, physical, and psychosocial risk factors, a significant zero-order correlation between avoidance/numbing symptoms and SD [2].

Partner relationship is the next prominent predictor of SD in veterans with PTSD. Results in the overall sample revealed that being in a partner relationship reduces the risk of DE, ED, HSD, IS, and OS. Being in a relationship has no predictive value for PE. Analysis in the sample of participants who were in a partner relationship indicated that a low level of relationship satisfaction was a significant predictor of DE, ED, HSD, and IS and OS. Relationship satisfaction was not a significant predictor of PE. The association of PTSD with impairments in romantic relationship satisfaction has been previously reported [11,19,20]. A recent meta-analysis of 23 studies found an association between the emotional numbing and avoidance symptom cluster and parent, child, family, and marital/partner functioning problems [48]. Sexual functioning and relationship satisfaction are also robustly, positively correlated in many different samples across a variety of adult populations, including those who are dating [49,50], in long-term relationships [51], and married [52,53]. A lower level of relationship satisfaction in our study sample was an independent predictor of SD and was not mediated by the severity of any PTSD cluster. Sexual functioning is one of the essential domains of relationship functioning. Association between SD and quality of relationship is bidirectional and reciprocal. Relationship problems caused by family stressors, economic reasons, lifestyle, etc. inevitably affect sexual functioning. Problems in sexual functioning may have an impact on all other domains of a relationship. In the context of PTSD, the quality of a relationship also depends on the accommodation capacities of the partner for mutual acceptance, which is important for healthy sexual functioning. Additionally, PTSD may affect relationship and sexual functioning indirectly through changes of behavioral patterns. For example, insomnia and nightmares are less likely to have a direct impact on sexual functioning than numbing symptoms. On the other hand, these symptoms may lead to sleeping in separate beds, allowing or encouraging the rituals and avoidant behavior that lessen the quality of a relationship and sexual functioning. This finding implies that therapeutic efforts directed to promoting relationship satisfaction in veterans with PTSD could have a positive effect on sexual functioning in most of its domains. Interestingly, being in a relationship and relationship satisfaction are not significant predictors of PE. This finding could be explained by considering PE symptoms as more of an individual than a relational problem, which in turn is not worsened or maintained by disturbances in a partner relationship.

Antidepressant use is a significant predictor of the impairment of orgasmic functioning and sexual desire, i.e., veterans with PTSD that use antidepressants have increased risk for DE and HSD. Surprisingly, antidepressant utilization did not show predictive values for ED and OS. Adverse sexual effects are frequent with commonly prescribed psychotropic drugs and are usually underestimated [24,54]. The recent clinical guidelines highlight antidepressants as first-line pharmacotherapeutic agents in the management of PTSD [55,56]. In spite of increasing rates of drug utilization (80%) among veterans with PTSD [57], some studies revealed a marked inconsistency with the current guidelines for treatment of PTSD, particularly in the post-conflict settings [58]. In that context, our finding of antidepressant use as a significant predictor of DE and HSD is important, bearing in mind that 41.5% of our participants have DE and 45.4% have HSD. The findings are consistent with a meta-analysis which revealed increased rates of SD among patients in treatment with antidepressants [54]. Furthermore, higher rates of total and specific-treatment emergent SD and specific phases of dysfunction were found for drugs with a predominantly serotonergic action, including selective serotonin reuptake inhibitors (SSRIs) and serotonin and norepinephrine reuptake inhibitors (SNRIs) [55,59]. Ejaculation-delaying effect of antidepressants on orgasmic function is, on the other hand, the basis for the use of either tricyclic antidepressant or SSRIs in treatment of PE. Among other medications from this pharmacological group, paroxetine has the most prominent ejaculation-delaying effect [60] caused by its impact on serotonergic receptors, cholinergic receptor blockade, and inhibition of nitric oxide synthase [61–64]. It is also supported by the results of this study, as antidepressants are not significant predictors of PE.

Arterial hypertension was a significant predictor of ED, DE, IS, and OS in the overall sample. It was a significant predictor of ED and DE in the sample of veterans in a relationship. These findings are consistent with those of numerous studies that emphasize high blood pressure as a risk factor for SD [65–67]. Actually, vasculogenic ED is considered part of a systemic vasculopathy and has a known relationship with cardiovascular risk factors such as hypertension, diabetes, dyslipidemia, and smoking [68]. A research that included 1255 male participants revealed that lower systolic and diastolic blood pressure were associated with better sexual functioning [67].

The significant predictor of PE in the overall sample and among participants in a relationship was DM. Patients with DM have higher rates of various SD directly related to the deleterious complications of their disease. [69–71]. DM is also indirectly related to SD through anxiety and depression that are often experienced by men with DM [72]. Of these, ED was most commonly reported [69–71]. Some studies reported higher rates of PE in patients with DM, indicating duration, severity, and poor metabolic control as the main risk factors for PE in diabetic patients. On the other hand, a close relationship between ED and PE exists. Some authors suggest that the longer the erectile problem, the worse the anxiety, and the more marked the PE [73]. Because of performance anxiety regarding their erectile reliability, patients could rush through an intercourse, with PE as a deleterious consequence [74].

AUD was a significant predictor of SD and OS in the overall sample and in those who patients were in a relationship. The results are consistent with the findings of a previous research and meta-analysis [65]. This finding is important in the context of populations of veterans with PTSD, as repeated heavy drinking is one of the common strategies to alleviate trauma symptoms that may lead to the development of AUD. The prevalence of AUD in PTSD is also high. For example, in the US, 42% of PTSD subjects met criteria for AUD diagnosis [75]. The prevalence of alcohol-induced sexual dysfunction is unclear, probably because of underreporting. Sexual disorders ranging from 8% to 95.2% have been reported in men with chronic alcohol use [76–80]. The common dysfunctions reported were lack of sexual desire [79,80], premature ejaculation [81,82], and erectile dysfunction [76,82–84].

Although the prevalence of the SD was not the main focus of this research, it is indicative that none of the participants reported being diagnosed with SD. Only one veteran with PTSD reported the utilization of a medication prescribed to treat ED (sildenafil). This finding is completely inconsistent with data from previous studies suggesting that SD is strongly related to PTSD, particularly war-related PTSD [1–5]. A backup check of medical records confirmed only one diagnosis of SD recorded in the study sample. Two widely used instruments for the assessment of the presence and severity of the different types of SD were applied with restrictive criteria for severity of SD symptoms, consistent with DSM-5 for diagnosis of SD (i.e., present in at least 75% of sexual activity occasions) in order to avoid over-diagnosing minor and potentially transient problems in sexual functioning. According to that criteria, the following rates were found: SD in 64.9% of patients, DE in 44%, ED in 46.2%, HSD in 44.6%, PE in 21.3%. The rates of SD differ across studies [6–10], mainly because of different methodological approaches. Predominantly, two methods for identifying SD have been used in research. In some studies, the estimation of SD diagnosis was based on reported patients' symptoms and problems in sexual functioning, with wide criteria for SD applied. In another study, the presence of SD was considered if SD diagnosis was recorded or medication for SD was used, which may be a more conservative approach. Both methods for identifying SD may be problematic. If we chose the second approach, we could conclude that veterans with PTSD in our sample had superior sexual functioning. Therefore, we chose the first approach, bearing in mind that self-reported symptoms in questionnaires can be used only for an estimation and provisional diagnosis of SD. Clinical interviews are irreplaceable and necessary to sufficiently diagnose SD if they are conducted by well-trained personnel, who are also trained about social stigmatization. Conversely, they may contribute to underreporting biases arising from personal concerns about social stigmatization and lack of privacy, particularly in older or less educated participants [85]. The rates of SD in this study confirm that the complete absence of SD diagnosis in our clinical setting could not be a consequence of non-clinically significant problems among veterans. A dramatically higher self-reported prevalence of SD suggests a number of veterans may be choosing not to disclose problems in sexual functioning with their healthcare providers because of embarrassment, discomfort, or lack of knowledge about treatment possibilities.

4.1. Strenghts

This study was primarily designed to assess SD in the population of veterans with PTSD. Veterans with PTSD were included regardless of their relationship status, as even those not in a current romantic relationship may engage in sexual behavior and are often overlooked in studies. Data related to military deployment, sociodemographic and relationship factors, psychiatric comorbidity, psychotropic and other medication, and medical conditions were systematically collected, as all these factors could be important contributors to SD. PTSD symptoms were assessed jointly, but, more importantly, the impact of each cluster of PTSD symptoms (according to DSM-5 classification) on sexual functioning was also assessed. In assessing SD, we applied a comprehensive approach covering a broader range of possible sexual health problems as well as perceived sexual satisfaction.

4.2. Limitations

This study has several limitations. Findings from this study may not be reflective of and generalisable to the broader veteran or nonveteran population. Because of the many variables tested, data analysis suffered from multiple comparisons, allowing for possible false positive effects/predictors. Health-care-seeking participants could suffer from more serious problems in each area covered by the research. Furthermore, the generalisability is limited by a gender-imbalanced sample, as only male veterans were included in the research. Because of the cross-sectional design, the temporality of the relationship between the different studied variables and sexual dysfunction could not be evaluated. The findings were based on self-reported symptoms from questionnaire measures. Self-reports of sexual activity and satisfaction may be under- or overreported because of stigmatization.

5. Conclusions

One of the most salient implications of the current study is the importance of sexual health assessment in veterans with PTSD. This study represents an advancement in our currently limited understanding of patterns of association of PTSD with different types of SD and of the predictors of that relationship. As veterans with PTSD are more likely to suffer from SD if they experience more D symptoms and if they are not in a relationship or are less satisfied with the relationship, future research should develop therapeutic interventions more focused on the negative appraisals, emotional numbness, and irritability and other negative cognitions and emotions, as well as interventions intended to improve relationship functioning with the aim to lessen the rates of SD in this population. Psychotherapy is strongly recommended as the first-line treatment approach in PTSD. Sex therapy is effective in the variety of the SD, and couple psychotherapy is an established approach for relationship problems and dissatisfaction. Psychotherapeutic treatments, which would comprehensively cover different aspects of the problems in patients with PTSD and SD comorbidity, could have greater compliance rates, less iatrogenic adverse effects, and better treatment effects. Psychotropic treatment with fewer adverse sexual effects and management of the treatment-emergent side effects are of utmost importance if pharmacotherapy is applied. Medical conditions, particularly those stress-related and frequent in study populations with diabetes and hypertension, carry an additional burden of increased risk for SD. Appropriate prevention, screening for those conditions, and their active treatment could improve the sexual life of veterans with PTSD.

Supplementary Materials: The following are available online at http://www.mdpi.com/2077-0383/8/4/432/s1, Material S1: Prevalence of comorbid disorders and drug use and association with SD, including Table S1: Comorbidity and drugs and differences according to the presence of sexual dysfunction; Table S2: Correlation coefficients; Table S3: Summary of the final step in hierarchical regression analysis for the overall sample; Table S4: Summary of the final step in hierarchical regression analysis for the subset sample of veterans in a relationship.

Author Contributions: Conceptualization, M.L.-C. and M.P.; methodology, M.L.-C., A.S., M.P., B.P., D.S.-Ž., and S.V.; software, A.S.; validation, M.L.-C. and A.S.; formal analysis, A.S.; investigation, M.P., M.L.-C., A.S., B.P., D.S.-Ž., and S.V.; resources, M.L.-C., A.S., M.P.; data curation, M.L.-C., A.S., M.P., B.P., D.S.-Ž., and S.V.; Writing—Original Draft preparation, M.L.-C., A.S., and M.P.; Writing—Review and Editing, M.L.-C., A.S., M.P., B.P., D.S.-Ž., and S.V.; visualization, M.L.-C. and A.S.; project administration, M.L.-C., A.S., and M.P.

Acknowledgments: The authors would like to thank the participants of the study, without whom this research could not have been undertaken. The authors would also like to thank their colleagues Tanja Frančišković, Ika Rončević-Gržeta, Jasna Grković, Tanja Grahovac-Juretić, Tomislav Lesica, Sandra Blažević-Zelić, Gordana Šikić, Zoran Šuković, Nada Kaurić-Raos, Tihomir Perić, Gavrilo Nešković, Vlatka Franjkutić, Andreja Korpar, and Alma Kranjc for their cooperation and support.

Conflicts of Interest: The authors declare no conflict of interest.

References

1. Hosain, G.M.; Latini, D.M.; Kauth, M.; Goltz, H.H.; Helmer, D.A. Sexual dysfunction among male veterans returning from Iraq and Afghanistan: Prevalence and correlates. *J. Sex. Med.* **2013**, *10*, 516–523. [CrossRef]
2. Badour, C.L.; Gros, D.F.; Szafranski, D.D.; Acierno, R. Problems in sexual functioning among male OEF/OIF veterans seeking treatment for posttraumatic stress. *Compr. Psychiatry* **2015**, *58*, 74–81. [CrossRef] [PubMed]
3. Yehuda, R.; Lehrner, A.; Rosenbaum, T.Y. PTSD and Sexual Dysfunction in Men and Women. *J. Sex. Med.* **2015**, *12*, 1107–1119. [CrossRef] [PubMed]
4. Breyer, B.N.; Cohen, B.E.; Bertenthal, D.; Rosen, R.C.; Neylan, T.C.; Seal, K.H. Sexual Dysfunction in Male Iraq and Afghanistan War Veterans: Association with Posttraumatic Stress Disorder and Other Combat-Related Mental Health Disorders: A Population-Based Cohort Study. *J. Sex. Med.* **2014**, *11*, 75–83. [CrossRef] [PubMed]
5. Bentsen, I.L.; Giraldi, A.G.; Kristensen, E.; Andersen, H.S. Systematic Review of Sexual Dysfunction Among Veterans with Post-Traumatic Stress Disorder. *Sex. Med. Rev.* **2015**, *3*, 78–87. [CrossRef]
6. Letourneau, E.J.; Schewe, P.A.; Frueh, B.C. Preliminary evaluation of sexual problems in combat veterans with PTSD. *J. Trauma. Stress* **1997**, *10*, 125–132. [CrossRef] [PubMed]
7. Cosgrove, D.J.; Gordon, Z.; Bernie, J.E.; Hami, S.; Montoya, D.; Stein, M.B.; Monga, M. Sexual dysfunction in combat veterans with post-traumatic stress disorder. *Urology* **2002**, *60*, 881–884. [CrossRef]
8. Riggs, D.S.; Byrne, C.A.; Weathers, F.W.; Litz, B.T. The quality of the intimate relationships of male Vietnam veterans: Problems associated with posttraumatic stress disorder. *J. Trauma. Stress* **1998**, *11*, 87–101. [CrossRef]
9. Cook, J.M.; Riggs, D.S.; Thompson, R.; Coyne, J.C.; Sheikh, J.I. Posttraumatic stress disorder and current relationship functioning among World War II ex-prisoners of war. *J. Fam. Psychol.* **2004**, *18*, 36–45. [CrossRef] [PubMed]
10. Dekel, R.; Solomon, Z. Marital relations among former prisoners of War: Contribution of posttraumatic stress disorder, aggression, and sexual satisfaction. *J. Fam. Psychol.* **2006**, *20*, 709–712. [CrossRef]
11. Nunnink, S.E.; Goldwaser, G.; Afari, N.; Nievergelt, C.M.; Baker, D.G. The role of emotional numbing in sexual functioning among veterans of the Iraq and Afghanistan wars. *Mil. Med.* **2010**, *175*, 424–428. [CrossRef] [PubMed]
12. Bhalla, A.; Allen, E.; Renshaw, K.; Kenny, J.; Litz, B. Emotional numbing symptoms partially mediate the association between exposure to potentially morally injurious experiences and sexual anxiety for male service members. *J. Trauma. Dissociation* **2018**, *19*, 417–430. [CrossRef] [PubMed]
13. Kotler, M.; Cohen, H.; Aizenberg, D.; Matar, M.; Loewenthal, U.; Kaplan, Z.; Miodownik, H.; Zemishlany, Z. Sexual dysfunction in male posttraumatic stress disorder patients. *Psychother Psychosom* **2000**, *69*, 309–315. [CrossRef] [PubMed]

14. Hirsch, K.A. Sexual dysfunction in male Operation Enduring Freedom/Operation Iraqi Freedom patients with severe post-traumatic stress disorder. *Mil. Med.* **2009**, *174*, 520–522. [CrossRef] [PubMed]
15. Yehuda, R.; Southwick, S.; Giller, E.L.; Ma, X.; Mason, J.W. Urinary catecholamine excretion and severity of PTSD symptoms in Vietnam combat veterans. *J. Nerv. Ment. Dis.* **1992**, *180*, 321–325. [CrossRef]
16. *American Psychiatric Association. Diagnostic and Statistical Manual of Mental Disorders: DSM-5^{TM}*, 5th ed.; American Psychiatric Publishing, Inc.: Arlington, VA, USA, 2013. [CrossRef]
17. Turchik, J.A.; Pavao, J.; Nazarian, D.; Iqbal, S.; McLean, C.; Kimerling, R. Sexually Transmitted Infections and Sexual Dysfunctions Among Newly Returned Veterans With and Without Military Sexual Trauma. *Int. J. Sex. Health* **2012**, *24*, 45–59. [CrossRef]
18. Cameron, R.P.; Mona, L.R.; Syme, M.L.; Clemency Cordes, C.; Fraley, S.S.; Chen, S.S.; Klein, L.S.; Welsh, E.; Smith, K.; Lemos, L. Sexuality among wounded veterans of Operation Enduring Freedom (OEF), Operation Iraqi Freedom (OIF), and Operation New Dawn (OND): Implications for rehabilitation psychologists. *Rehabil. Psychol.* **2011**, *56*, 289–301. [CrossRef] [PubMed]
19. Taft, C.T.; Watkins, L.E.; Stafford, J.; Street, A.E.; Monson, C.M. Posttraumatic stress disorder and intimate relationship problems: A meta-analysis. *J. Consult. Clin. Psychol.* **2011**, *79*, 22–33. [CrossRef]
20. Lambert, J.E.; Engh, R.; Hasbun, A.; Holzer, J. Impact of posttraumatic stress disorder on the relationship quality and psychological distress of intimate partners: A meta-analytic review. *J. Fam. Psychol.* **2012**, *26*, 729–737. [CrossRef]
21. Pereira, M.G.; Pereira, D.; Pedras, S. PTSD, psychological morbidity and marital dissatisfaction in colonial war veterans. *J. Ment. Health* **2019**, *19*, 1–8. [CrossRef] [PubMed]
22. Perelman, M.A. The sexual tipping point: A mind/body model for sexual medicine. *J. Sex. Med* **2009**, *6*, 629–632. [CrossRef] [PubMed]
23. Reed, G.M.; Drescher, J.; Krueger, R.B.; Atalla, E.; Cochran, S.D.; First, M.B.; Cohen-Kettenis, P.T.; Arango-de Montis, I.; Parish, S.J.; Cottler, S.; et al. Disorders related to sexuality and gender identity in the ICD-11: Revising the ICD-10 classification based on current scientific evidence, best clinical practices, and human rights considerations. *World Psychiatry* **2016**, *15*, 205–221. [CrossRef] [PubMed]
24. Montejo, A.L.; Montejo, L.; Baldwin, D.S. The impact of severe mental disorders and psychotropic medications on sexual health and its implications for clinical management. *World Psychiatry* **2018**, *17*, 3–11. [CrossRef] [PubMed]
25. Letica-Crepulja, M.; Grahovac-Juretić, T.; Katalinić, S.; Lesica, T.; Rončević-Gržeta, I.; Frančišković, T. Posttraumatic Stress Disorder and Comorbid Sexual Dysfunctions. *Psychiatr. Danub.* **2017**, *29*, 221–225. [CrossRef]
26. Antičević, V.; Britvić, D. Sexual Functioning in War Veterans with Posttraumatic Stress Disorder. *Croat. Med. J.* **2008**, *49*, 499–505. [CrossRef] [PubMed]
27. Arbanas, G. Does post-traumatic stress disorder carry a higher risk of sexual dysfunctions? *J. Sex. Med.* **2010**, *7*, 1816–1821. [CrossRef]
28. Sheehan, D.V.; Lecrubier, Y.; Harnett-Sheehan, K.; Janavs, J.; Weiller, E.; Bonara, L.I.; Keskiner, A.; Schinka, J.; Knapp, E.; Sheehan, M.F.; et al. Reliability and Validity of the MINI International Neuropsychiatric Interview (M.I.N.I.): According to the SCID-P and its reliability. *Eur. Psychiatry* **1997**, *12*, 232–241. [CrossRef]
29. Weathers, F.W.; Litz, B.T.; Keane, T.M.; Palmieri, P.A.; Marx, B.P.; Schnurr, P.P. The PTSD Checklist for DSM-5 (PCL-5). National Center for PTSD. Available online: www.ptsd.va.gov (accessed on 15 October 2018).
30. Blevins, C.A.; Weathers, F.W.; Davis, M.T.; Witte, T.K.; Domino, J.L. The Posttraumatic Stress Disorder Checklist for DSM-5 (PCL-5): Development and initial psychometric evaluation. *J. Trauma. Stress* **2015**, *28*, 489–498. [CrossRef] [PubMed]
31. Sveen, J.; Bondjers, K.; Willebrand, M. Psychometric properties of the PTSD Checklist for DSM-5: A pilot study. *Eur J Psychotraumatol* **2016**, *7*, 30165. [CrossRef] [PubMed]
32. Bovin, M.J.; Marx, B.P.; Weathers, F.W.; Gallagher, M.W.; Rodriguez, P.; Schnurr, P.P.; Keane, T.M. Psychometric properties of the PTSD Checklist for Diagnostic and Statistical Manual of Mental Disorders-Fifth Edition (PCL-5) in Veterans. *Psychol. Assess.* **2015**, *28*, 1379–1391. [CrossRef] [PubMed]
33. Wortmann, J.H.; Jordan, A.H.; Weathers, F.W.; Resick, P.A.; Dondanville, K.A.; Hall-Clark, B.; Foa, E.B.; Young-McCaughan, S.; Yarvis, J.; Hembree, E.A.; et al. Psychometric analysis of the PTSD Checklist-5 (PCL-5) among treatment-seeking military service members. *Psychol. Assess.* **2016**, *28*, 1392–1403. [CrossRef] [PubMed]

34. Rosen, R.C.; Riley, A.; Wagner, G.; Osterloh, I.H.; Kirkpatrick, J.; Mishra, A. The international index of erectile function (IIEF): A multidimensional scale for assessment of erectile dysfunction. *Urology* **1997**, *49*, 822–830. [CrossRef]
35. Rosen, R.C.; Cappelleri, J.C.; Gendrano, N. 3rd. The International Index of Erectile Function (IIEF): A state-of-the science review. *Int. J. Impot. Res.* **2002**, *14*, 226–244. [CrossRef] [PubMed]
36. Cappelleri, J.C.; Rosen, R.C.; Smith, M.D.; Mishra, A.; Osterloh, I.H. Diagnostic evaluation of the erectile function domain of the International Index of Erectile Function. *Urology* **1999**, *54*, 346–351. [CrossRef]
37. Cappelleri, J.C.; Siegel, R.L.; Osterloh, I.H.; Rosen, R.C. Relationship between patient self-assessment of erectile function and the erectile function domain of the International Index of Erectile Function. *Urology* **2000**, *56*, 477–481. [CrossRef]
38. Symonds, T.; Perelman, M.A.; Althof, S.; Giuliano, F.; Martin, M.; May, K.; Abraham, L.; Crossland, A.; Morris, M. Development and validation of a premature ejaculation diagnostic tool. *Eur. Urol.* **2007**, *52*, 565–573. [CrossRef]
39. Pakpour, A.H.; Yekaninejad, M.S.; Nikoobakht, M.R.; Burri, A.; Fridlund, B. Psychometric properties of the Iranian version of the Premature Ejaculation Diagnostic Tool. *Sex. Med.* **2014**, *2*, 31–40. [CrossRef]
40. Hendrick, S.S. A generic measure of relationship satisfaction. *J. Marriage Fam.* **1988**, *50*, 93–98. [CrossRef]
41. Hendrick, S.S. Self-disclosure and marital satisfaction. *J. Pers. Soc. Psychol.* **1981**, *40*, 1150–1159. [CrossRef]
42. WHO Collaborating Centre for Drug Statistics Methodology. *ATC Index and DDDs*; Norwegian Institute of Public Health: Oslo, Norway, 2008.
43. Peduzzi, P.; Concato, J.; Kemper, E.; Holford, T.R.; Feinstein, A.R. A simulation study of the number of events per variable in logistic regression analysis. *J. Clin. Epidemiol.* **1996**, *49*, 1373–1379. [CrossRef]
44. Elhai, J.D.; Palmieri, P.A. The factor structure of posttraumatic stress disorder: A literature update, critique of methodology, and agenda for future research. *J. Anxiety Disord.* **2011**, *25*, 849–854. [CrossRef] [PubMed]
45. Yufik, T.; Simms, L.J. A meta-analytic investigation of the structure of posttraumatic stress disorder symptoms. *J. Abnorm. Psychol.* **2010**, *119*, 764–776. [CrossRef] [PubMed]
46. King, D.W.; Leskin, G.A.; King, L.A.; Weathers, F.W. Confirmatory factor analysis of the clinician-administered PTSD Scale: Evidence for the dimensionality of posttraumatic stress disorder. *Psychol. Assess.* **1998**, *10*, 90–96. [CrossRef]
47. Armour, C.; Műllerová, J.; Elhai, J.D. A systematic literature review of PTSD's latent structure in the Diagnostic and Statistical Manual of Mental Disorders: DSM-IV to DSM-5. *Clin. Psychol. Rev.* **2016**, *44*, 60–74. [CrossRef]
48. Birkley, E.L.; Eckhardt, C.I.; Dykstra, R.E. Posttraumatic Stress Disorder Symptoms, Intimate Partner Violence, and Relationship Functioning: A Meta-Analytic Review. *J. Trauma. Stress* **2016**, *29*, 397–405. [CrossRef]
49. Byers, E.S.; MacNeil, S. Further validation of the interpersonal exchange model of sexual satisfaction. *J. Sex Marital Ther.* **2006**, *32*, 53–69. [CrossRef]
50. Sprecher, S. Sexual satisfaction in premarital relationships: Associations with satisfaction, love, commitment, and stability. *J. Sex Res.* **2002**, *39*, 190–196. [CrossRef] [PubMed]
51. Blumstein, P.; Schwartz, P. *American Couples: Money, Work, Sex*; William Morrow: New York, NY, USA, 1983.
52. Butzer, B.; Campbell, L. Adult attachment, sexual satisfaction, and relationship satisfaction: A study of married couples. *Pers. Relatsh.* **2008**, *15*, 141–154. [CrossRef]
53. Yeh, H.C.; Lorenz, F.O.; Wickrama, K.A.S.; Conger, R.D.; Elder, G.H., Jr. Relationships among sexual satisfaction, marital quality, and marital instability at midlife. *J. Fam. Psychol.* **2006**, *20*, 339–343. [CrossRef]
54. Serretti, A.; Chiesa, A. Sexual side effects of pharmacological treatment of psychiatric diseases. *Clin. Pharmacol. Ther.* **2011**, *89*, 142–147. [CrossRef]
55. National Institute for Clinical Excellence (NICE). Post-traumatic stress disorder. The management of PTSD in adults and children in primary and secondary care. National Clinical Practice Guideline number 116. Available online: https://www.nice.org.uk/guidance/ng116 (accessed on 15 January 2019).
56. US Department of Veterans Affairs. VA/DOD Clinical Practice Guideline for the Management of posttraumatic stress disorder and acute stress disorder. Available online: https://www.healthquality.va.gov/guidelines/MH/ptsd/VADoDPTSDCPGFinal012418.pdf (accessed on 10 October 2018).
57. Bernardy, N.C.; Lund, B.C.; Alexander, B.; Friedman, M.J. Prescribing trends in veterans with posttraumatic stress disorder. *J. Clin. Psychiatry* **2012**, *73*, 297–303. [CrossRef]

58. Letica-Crepulja, M.; Korkut, N.; Grahovac, T.; Curać, J.; Lehpamer, K.; Frančišković, T. Drug Utilization Trends in Patients With Posttraumatic Stress Disorder in a Postconflict Setting: Consistency With Clinical Practice Guidelines. *J. Clin. Psychiatry* **2015**, *76*, e1271–e1276. [CrossRef]
59. Angst, J. Sexual problems in healthy and depressed persons. *Int. Clin. Psychopharmacol.* **1998**, *6*, S1–S4. [CrossRef]
60. Segraves, R.T. Rapid ejaculation: A review of nosology, prevalence and treatment. *Int. J. Impot. Res.* **2006**, *18*, 24–32. [CrossRef]
61. Waldinger, M.D.; Hengeveld, M.W.; Zwinderman, A.H.; Olivier, B. Effect of SSRI antidepressants on ejaculation: A double-blind randomized placebo-controlled study with fluoxetine, fluvoxamine, paroxetine and sertraline. *J. Clin. Psychopharmacol.* **1998**, *18*, 274–281. [CrossRef] [PubMed]
62. Waldinger, M.D.; Olivier, B. Animal models of premature and retarded ejaculation. *World J. Urol.* **2005**, *23*, 115–118. [CrossRef] [PubMed]
63. Waldinger, M.D. The neurobiological approach to premature ejaculation. *J. Urol.* **2002**, *168*, 2359–2367. [CrossRef]
64. Rowland, D.; McMahon, C.G.; Abdo, C.; Chen, J.; Jannini, E.; Waldinger, M.D.; Ahn, T.Y. Disorders of Orgasm and Ejaculation in Men. *J. Sex. Med.* **2010**, *7*, 1668–1686. [CrossRef] [PubMed]
65. Foy, C.G.; Newman, J.C.; Berlowitz, D.R.; Russell, L.P.; Kimmel, P.L.; Wadley, V.G.; Thomas, H.N.; Lerner, A.J.; Riley, W.T.; SPRINT Study Research Group. Blood Pressure, Sexual Activity, and Dysfunction in Women With Hypertension: Baseline Findings From the Systolic Blood Pressure Intervention Trial (SPRINT). *J. Sex. Med.* **2016**, *13*, 1333–1346. [CrossRef] [PubMed]
66. Lunelli, R.P.; Irigoyen, M.C.; Goldmeier, S. Hypertension as a risk factor for female sexual dysfunction: Cross-sectional study. *Rev. Bras. Enferm.* **2018**, *71*, 2477–2482. [CrossRef] [PubMed]
67. Foy, C.G.; Newman, J.C.; Berlowitz, D.R.; Russell, L.P.; Kimmel, P.L.; Wadley, V.G.; Thomas, H.N.; Lerner, A.J.; Riley, W.T.; SPRINT Study Research Group. Blood Pressure, Sexual Activity, and Erectile Function in Hypertensive Men: Baseline Findings from the Systolic Blood Pressure Intervention Trial (SPRINT). *J. Sex. Med.* **2019**, *16*, 235–247. [CrossRef]
68. Javaroni, V.; Neves, M.F. Erectile Dysfunction and Hypertension: Impact on Cardiovascular Risk and Treatment. *Int. J. Hypertens* **2012**, *2012*, 627278. [CrossRef]
69. Phé, V.; Rouprêt, M. Erectile dysfunction and diabetes: A review of the current evidence-based medicine and a synthesis of the main available therapies. *Diabetes Metab.* **2012**, *38*, 1–13. [CrossRef] [PubMed]
70. Hackett, G.; Krychman, M.; Baldwin, D.; Bennett, N.; El-Zawahry, A.; Graziottin, A.; Lukasiewicz, M.; McVary, K.; Sato, Y.; Incrocci, L. Coronary Heart Disease, Diabetes, and Sexuality in Men. *J. Sex. Med.* **2016**, *13*, 887–904. [CrossRef]
71. Malavige, L.S.; Levy, J.C. Erectile dysfunction in diabetes mellitus. *J. Sex. Med.* **2009**, *6*, 1232–1247. [CrossRef] [PubMed]
72. Eriksson, M.A.; Rask, E.; Johnson, O.; Carlström, K.; Ahrén, B.; Eliasson, M.; Boman, K.; Söderberg, S. Sex-related differences in the associations between hyperleptinemia, insulin resistance and dysfibrinolysis. *Blood Coagul Fibrinolysis* **2008**, *19*, 625–632. [CrossRef]
73. Oztürk, B.; Cetinkaya, M.; Saglam, H.; Adsan, O.; Akin, O.; Memis, A. Erectile dysfunction in premature ejaculation. *Arch. Ital. Urol. Androl.* **1997**, *69*, 133–136. [PubMed]
74. Majzoub, A.; Arafa, M.; Al-Said, S.; Dabbous, Z.; Aboulsoud, S.; Khalafalla, K.; Elbardisi, H. Premature ejaculation in type II diabetes mellitus patients: Association with glycemic control. *Transl. Androl. Urol.* **2016**, *5*, 248–254. [CrossRef]
75. Pietrzak, R.H.; Goldstein, R.B.; Southwick, S.M.; Grant, B.F. Prevalence and Axis I comorbidity of full and partial posttraumatic stress disorder in the United States: Results from wave 2 of the National Epidemiologic Survey on alcohol and related conditions. *J. Anxiety Disord.* **2011**, *25*, 456–465. [CrossRef]
76. Prabhakaran, D.K.; Nisha, A.; Varghese, P.J. Prevalence and correlates of sexual dysfunction in male patients with alcohol dependence syndrome: A cross-sectional study. *Indian J. Psychiatry* **2018**, *60*, 71–77. [CrossRef]
77. Dişsiz, M.; Oskay, Ü.Y. Evaluation of sexual functions in Turkish alcohol-dependent males. *J. Sex. Med.* **2011**, *8*, 3181–3187. [CrossRef]
78. Graham, C.A.; Bancroft, J. The sexual dysfunction. In *New Oxford Textbook of Psychiatry*, 2nd ed.; Gelder, M.G., Andreasen, C.N., Lopez-Ibor, J.J., Geddes, J.R., Eds.; Oxford University Press: Oxford, UK, 2009; pp. 821–832.
79. Vijayasenan, M.E. Alcohol and sex. *N Z Med. J.* **1981**, *93*, 18–20. [PubMed]

80. Jensen, S.B. Sexual customs and dysfunction in alcoholics: Part I. *Br. J. Sex. Med.* **1979**, *6*, 29–32.
81. Arackal, B.S.; Benegal, V. Prevalence of sexual dysfunction in male subjects with alcohol dependence. *Indian J. Psychiatry* **2007**, *49*, 109–112. [CrossRef] [PubMed]
82. Dachille, G.; Lamuraglia, M.; Leone, M.; Pagliarulo, A.; Palasciano, G.; Salerno, M.T.; Ludovico, G.M. Erectile dysfunction and alcohol intake. *Urologia* **2008**, *75*, 170–176. [CrossRef] [PubMed]
83. Pandey, A.K.; Sapkota, N.; Tambi, A.; Shyangwa, P.M. Clinico-demographic profile, sexual dysfunction and readiness to change in male alcohol dependence syndrome inpatients in a tertiary hospital. *Nepal Med. Coll. J.* **2012**, *14*, 35–40. [PubMed]
84. Grover, S.; Mattoo, S.K.; Pendharkar, S.; Kandappan, V. Sexual dysfunction in patients with alcohol and opioid dependence. *Indian J. Psychol. Med.* **2014**, *36*, 355–365. [CrossRef]
85. Laumann, E.O.; Youm, Y. Racial/ethnic group differences in the prevalence of sexually transmitted diseases in the United States: A network explanation. *Sex. Transm. Dis.* **1999**, *26*, 250–261. [CrossRef] [PubMed]

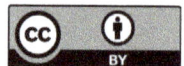

© 2019 by the authors. Licensee MDPI, Basel, Switzerland. This article is an open access article distributed under the terms and conditions of the Creative Commons Attribution (CC BY) license (http://creativecommons.org/licenses/by/4.0/).

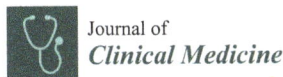

Article

Sexual Dysfunctions and Their Association with the Dual Control Model of Sexual Response in Men and Women with High-Functioning Autism

Daniel Turner [1,2,*], Peer Briken [2] and Daniel Schöttle [2,3]

1. Department of Psychiatry and Psychotherapy, University Medical Center Mainz, 55131 Mainz, Germany
2. Institute for Sex Research and Forensic Psychiatry, University Medical Center Hamburg-Eppendorf, 20246 Hamburg, Germany; briken@uke.de (P.B.); d.schoettle@uke.de (D.S.)
3. Department of Psychiatry and Psychotherapy, University Medical Center Hamburg-Eppendorf, 20246 Hamburg, Germany
* Correspondence: daniel.turner@unimedizin-mainz.de; Tel.: +49-6131-17-2920

Received: 20 February 2019; Accepted: 22 March 2019; Published: 28 March 2019

Abstract: Adults with an Autism Spectrum Disorder (ASD) are characterized by impairments in social interaction and communication, repetitive and stereotyped interests and behaviours as well as hyper- and/or hyposensitivities. These disorder specific symptoms could be associated with the development of sexual disorders. The Dual Control Model of Sexual Response presents one approach that is frequently used to explain the emergence of sexual dysfunctions. The aim of the present study was to assess the extent of symptoms of sexual dysfunctions in men and women with ASD and to evaluate their association with the individual propensity of sexual excitation and inhibition as defined by the Dual Control Model. Both men and women with ASD were more likely to report about sexual dysfunctions than individuals from the control group. In men with ASD, sexual inhibition was significantly correlated with the emergence of sexual dysfunctions, while there was no association between sexual functioning and sexual excitation. In women, the opposite pattern was found. Especially the peculiarities in sensitive perception could be responsible for the observed problems with sexual functioning in individuals with ASD. The present findings highlight the great need for specialized treatment programs addressing the frequently observed sexuality-related problems in individuals with ASD. However, up to now such treatment programs are lacking.

Keywords: sexual dysfunction; autism; erectile dysfunction; sexual satisfaction; Asperger syndrome; sexual desire; lubrication; sexual intercourse; sexual excitation; sexual inhibition

1. Introduction

Autism Spectrum Disorder (ASD) is characterized by impairments in social interaction and communication, as well as repetitive and stereotyped interests and behaviours [1]. It is estimated that up to 1.7% of the population are affected by ASD [2,3]. About 50% of individuals with ASD have average intellectual functioning and in the meantime more and more adults are being diagnosed in later life [4]. Just like in other neurodevelopmental disorders, there is a male preponderance in ASD and the male to female ratio is estimated to be around 3–4:1 [5,6]. However, these reported gender differences are currently subject of a controversial discussion and it is suggested that this effect might be largely attributable to the possible gender-biased artefact of a male-symptomatic based diagnostic system with later diagnosed females requiring heavier symptom loads for diagnosis [7].

Nevertheless, all individuals with ASD have in common that they have (in varying degrees) difficulties in interpreting non-verbal cues, such as decoding and interpreting facial expressions and have limited capabilities in theory of mind skills [1]. When throughout development social interactions become more complex and romantic and sexual relationships become increasingly important, the learned social skills often cannot keep up with the social demands needed for the initiation and maintenance of romantic peer-relationships [8]. Thus, many stereotypes around individuals with ASD concerning sexuality related issues have arisen, such as, ASD individuals are seen as being only sparsely interested in sexual and romantic relationships or as being mainly asexual [9,10]. Contrary to these stereotypes, however, in recent years a growing body of research has accumulated showing that most individuals with ASD report a general interest in solitary and dyadic sexual behaviours and show the full range of sexual behaviours, just like their clinically non-affected counterparts [11–14]. Nevertheless, the deficits in intuitively understand social and nonverbal communication cues, difficulties in perspective-taking, inflexibility, affective dysregulation, repetitive and stereotyped interests and peculiarities in sensitive perception leading to either over- or underreactions to sensory stimuli can hamper the development of romantic and sexual relationships, can be associated with impaired sexual functioning and sometimes also with the development of sexual disorders [15–17].

In a first study of our working group, focusing on paraphilias and hypersexuality in high-functioning men and women with ASD, it was found that high-functioning ASD men reported more frequently about masochistic, sexually sadistic, voyeuristic, frotteuristic and paedophilic fantasies and more frequently about frotteuristic behaviours compared to men from a control group. Furthermore, more men with ASD reported about hypersexual fantasies and behaviours than their non-affected peers. High-functioning ASD women reported more frequently about masochistic behaviours than healthy women, while no other differences occurred [18]. Men with ASD usually show a more pronounced ASD symptomatology regarding for example, repetitive behaviours or hypo- and hypersensitivities, which could be one possible explanation for the higher prevalence of hypersexual and paraphilic fantasies and behaviours in ASD men compared to ASD women [18,19]. Thereby, the more frequently observed repetitive behaviours and obsessive interests could translate into sexualized interests and behaviours, which result in a faster habituation leading the individual to seek novel sexual activities, for example, paraphilic sexual activities.

Besides paraphilic and hypersexual behaviours, the disorder-inherent deficits and symptoms could also be accompanied by sexual dysfunctions in ASD men and women. Sexual dysfunctions are disorders characterized by a clinically significant disturbance in a person's ability to respond sexually or to experience sexual pleasure [1]. Sexual dysfunctions are usually classified in accordance with the four phases of the sexual reaction cycle: disorders of sexual appetence (e.g., female sexual interest/arousal disorder), disorders of sexual desire (e.g., erectile disorder, male hypoactive sexual desire disorder), orgasm disorders (e.g., premature (early) ejaculation and delayed ejaculation, female orgasmic disorder) and sexual pain disorders. (e.g., genito-pelvic pain/penetration disorder). In the general population it is estimated that about 40% to 50% of all women report at least one sexual dysfunction throughout their lifetime, while the life-time prevalence in men is estimated to be about 20% to 40% [20–22].

Bancroft and Janssen have developed a theoretical model, which could help to explain some aspects of the emergence of sexual dysfunctions in both men and women: the Dual Control Model of Sexual Response [23]. The Dual Control Model postulates that whether or not a sexual response occurs in a particular situation depends on the interaction between an excitatory and an inhibitory neuroanatomical and neuroendocrinological network [23,24]. Individuals high in sexual inhibition and low in sexual excitation are more likely to develop sexual dysfunctions [23,25,26].

Based on these findings we aimed at assessing symptoms of sexual dysfunctions in men and women with ASD using standardized assessment scales and at evaluating the association between the individual propensity of sexual excitation and inhibition and sexual dysfunctions in both ASD individuals and healthy controls. Due to the above-stated ASD specific symptoms we hypothesized that (1.) both men and women with ASD would show more signs of sexual dysfunctions than healthy controls and (2.) that in individuals with ASD as well as in healthy controls higher sexual excitation and lower sexual inhibition scores would be related with less signs of sexual dysfunctions.

2. Materials and Methods

2.1. Participants

The present study included $n = 96$ adults with high-functioning Autism or Asperger syndrome who were compared to $n = 96$ healthy controls. In order to control for the influence of age and education on the sexual outcome measures the participants were matched concerning these variables (Table 1). All patients with ASD self-reported that they had been diagnosed by an experienced psychiatrist or psychologist. However, due to data protection regularities we did not gather any more information from the diagnosing clinicians about the diagnostic procedures. In Germany, mental disorders are usually diagnosed based on the diagnostic criteria of the International Classification of Diseases, 10th version (ICD-10) of the World Health Organization (WHO) and thus it could be assumed that all diagnoses of our study participants were made according to the ICD-10. Mean age at which patients received their ASD diagnosis was 35.7 years (SD = 9.1 years; range = 17 to 55 years). To assess the extent of autism symptoms all participants rated the German version of the Autism Spectrum Quotient-Short Form (AQ-SF) [27]. ASD patients had significantly higher scores on the AQ-SF than the healthy controls (Table 1). While all of the ASD patients scored above the proposed cut-off value of 17 points in the AQ-SF, none of the healthy controls did so. Both, the ASD individuals as well as our control participants had on average 12 years of school education suggesting that all of them had at least average intellectual functioning.

Table 1. Sociodemographic and clinical characteristics of study participants.

	ASD ($n = 96$)	HCs ($n = 96$)
Male (n, %)	56 (58.3%)	57 (59.4%)
Age (years, SD)	39.2 (9.5)	37.9 (9.7)
School education (years, SD)	11.9 (1.5)	12.4 (1.3)
AQ sum score (M, SD)	26.7 (4.9)	6.4 (3.3)
Regular use of alcohol (n, %)	21 (21.9%)	50 (52.1%) **
Regular use of illegal drugs (n, %)	7 (7.3%)	12 (12.5%)
Any psychiatric disorders other than ASD	34 (35.4%) **	0
Endocrine disorders	5 (5.2%)	0
Genital abnormalities	0	0
Regular medication intake	57 (59.4%) **	16 (16.7%)
Regular intake of psychopharmacological drugs	30 (31.3%) **	2 (2.1%)
Hormone replacement therapy	4 (4.2%)	2 (2.1%)

ASD = Autism Spectrum Disorder; HCs = Healthy Controls. Regular intake is defined as at least three times a week. ** $p \leq 0.01$.

Of the ASD patients 78.2% ($n = 75$) indicated being exclusively or predominantly heterosexual, 10.4% ($n = 10$) being exclusively or predominantly homosexual, 8.3% ($n = 8$) being equally hetero- and homosexual and 3.1% ($n = 3$) indicated having no sexual orientation. In contrast, all healthy controls (HCs) were exclusively or predominantly heterosexual. Sexual orientation was assessed using the Kinsey scale [28]. More HCs ($n = 78$, 81.3%) were currently in a relationship than individuals with ASD ($n = 27$, 28.1%; $p < 0.001$) and more HCs ($n = 96$, 100%) indicated that they had previously been in a relationship lasting more than three month than individuals with ASD ($n = 60$; 62.5%; $p < 0.001$).

The control participants consumed alcoholic beverages on a more regular basis than the ASD individuals. On the other side more individuals with an ASD reported about psychiatric comorbidities, about regular medication intake in general and intake of psychopharmacological drugs in specific.

2.2. Procedure

All information about study participants were gathered using self-report questionnaires. These could be answered at home. Individuals diagnosed with ASD were recruited via self-help groups throughout Germany and through the Autism outpatient centre at the University Medical Center Hamburg-Eppendorf, Germany. Healthy controls were recruited through advertisements at the University Medical Center Hamburg-Eppendorf, at the University Medical Center Mainz, at local shopping malls and through personal contacts of the principal investigators.

The ethical review board of the Hamburg Medical Council approved the study protocol of the present study (PV4380).

2.3. Measures

2.3.1. International Index of Erectile Function (IIEF)

The IIEF consists of 15 items and assesses the extent of sexual problems in male respondents. Thereby, sexual functioning is measured on five subscales: erectile functioning, orgasmic functioning, sexual desire, satisfaction with sexual intercourse and overall sexual satisfaction. Lower scores on each subscale represent more problems. The guidelines on the clinical application of the IIEF recommend that patients with a score below 14 out of 30 points on the erectile functioning subscale should be considered for treatment with Sildenafil [29]. Internal consistency for the total score as well as for all subscales of the original version of the IIEF was between $\alpha = 0.73$ and 0.91 [29]. In the validation study of the German version of the questionnaire internal validity of the total score was $\alpha = 0.95$, however, in contrast to the English version only a four-factorial solution was found [30]. In a follow-up study with 261 German men the original five factor structure could be replicated by confirmatory factor analysis, although a four-factor model represented an acceptable fit as well [31]. Nevertheless, in the present study we followed the original five-factor model of the questionnaire.

2.3.2. Female Sexual Function Index (FSFI)

The FSFI consists of 19 items and assesses the extent of sexual problems in women on six domains: sexual desire, sexual arousal, lubrication, orgasm, sexual satisfaction and sexual pain. Lower scores represent more problems. Internal consistency for the total score as well as for all subscales of the original version of the IIEF was above $\alpha = 0.82$ and test-retest reliabilities were between $r = 0.79$ and 0.86 for the subscales [32]. The German validation study was performed using an online sample of 1243 German women and supported the six factorial design of the original version. Internal consistencies were between $\alpha = 0.75$ and 0.95 for the total score and the scores of the subscales [33].

2.3.3. Sexual Inhibition/Sexual Excitation Scales-Short Form (SIS/SES-SF)

Based on the Dual Control Model of Sexual Response the SIS/SES-SF is a 14-item questionnaire that assesses participants' reactions in sexual situations on three subscales: one sexual excitation subscale (SES) and two sexual inhibition subscales (SIS1 and SIS2) [34]. While SIS1 measures sexual inhibition due to a threat of performance failure, SIS2 assesses sexual inhibition due to a threat of performance consequences, for example, unwanted pregnancy or sexually transmitted diseases [35]. In a first validation study of the German version of the SIS/SES-SF, internal consistencies of $\alpha = 0.82$ for SES, $\alpha = 0.60$ for SIS1 and $\alpha = 0.70$ for SIS 2 were reported [36].

3. Results

3.1. Relationship and Sexual Satisfaction

While more women from the control group viewed sexuality as an important part in their lives (HCs: 53.8% vs. ASD: 20%), no differences occurred concerning relationship and sexual satisfaction between women with ASD and women from the control group. Moreover, more female controls rated themselves as being sexually attractive (HCs: 53.8% vs. ASD: 20%).

When comparing ASD men to men from the control group, it was found that more male controls were satisfied with their current relationship (HCs: 63.8% vs. ASD: 11.1%) and sexual life (HCs: 59.6% vs. ASD: 10.7%). Furthermore, more male controls viewed themselves as being sexually attractive (HCs: 73.7% vs. ASD: 3.6%), while no differences occurred concerning the importance of sexuality.

Finally, when comparing ASD women with ASD men it was found that more ASD women were currently in a relationship (women: 46.2% vs. men: 16.1%), more ASD women were satisfied with their current relationship (women: 44.4% vs. men: 11.1%) and ASD women viewed themselves as more sexually attractive than ASD men (women: 20.0% vs. men: 3.6%). On the other side more ASD men viewed sexuality as an important part in their life (women: 20.0% vs. men: 50.0%). No differences occurred concerning sexual satisfaction.

3.2. Sexual Dysfunctions

The female controls scored significantly higher on all FSFI subscales indicating that they reported less problems with sexual desire, sexual arousal and sexual satisfaction, lubrication, orgasm quality and less sexual pain compared to the women with ASD (Table 2). The male controls also reported about significantly better overall sexual functioning than the ASD men. However, when assessing the IIEF subscales this accounted only for erectile functioning and sexual intercourse satisfaction, while no differences were found concerning orgasmic functioning and sexual desire. Furthermore, more ASD men than male controls were below the cut off for erectile functioning problems justifying the use of medication to treat these problems, however, this difference only closely approached the intended level of significance (Table 2).

Table 2. Average questionnaire sum and subscale scores compared between autism spectrum disorder (ASD) patients and healthy controls (HCs).

	ASD	HCs	t/χ^2	p
Women				
SES	10.06 (SD = 4.14)	14.6 (SD = 2.67)	3.66	0.001
SIS1	11.94 (SD = 1.80)	9.53 (SD = 1.41)	−4.23	0.0001
SIS2	14.22 (SD = 1.66)	12.71 (SD = 1.94)	−2.37	0.03
FSFI Sum score (max. 95)	38.21 (SD = 22.65)	78.67 (SD = 9.48)	10.31	0.0001
FSFI Desire (max. 10)	3.3 (SD = 1.95)	6.27 (SD = 1.53)	7.52	0.0001
FSFI Arousal (max. 20)	8.5 (SD = 6.05)	16.87 (SD = 2.42)	8.03	0.0001
FSFI Lubrication (max. 20)	10.1 (SD = 7.83)	18.33 (SD = 1.68)	6.42	0.0001
FSFI Orgasm (max. 15)	6.45 (SD = 4.97)	12.80 (SD = 2.51)	7.14	0.0001
FSFI Satisfaction (max. 15)	6.95 (SD = 3.47)	11.93 (SD = 2.46)	7.34	0.0001
FSFI Pain (max. 15)	4.25 (SD = 6.49)	12.47 (SD = 4.19)	6.67	0.0001
Men				
SES	17.5 (SD = 3.20)	13.89 (SD = 2.53)	−4.56	0.0001
SIS1	10.04 (SD = 2.25)	9.56 (SD = 1.85)	−0.86	0.40
SIS2	12.67 (SD = 2.75)	11.96 (SD = 2.46)	−0.97	0.34
IIEF sum score (max. 75)	39.96 (SD = 14.35)	55.70 (SD = 19.11)	6.89	0.0001
IIEF erectile function (max. 30)	15.54 (SD = 7.56)	23.19 (SD = 9.50)	4.73	0.0001
IIEF orgasmic function (max. 10)	8.0 (SD = 3.19)	8.3 (SD = 3.12)	0.05	0.61
IIEF sexual desire (max. 10)	6.69 (SD = 1.98)	7.07 (SD = 1.57)	1.13	0.26
IIEF intercourse satisfaction (max. 15)	2.12 (SD = 4.11)	9.52 (SD = 4.58)	9.03	0.0001
IIEF overall satisfaction (max. 10)	4.65 (SD = 1.83)	7.63 (SD = 2.36)	7.49	0.0001
Below cut off for erectile function problems (<14)	12 (21.4%)	5 (8.8%)	3.54	0.06

FSFI = Female Sexual Function Index, IIEF = International Index of Erectile Functioning.

In order to address the impact of the assessed clinical characteristics on sexual functioning in our ASD participants, we calculated two linear logistic regression analyses (one for the male ASD participants and one for the female ASD participants) with overall sexual functioning (IIEF sum score in men and FSFI sum score in women) as the outcome variable and regular alcohol or illegal drug intake, any psychiatric disorders, any endocrine disorders, genital abnormalities, regular intake of psychopharmacological agents and hormone replacement therapy as predictors. Table 3 gives an overview about the results of the logistic regression analyses showing that neither in ASD men nor in ASD women any of the additionally assessed clinical features had a significant influence on the overall sexual functioning scores.

Table 3. Linear logistic regression addressing the relationship between clinical factors and sexual dysfunctions in individuals with Autism Spectrum Disorder (ASD).

	Coefficients				
	b	SE	p	Exp(B)	95% CI
ASD Men					
Regular alcohol intake	0.01	7.14	0.96	0.37	−14.53–15.26
Regular intake of illegal drugs	0.25	11.55	0.27	13.02	−11.07–37.10
Any other psychiatric disorder	0.04	6.43	0.86	1.15	−12.25–14.56
Regular intake of drugs	0.01	6.87	0.99	0.06	−14.28–14.40
Regular intake of psychopharmacological drugs	−0.51	8.19	0.08	−15.15	−32.24–1.94
ASD Women					
Regular alcohol intake	0.1	19.51	0.79	5.21	−37.74–48.16
Regular intake of illegal drugs	0.24	25.44	0.51	17.32	−38.68–73.32
Any other psychiatric disorder	0.03	14.58	0.93	1.40	−30.70–33.50
Endocrinological disorders	−0.50	22.86	0.21	−30.30	−80.61–20.02
Regular intake of drugs	0.37	20.34	0.30	22.36	−22.40–67.13
Regular intake of psychopharmacological drugs	−0.46	16.26	0.23	−20.65	−56.43–15.13
Hormone replacement therapy	−0.08	14.88	0.81	−3.76	−36.51–28.99

3.3. Sexual Excitation and Sexual Inhibition

Table 2 also provides an overview about the SIS/SES-SF scores in ASD women and men compared to the HCs. While ASD women had significantly lower scores in sexual excitation compared to their non-ASD counterparts, ASD men had significantly higher scores on the sexual excitation subscale. Furthermore, women with ASD also had higher scores in SIS1 and SIS2, while no differences occurred between ASD men and the HCs.

3.4. Correlational Analyses

Women with ASD scoring higher on SES reported fewer overall problems with sexual functioning (Table 4). More specifically, higher SES scores were correlated with fewer problems with sexual desire, sexual arousal, lubrication and orgasm. No significant correlations were found between SIS1 and SIS2 and any of the FSFI subscales in ASD women. Comparably, in healthy women SES was also positively correlated with overall sexual functioning. Furthermore, SIS2 was negatively correlated with sexual desire and sexual arousal, meaning that those with higher SIS2 scores reported about more problems with sexual desire and sexual arousal.

In the male controls higher scores in SES were correlated with higher scores with overall sexual functioning, erectile functioning, sexual desire and overall sexual satisfaction (Table 5). In contrast, no association was found between SES and any of the IIEF subscales in ASD men, however, SIS1 and SIS2 were negatively correlated with overall sexual functioning as well as most of the IIEF subscales.

Table 4. Correlational analysis between the sexual inhibition/sexual excitation scales short form (SIS/SES) and female sexual functioning assessed with the female sexual function index (FSFI).

	FSFI Sum Score	FSFI Desire	FSFI Arousal	FSFI Lubrication	FSFI Orgasm	FSFI Satisfaction	FSFI Pain
			ASD				
SES	0.40 **	0.48 **	0.56 **	0.43 **	0.51 **	−0.16	0.11
SIS1	−0.19	−0.19	−0.27	−0.26	−0.29	0.20	−0.14
SIS2	−0.26	−0.11	−0.20	−0.20	−0.09	0.06	−0.14
			Healthy controls				
SES	0.58 **	0.50 **	0.30	0.13	0.45 **	0.64 **	0.63 **
SIS1	−0.27	−0.04	−0.13	−0.26	−0.15	−0.13	−0.26
SIS2	−0.12	−0.46 **	−0.43 **	−0.12	−0.03	−0.07	0.22

** $p < 0.01$.

Table 5. Correlational analysis between the SIS/SES and male sexual functioning assessed with the IIEF.

	IIEF Sum Score	IIEF Erectile Function	IIEF Orgasmic Function	IIEF Sexual Desire	IIEF Intercourse Satisfaction	IIEF Overall Satisfaction
			ASD			
SES	0.19	0.21	0.17	0.10	0.18	0.01
SIS1	−0.37 **	−0.40 **	−0.31 *	−0.10	−0.37 **	−0.16
SIS2	−0.34 **	−0.36 **	−0.26 *	−0.37 **	−0.34 **	−0.04
			Healthy controls			
SES	0.43 **	0.45 **	0.10	0.46 **	−0.01	0.30 *
SIS1	−0.01	−0.03	−0.23	0.06	0.14	0.07
SIS2	0.02	0.06	−0.21	−0.05	0.17	−0.03

* $p < 0.05$; ** $p < 0.01$.

4. Discussion

To our knowledge, this is the first study to explore symptoms of sexual dysfunctions using self-report scales in a cohort of women and men with high-functioning ASD in comparison with a matched control group. In line with previous research, significantly less ASD men and women were currently in a romantic relationship compared to the HCs [37,38]. As was suggested in the introduction the disorder-specific symptoms like deficits in intuitively understanding social and nonverbal communication cues, difficulties in perspective-taking, cognitive and behavioural inflexibility as well as affective dysregulation, might hamper the initiation of romantic relationships in ASD individuals. Furthermore, both men and women with ASD reported lower relationship and sexual satisfaction than the HCs [39]. Within the present study we did not evaluate whether or not the current spouse of our study participants was diagnosed with ASD as well, however, this seems to be quite important, because it was shown that having a relationship with another autistic individual leads to an improved relationship satisfaction [13]. Women with ASD often have better social learning abilities, share more common interests with their peer group, have more advanced coping strategies and show less overt restricted interests and repetitive behaviours [40,41]. Thus, their problems in initiating and maintaining a romantic relationship are often not as pronounced as in ASD men, explaining why more women with ASD than men within the present study were in a romantic relationship [42]. Although fewer men with ASD were in a relationship compared to female ASD individuals, more men reported that sexuality was an important part in their life. These unfulfilled sexual desires could indicate that overall ASD men experience more distress concerning their own sexuality than ASD women.

Concerning sexual functioning it was found that men with ASD reported more problems with erectile functioning than the HCs. However, despite the findings of previous research that men with erectile dysfunctions from the general population usually have lower SES scores than those without erectile dysfunctions, the ASD men had significantly higher scores in sexual excitation than their non-affected counterparts [23,25,26]. This quite unexpected result could be the consequence of the peculiarities in sensitive perception in ASD men. On the one side the hypersensitivities experienced by many ASD men could cause that discrete (and even non-sexual) cues could be perceived as quite intense and sexually arousing, meaning that ASD men get sexually aroused more easily. In terms of the Dual Control Model this could be translated to a higher sexual excitation (e.g., Item 1 of the SIS/SES-SF: "When a sexually attractive stranger accidentally touches me, I easily become aroused"). On the other side, as quickly as sexual arousal might arise in ASD men, it could also decline again because due to the pronounced hypersensitivity a constant and increasingly strong stimulation is necessary in order to hold sexual arousal on an adequate level. This in many cases might not be possible and thus in the long run men with ASD experience more problems with erectile functioning because of the possibly more rapidly decreasing sexual arousal during (sexual) stimulation. Supporting this line of argument, the individual propensity of sexual excitation did not correlate neither with the IIEF sum score nor with any of the IIEF subscales, suggesting that sexual excitation might refer to a different kind of behaviour in ASD men compared to healthy men. A further possible explanation could be that ASD men have difficulties in recognizing and classifying signs of excitement and therefore answered the questions regarding excitement in a different manner than the male controls. Concerning the individual propensity of sexual inhibition, no differences were found between ASD men and the male controls. Furthermore, medium to large correlations in the expected direction were found between both sexual inhibition factors and the IIEF sum score and most of the IIEF subscales in the male ASD sample. These findings indicate that just like their non-affected counterparts, ASD men with a stronger propensity of sexual inhibition due to a threat of performance failure or due to a threat of performance consequences report about more sexual dysfunctions [23,26].

Comparably to the ASD men, the ASD women also reported significantly more sexual dysfunctions across all of the FSFI domains compared to the female controls. Just like in the ASD men this could be the consequence of the peculiarities in sensitive perception. However, the significantly lower sexual excitation and significantly higher sexual inhibition scores suggest that while in men hypersensitivities might be more important in the aetiology of sexual dysfunctions, in women it might rather be hyposensitivities. Women with ASD might need more intense sexual stimulation to become and stay sexually aroused during having sex and to reach an orgasm, explaining the lower sexual excitation scores. However, the ASD women in the present study also reported more frequently about sexual pain problems, suggesting that not only hyposensitivities but also hypersensitivities could be of relevance and it could be possible that normotypical sexual intercourse is perceived as painful by some ASD women. Both women with ASD and female controls scoring higher on sexual excitation reported better sexual functioning. Comparably, previous research found that in women from the general population higher SES scores were positively correlated with a more positive attitude towards sexuality, higher overall sexual functioning, higher sexual desire, higher sexual arousal, less problems with lubrication and higher orgasm quality [36,43,44]. Although women with ASD had significantly lower sexual inhibition scores than female HCs, no association was found between sexual inhibition and sexual functioning in the ASD women. ASD women have an up to three times increased risk to be sexually victimized than non-ASD women, which could explain the higher sexual inhibition scores. It could have been expected that those individuals with an especially pronounced propensity of sexual inhibition would also show more sexual dysfunctions, however, this was obviously not the case [45].

The findings of the present study are limited because diagnoses were assessed via self-report and one cannot be sure that all participants were diagnosed by a trained psychologist or psychiatrist. Due to data protection regulations we were not allowed to contact the diagnosing clinicians in order to verify the diagnoses of our study participants. We tried to reduce false positives by using the well-established cut-off of the German version of the AQ-SF, which proved in other studies to be sufficiently sensitive and specific to assess autistic symptomatology [27]. Nevertheless, future studies should choose a more standardized assessment approach concerning the verification of clinical diagnoses, for example by conducting a clinical interview. Furthermore, all participants were recruited through ASD self-help groups or ASD outpatient care centres, indicating that their contact with the medical system was due to their symptomatology. Although we assessed comorbid psychiatric disorders in general, we did not evaluate specific disorders, such as depressive or anxiety disorders, which are highly prevalent in autistic individuals and could affect sexual well-being and functioning. Using diagnostic interviews in future studies could help to also prevent this shortcoming. Furthermore, we did not assess intellectual functioning of our participants (e.g., by assessing IQ scores), however, as our study participants had on average 12 years of school education it can be assumed that all participants possessed at least average intellectual abilities. It is possible that especially individuals with a higher interest in sexuality-related issues and perhaps also with more sexual problems, were more likely to volunteer to participate in the present study leading to a sampling bias and an overestimation of sexual problems. However, it is likely that this should have also accounted for the individuals in the control group, thereby equalizing a possible overestimation of the actual rate of sexual dysfunctions in the ASD group at least to some degree. Our results are further limited by the fact that we did not evaluate whether or not the spouses of our ASD individuals were diagnosed with ASD as well. As stated above previous research has suggested higher sexual and relationship satisfaction when both companions are diagnosed with ASD. Thus, future studies addressing sexual functioning of ASD individuals should definitely consider this point. Finally, we did not evaluate hormonal profiles of our study participants, although differences in hormone serum concentrations could have a great impact on sexual functioning as well. Future studies should therefore assess the hormonal profiles of ASD individuals in order to find out if the increased prevalence of sexual dysfunctions found in ASD individuals is due to somatic or psychiatric reasons or both. At least though we did not find any differences in the self-reported frequency of endocrine disorders, genital abnormalities or hormonal substitution treatment.

The present study has shown that a considerable number of individuals with ASD report about a general relationship and sexual dissatisfaction and about sexual dysfunctions. Furthermore, the sexual problems are probably to a large part attributable to the disorder-specific symptoms, such as impaired social and interpersonal skills, difficulties in perspective taking and theory of mind and the peculiarities in sensitive perception. This points out that there is a great need for specialized treatment programs teaching individuals with ASD how they can, despite their disorder, have a fulfilling and satisfying sexual life. Unfortunately, such treatment programs are almost non-existent up to now, at least for adults with high-functioning ASD.

Author Contributions: Conceptualization, D.T., P.B. and D.S.; methodology, D.T., P.B. and D.S.; validation, D.T., P.B. and D.S.; formal analysis, D.T.; investigation, D.T. and D.S.; resources, D.T., P.B. and D.S.; data curation, D.T. and D.S.; writing—original draft preparation, D.T.; writing—review and editing, P.B. and D.S.; supervision, P.B.; project administration, D.T. and D.S.

Acknowledgments: The present study was part of the doctoral thesis of Stefanie Schmidt, therefore we want to thank Stefanie Schmidt for her assistance in collecting the data.

Conflicts of Interest: The authors declare no conflict of interest.

References

1. American Psychiatric Association. *Diagnostic and Statistical Manual of Mental Disorders (DSM-5)*; American Psychiatric Publishing: Washington, DC, USA, 2013.
2. Elsabbagh, M.; Divan, G.; Koh, Y.; Kim, Y.S.; Kauchali, S.; Marcín, C.; Montiel-Nava, C.; Patel, V.; Paula, C.S.; Wang, C.; et al. Global prevalence of Autism and other pervasive developmental disorders. *Autism Res.* **2012**, *5*, 160–179. [CrossRef] [PubMed]
3. Baio, J.; Wiggins, L.; Christensen, D.L.; Maenner, M.J.; Daniels, J.; Warren, Z.; Kurzius-Spencer, M.; Zahorodny, W.; Robinson Rosenberg, C.; White, T.; et al. Prevalence of Autism Spectrum Disorder among children aged 8 years. *MMWR Surveill. Summ.* **2018**, *67*, 1–23. [CrossRef] [PubMed]
4. Fombonne, E. Epidemiology of pervasive developmental disorders. *Pediatr. Res.* **2009**, *65*, 591–598. [CrossRef] [PubMed]
5. Lai, M.C.; Lombardo, M.V.; Auyeung, B.; Chakrabarti, B.; Baron-Cohen, S. Sex/Gender differences and Autism: Setting the scene for future research. *J. Am. Acad. Child Adolesc. Psychiatry* **2015**, *54*, 11–24. [CrossRef] [PubMed]

6. Idring, S.; Rai, D.; Dal, H.; Dalman, C.; Sturm, H.; Zander, E.; Lee, B.K.; Serlachius, E.; Magnusson, C. Autism spectrum disorders in the Stockholm Youth Cohort: Design, prevalence and validity. *PLoS ONE* **2012**, *7*, e41280. [CrossRef]
7. Loomes, R.; Hull, L.; Mandy, W.P.L. What is the male-to-female ratio in Autism spectrum disorder? A systematic review and meta-analysis. *J. Am. Acad. Child Adolesc. Psychiatry* **2017**, *56*, 466–474. [CrossRef]
8. Seltzer, M.M.; Krauss, M.W.; Shattuck, P.T.; Orsmond, G.; Swe, A.; Lord, C. The symptoms of Autism spectrum disorders in adolescence and adulthood. *J. Autism Dev. Disord.* **2003**, *33*, 565–581. [CrossRef]
9. Koller, R. Sexuality and adolescents with Autism. *Sex. Disabil.* **2000**, *18*, 125–135. [CrossRef]
10. Konstantareas, M.M.; Lunsky, Y.J. Sociosexual knowledge, experience, attitudes and interests of individuals with autistic disorder and developmental delay. *J. Autism Dev. Disord.* **1997**, *27*, 397–413. [CrossRef]
11. Dewinter, J.; Vermeiren, R.; Vanwesenbeeck, I.; Van Nieuwenhuizen, C. Adolescent boys with autism spectrum disorder growing up: Follow-up of self-reported sexual experience. *Eur. Child Adolesc. Psychiatry* **2016**, *25*, 969–978. [CrossRef]
12. Byers, E.S.; Nichols, S.; Voyer, S.D. Challenging stereotypes: Sexual functioning of single adults with high functioning Autism spectrum disorder. *J. Autism Dev. Disord.* **2013**, *43*, 2617–2627. [CrossRef] [PubMed]
13. Strunz, S.; Schermuck, C.; Ballerstein, S.; Ahlers, C.J.; Dziobek, I.; Roepke, S. Romantic relationships and relationship satisfaction among adults with Asperger syndrome and high-functioning Autism. *J. Clin. Psychol.* **2017**, *73*, 113–125. [CrossRef] [PubMed]
14. Turner, D.; Briken, P.; Schöttle, D. Autism-spectrum disorders in adolescence and adulthood: Focus on sexuality. *Curr. Opin. Psychiatry* **2017**, *30*, 409–416. [CrossRef]
15. Stokes, M.; Kaur, A. High-functioning autism and sexuality: A parental perspective. *Autism* **2005**, *9*, 266–289. [CrossRef]
16. Howlin, P.; Mawhood, L.; Rutter, M. Autism and developmental receptive language disorder—A follow-up comparison in early adult life. II: Social, behavioural and psychiatric outcomes. *J. Child Psychol. Psychiatry* **2000**, *41*, 561–578. [CrossRef]
17. Aston, M. Asperger syndrome in the bedroom. *Sex. Relatsh. Ther.* **2012**, *27*, 73–79. [CrossRef]
18. Schöttle, D.; Briken, P.; Tüscher, O.; Turner, D. Sexuality in autism: Hypersexual and paraphilic behavior in women and men with high-functioning Autism spectrum disorder. *Dialogues Clin. Neurosci.* **2017**, *19*, 381–393. [PubMed]
19. Van Wijngaarden-Cremers, P.J.M.; van Eeten, E.; Groen, W.B.; van Deurzen, P.A.; Oosterling, I.J.; van der Gaag, R. Gender and age differences in the core triad of impairments in Autism spectrum disorders: A systematic review and meta-analysis. *J. Autism Dev. Disord.* **2014**, *44*, 627–635. [CrossRef] [PubMed]
20. McCabe, M.P.; Sharlip, I.D.; Lewis, R.; Atalla, E.; Balon, R.; Fisher, A.D.; Laumann, E.; Lee, S.W.; Segraves, R.T. Incidence and prevalence of sexual dysfunction in women and men: A consensus statement from the Fourth International Consultation on Sexual Medicine 2015. *J. Sex. Med.* **2016**, *13*, 144–152. [CrossRef]
21. Nappi, R.E.; Cucinella, L.; Martella, S.; Rossi, M.; Tiranini, L.; Martini, E. Female sexual dysfunction (FSD): Prevalence and impact on quality of life (QoL). *Maturitas* **2016**, *94*, 87–91. [CrossRef]
22. Corona, G.; Rastrelli, G.; Limoncin, E.; Sforza, A.; Jannini, E.A.; Maggi, M. Interplay between premature ejaculation and erectile dysfunction: A systematic review and meta-analysis. *J. Sex. Med.* **2015**, *12*, 2291–2300. [CrossRef]
23. Bancroft, J.; Janssen, E. The dual control model of male sexual response: A theoretical approach to centrally mediated erectile dysfunction. *Neurosci. Biobehav. Rev.* **2000**, *24*, 571–579. [CrossRef]
24. Bancroft, J.; Graham, C.; Janssen, E.; Sanders, S. The dual control model: Current status and future directions. *J. Sex. Res.* **2009**, *46*, 121–142. [CrossRef]
25. Bancroft, J.; Carnes, L.; Janssen, E.; Goodrich, D.; Long, J.S. Erectile and ejaculatory problems in gay and heterosexual men. *Arch. Sex. Behav.* **2005**, *34*, 285–297. [CrossRef] [PubMed]
26. Janssen, E.; Bancroft, J. The dual control model: The role of sexual inhibition & excitation in sexual arousal and behavior. In *The Psychophysiology of Sex*; Janssen, E., Ed.; Indiana University Press: Bloomington, IN, USA, 2007.
27. Freitag, C.M.; Retz-Junginger, P.; Retz, W.; Seitz, C.; Palmason, H.; Meyer, J.; Rösler, M.; von Gontard, A. Evaluation der deutschen Version des Autismus-Spektrum-Quotienten (AQ)—Die Kurzversion AQ-k. *Klin. Psychol. Psychother.* **2007**, *36*, 280–289. [CrossRef]

28. Kinsey, A.C.; Pomeroy, W.B.; Martin, C.E.; Sloan, S. *Sexual Behavior in the Human Male*; Indiana University Press: Bloomington, IN, USA, 1948.
29. Rosen, R.C.; Riley, A.; Wagner, G.; Osterloh, I.H.; Kirkpatrick, J.; Mishra, A. The international index of erectile function (IIEF): A multidimensional scale for assessment of erectile dysfunction. *Urology* **1997**, *49*, 822–830. [CrossRef]
30. Wiltink, J.; Hauck, E.W.; Phädayanon, M.; Weidner, W.; Beutel, M.E. Validation of the German version of the International Index of Erectile Function (IIEF) in patients with erectile dysfunction, Peyronie's disease and controls. *Int. J. Impot. Res.* **2003**, *15*, 192–197. [CrossRef] [PubMed]
31. Kriston, L.; Günzler, C.; Harms, A.; Berner, M. Confirmatory factor analysis of the German version of the International Index of Erectile Function (IIEF): A comparison of four models. *J. Sex. Med.* **2008**, *5*, 92–99. [CrossRef]
32. Rosen, R.; Brown, C.; Heiman, J.; Leiblum, S.; Meston, C.; Shabsigh, R.; Ferguson, D.; D'Agostino, R. The female sexual function index (FSfI): A multidimensional self-report instrument for the assessment of female sexual function. *J. Sex. Marital Ther.* **2000**, *26*, 191–205. [CrossRef]
33. Berner, M.M.; Kriston, L.; Zahradnik, H.P.; Härter, M.; Rohde, A. Überprüfung der Gültigkeit und Zuverlässigkeit des Deutschen Female Sexual Function Index (FSFI-d). *Geburtshilfe Frauenheilkd.* **2004**, *64*, 293–303.
34. Reid, R.C.; Garos, S.; Carpenter, B.N. Reliability, validity and psychometric development of the Hypersexual Behavior Inventory in an outpatient sample of men. *Sex. Addict. Compulsivity* **2011**, *18*, 30–51. [CrossRef]
35. Janssen, E.; Vorst, H.; Finn, P.; Bancroft, J. The Sexual Inhibition (SIS) and Sexual Excitation (SES) Scales: I. Measuring sexual inhibition and excitation proneness in men. *J. Sex. Res.* **2002**, *39*, 114–126. [CrossRef] [PubMed]
36. Velten, J.; Scholten, S.; Margraf, J. Psychometric properties of the Sexual Excitation/Sexual Inhibition Inventory for Women and Men (SESII-W/M) and the Sexual Excitation Scales/Sexual Inhibition Scales short form (SIS/SES-SF) in a population-based sample in Germany. *PLoS ONE* **2018**, *13*, e0193080. [CrossRef] [PubMed]
37. Dewinter, J.; De Graaf, H.; Begeer, S. Sexual orientation, gender identity and romantic relationships in adolescents and adults with Autism spectrum disorder. *J. Autism Dev. Disord.* **2017**, *47*, 2917–2934. [CrossRef] [PubMed]
38. Holmes, L.G.; Himle, M.B.; Strassberg, D.S. Parental romantic expectations and parent—Child sexuality communication in autism spectrum disorders. *Autism* **2016**, *20*, 687–699. [CrossRef]
39. Hannah, L.A.; Stagg, S.D. Experiences of sex education and sexual awareness in young adults with Autism spectrum disorder. *J. Autism Dev. Disord.* **2016**, *46*, 3678–3687. [CrossRef]
40. Frazier, T.W.; Georgiades, S.; Bishop, S.L.; Hardan, A.Y. Behavioral and cognitive characteristics of females and males with Autism in the Simons Simplex Collection. *J. Am. Acad. Child Adolesc. Psychiatry* **2014**, *53*, 329–340. [CrossRef]
41. Baron-Cohen, S.; Cassidy, S.; Auyeung, B.; Allison, C.; Achoukhi, M.; Robertson, S.; Pohl, A.; Lai, M.C. Attenuation of typical sex differences in 800 adults with Autism vs. 3900 controls. *PLoS ONE* **2014**, *9*, e102251. [CrossRef]
42. Byers, E.S.; Nichols, S.; Voyer, S.D.; Reilly, G. Sexual well-being of a community sample of high-functioning adults on the autism spectrum who have been in a romantic relationship. *Autism* **2013**, *17*, 418–433. [CrossRef]
43. Carpenter, D.; Janssen, E.; Graham, C.A.; Vorst, H.; Wicherts, J. Women's scores on the Sexual Inhibition/Sexual Excitation Scales (SIS/SES): Gender similarities and differences. *J. Sex. Res.* **2008**, *45*, 36–48. [CrossRef]
44. Gomes, A.L.Q.; Janssen, E.; Santos-Iglesias, P.; Pinto-Gouveia, J.; Fonseca, L.M.; Nobre, P.J. Validation of the Sexual Inhibition and Sexual Excitation Scales (SIS/SES) in Portugal: Assessing gender differences and predictors of sexual functioning. *Arch. Sex. Behav.* **2018**, *47*, 1721–1732. [CrossRef] [PubMed]
45. Brown-Lavoie, S.M.; Viecili, M.A.; Weiss, J.A. Sexual knowledge and victimization in adults with Autism spectrum disorders. *J. Autism Dev. Disord.* **2014**, *44*, 2185–2196. [CrossRef] [PubMed]

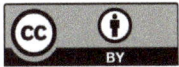

© 2019 by the authors. Licensee MDPI, Basel, Switzerland. This article is an open access article distributed under the terms and conditions of the Creative Commons Attribution (CC BY) license (http://creativecommons.org/licenses/by/4.0/).

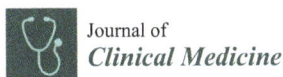

Journal of
Clinical Medicine

Article

Mental Health and Proximal Stressors in Transgender Men and Women

Noelia Fernández-Rouco [1], Rodrigo J. Carcedo [2,*], Félix López [2] and M. Begoña Orgaz [2]

1. Department of Education, Faculty of Education University of Cantabria, Av. de Los Castros s/n, 39005 Santander, Spain; fernandezrn@unican.es
2. Department of Developmental and Educational Psychology, Faculty of Psychology, University of Salamanca, Av. Merced 109-131, 37005 Salamanca, Spain; flopez@usal.es (F.L.); borgaz@usal.es (M.B.O.)
* Correspondence: rcarcedo@usal.es; Tel.: +34-92-329-4400 (ext. 5668)

Received: 1 March 2019; Accepted: 20 March 2019; Published: 25 March 2019

Abstract: This paper explores the subjective perception of some personal and interpersonal aspects of the lives of transgender people and the relationship they have with their mental health. One hundred and twenty transgender people (60 men and 60 women) participated in semi-structured interviews. Following quantitative methodology, analysis highlighted that social loneliness is the main predictor of lower levels of mental health (anxiety and depression) for both genders and recognized romantic loneliness as the strongest factor among transgender men. In both cases, higher levels of loneliness were associated with lower levels of mental health. The results have guided us to improve institutional and social responses and have provided an opportunity to promote the mental health of transgender people.

Keywords: transgender; anxiety; depression; social loneliness; romantic loneliness

1. Introduction

The mental health of transgender people is frequently disturbed in several spheres [1]. According to this, the Minority Stress Model asserts that mental health distress is often the result of a hostile or stressful social environment [2]. This model describes the processes by which sexual and gender minorities are subjected to minority stress: (a) distal or external stressors (environmental), such as exposure to discrimination and violence; (b) proximal interpersonal stressors such as feelings or expectations that external stressors will occur and the need to protect oneself from these external stressors; and (c) proximal personal stressors that reflect an internalization of negative attitudes and prejudice from society. Conversely, interactive and internalized proximal resilience is also possible, with internalization of positive self-image, use of adaptive coping skills and community attachments. Interactive and internalized proximal stressors are frequently described as distressing. The cumulative stressors can serve to overwhelm themselves and to lead to poor mental health outcomes [3].

Over the last decades, several studies have been focused on transgender people's mental health and other personal and interpersonal variables (stressors) including self-esteem and body image [4], coping skills [5], social and emotional loneliness [6], sexual satisfaction [7] or anxiety and depression [8], yet there are no studies in Spain analysing how all these topics are able to explain the state of transgender people's mental health.

This work focuses on internalized proximal stressors (self-esteem, body image and coping skills) and interpersonal ones (social and emotional loneliness and sexual satisfaction), as well as the associations occurring in transgender people's mental health (anxiety and depression). To improve the empowerment and mental health of transgender people, proximal stressors (more modifiable taking into account personal aspects) need to be identified, which would provide both transgender people and professionals the opportunity to intervene.

1.1. Mental Health: Anxiety and Depression in Transgender People

The concepts of mental health and the specific nature of the relationship between anxiety and depression have been much debated. Research from the past decades has been reviewed to assess whether there is a quantitative or qualitative difference between anxiety and depression. Anxiety and depression syndromes have been studied both separately and combined to determine whether a quantitative or qualitative difference exists between them [9]. In the end, although there are several studies supporting comorbidity between anxiety and depression [10], they are commonly perceived as different; depressed disorders are characterized by a devaluation of self and negative attitudes toward the past and future, whereas anxiety disorders are marked by themes of danger and anticipated harm [11].

Although mental health problems may be self-limiting or may respond to self-help or to lay-help [12], delaying or avoiding formal care can result in problematic consequences. Too, the duration of untreated illness is associated with worsened outcomes in mental health problems such as major depressive and anxiety disorders [13]. The stigma resulting from a context in which power is exercised to the detriment of members of a social group [14], in this case, transgender people, includes such behaviours as labelling, separation, stereotype awareness and prejudice and discrimination. This stigma, along with mental health problems, is an important factor which prevents people from seeking help [15]. Additionally, this stigma plays an important role in limiting the opportunities and access to resources of transgender people in a number of critical domains (e.g., employment, healthcare, etc.), while continuously having a detrimental effect on their mental health [16]. A large body of literature points out that transgender people experience greater mental health problems, such as depression and anxiety [17,18] than do cisgender individuals (cisgender refers to those who are not transgender). Concretely, transgender people experience greater quantities of stressors from childhood which result in an increase of mental health problems such as depression and anxiety [19]. Transgender individuals, too, face a host of minority stressors specific to their sexual and gender minority identities. Viewed from a broader perspective, stigmatized people may be more susceptible to mental health problems due to the accumulation of stressors experienced over the course of a lifetime, as opposed to simply experiencing those stressors in isolated, discrete moments [18].

In addition, many community-based surveys have found that women (with no differences between cisgender and transgender), on average, experience depressed moods more frequently than men, as measured by self-report scales [20]. Women also self-report higher levels of anxiety [21]. Too, though the range of anxiety being studied varies, findings show that transgender men experience anxiety more frequently than transgender women [8,22,23].

1.2. Proximal Stressors in Transgender People

Transgender people have been found to face multiple difficulties and interpersonal challenges [24]. Forms of rejection from family and loved ones [25], low levels of self-esteem [26] and body image problems resulting from an attempt to reject those body parts that they do not identify with [27], are all examples of such challenges. Furthermore, although the association between transgender status and sexuality is commonly taken for granted and though research exists regarding improvements in sexual functioning after transition [28] and the importance of sexual life for humans in general [29], there is no substantial evidence pointing to sexual satisfaction in this population but rather to an unsatisfactory sex life [30]. In any case, the importance of social relations is not unique to the transgender population; humans are social beings who form attachments from the moment they are born [31]. They have a fundamental, adaptive need to belong [32]. Additionally, coping skills are vital to living a successful life and to maintaining a healthy mental health state [33,34]. Coping mechanisms, therefore, have been theorized to buffer the effects of mental health problems which result from stigmatization [2].

The impact that stressors have on both physical and mental health have been summarized in previous studies [3]. This literature, however, does not take gender into account when studying transgender status, nor have previous studies looked at transgender men or women individually.

Finally, although certain stressors were studied both separately and jointly, no comprehensive studies yet exist in which proximal stressors are examined, including that of self-esteem, body image, coping skills, loneliness (social, family and romantic) and sexual satisfaction.

1.3. Associations Between Proximal Stressors and Mental Health for Transgender People

Much research exists linking different stressors to anxiety and depression. A large body of literature exists in which the relationship between self-esteem and depression is discussed. Furthermore, there is a growing body of longitudinal studies which indicate low levels of self-esteem predetermine depression; and correspondingly, people with high levels of self-esteem appear to have a lesser risk of suffering from depression [35]. In the same line, several theories postulate that a higher level of self-esteem serves as a buffer against anxiety [36]. This association was found within the transgender population as well, in relation to both anxiety and depression [37,38].

Body image is yet another factor that plays an important role in mental health [39]. Dissatisfaction with body image has been associated with an increase in mental health problems [40], a fact which holds true in the case of the transgender population [41]. The reinforcement of coping strategies, on the other hand, has proven effective in the management of issues encountered in the day to day, specifically in the prevention of problems related to mental health [42]. In fact, problem-focused coping predicted positive mental health outcomes among transgender youth [43] and the application of avoidant coping strategies during transitioning to manage gender-related stress has been associated with both depression and anxiety [8].

Interpersonal context has shown to be a major theme in the prevention or reduction of mental health problems. General loneliness was found to be an important variable for mental health [44]. Some authors have demonstrated that the emotional loneliness resulting from being cut-off from one's family is the strongest variable related to issues in mental health [45]. A large percentage of transgender individuals experience family rejection, social isolation and loneliness, which can result in a number of negative issues including mental health problems [46].

Sexuality is also a central topic for human development [47]. Specifically, there is a reciprocal relationship between certain mental problems such as anxiety and depression and sex problems [48]. Some studies in which other excluded populations were subjects, discovered that sexual satisfaction predicts positive mental health [49–52]. In terms of the transgender population, most studies which investigate sexual function are focused only on post-surgical outcomes [53].

Previous work studies the relationship that exists between different stressors and mental health but does not take into account the role that gender may play in this relationship owing to the fact that men and women are usually studied together [54], nor are the ways in which gender could affect the associations between stressors and mental health yet determined.

In summary, existing research has demonstrated that self-esteem, body image, coping skills, loneliness and sexual satisfaction are predictors of depression and anxiety. However, existing studies have not yet examined the relationships that exist between each of these variables and how gender moderates these relationships. The purpose of this study, therefore, is to examine the pattern of connections among each of these variables as they relate to transgender individuals, both transgender men and women. The current study aims to investigate (1) whether higher levels of self-esteem, body image, proactive coping skills, sexual satisfaction and lower levels of loneliness will be associated to better mental health and (2) whether differences exist between men and women.

2. Experimental Section

2.1. Participants

The sample consisted of 120 transgender people residing within Spain (93.3% Spanish and 6.7% foreigners, all from South America), 60 men (female-to-male) and 60 women (male-to-female). Participants were recruited in different cities and villages by this article's authors. Contact was made via phone call or emails sent to people in LGTB or Transgender non-profit organizations and internet forums on websites aimed at LGTB or transgender information. The age range of the sample was 18 to 63 years old (M = 33.8; S.D. = 10.1). Of the participants, 19.1% had primary studies, 15% finished secondary school, 38.3% finished professional training and 27.5% finished university. We selected participants while maintaining a balanced number of men and women in three different reassignment moments (i.e., persons who assumed gender without any hormonal or surgery treatment, persons in hormonal treatment, persons in surgery reassignment process and persons who fully reassigned their sex). After stratifying by gender and reassignment moments, they were selected under a "snowball" sampling scheme [55].

2.2. Procedure

The people who responded positively to the recruitment method were given a standard description of the study and were evaluated for their eligibility to participate which consisted of the following criteria: individuals had to identify themselves as exclusively transgender at the time of the interview, did not have any mental health problem diagnosis or current state that impede to answer accurately to an interview (e.g., schizophrenia or being under the influence of drugs, etc.), expressed a consistent desire to have reassignment surgery and were 18 years of age or older. Eligible participants who expressed an interest in participating in the study were interviewed in-person at a location of their choosing (e.g., home, cafeteria, etc.). Individuals participating in the study did so voluntarily and there were no incentives in exchange for participation. The study was conducted in Spanish.

Face to face interviews lasting about 90 min were conducted in which each participant was orally asked all the questions in order to assure that everything was fully understood, taking into account the modest educational level of a considerable percentage of participants. First author of this paper introduced herself as member of the university staff and expressed our interest in the experiences of transgender people. Only upon establishing rapport, informing participants that they were free to leave the study whenever they wished and that their participation was confidential and voluntary and explicitly obtaining informed consent, did interviews commence. Upholding these ethical standards is vital for the collection of good quality data. The Good Practice Manual for Research of CSIC (2011) was followed regarding ethical standards [56]. In addition, this study respected the norms of the Declaration of Helsinki.

2.3. Measures

2.3.1. Predictor Variables

Self-esteem. The instrument used was the Tennessee Self-Concept Scale 2nd Edition (TSCS:2) developed by Fitts and Warren as a review of Tennessee Self-Concept Scale [57,58]. The complete scale consists of 82 statements. The items are classified into three dimensions: (1) identity and self-concept: how does the individual see him/herself (30 items); (2) self-satisfaction or self-esteem: how does the individual accept him/herself (30 items); (3) self-behaviour: how does the individual behave towards him/herself (30 items). The short form is used with the first 20 questions and gives an indication of whether a person tends to see him/herself as generally positive and consistent or negative and variable. Scores from 1 (always false) to 5 (always true) are used, with higher scores reflecting higher levels of self-esteem. This instrument was chosen because it is standardized, easy to administer and has presented a good validity showing high correlations with other self-esteem scales [57]. Cronbach's alpha in this study was 0.83.

Body Image. The Body Image Scale [59] was used. A higher score indicates higher levels of dissatisfaction. On the 14-item Appraisal of Appearance Inventory (AAI), three independent observers (the diagnostician, a nurse from the gender team and the researcher) rated their subjective appraisal of the appearance of the subject on a 5-point scale of femininity/masculinity. Higher scores indicate higher levels of incompatibility with the appearance of the new gender. Cronbach's alpha in this study was 0.93.

Coping Skills. The Coping Skills Scale summarizes the dimensions described by Lazarus and Folkman [60,61]. It is a multidimensional instrument that assesses active coping, social support coping, avoidant coping cognitive passivity and repression and avoidant coping behaviour or refusal.

Certain items were eliminated from the scale for use in this study as they were not considered to be adequate indicators of the coping strategy. The scale has been adapted according to the characteristics of the participating sample and by combining the two avoidance coping subscales into one. The response format, however, was not altered: a scale from 1 (I have never faced a situation like that) to 4 (I have come into contact with a situation like that many times) was applied. An exploratory factor analysis was conducted in order to pinpoint these modifications, yielding five factors (66.95% variance explained) that ultimately were grouped into three factors to rule out the items in our sample did not indicate the use of the strategy for coping in the original scale: active coping strategy, coping strategies and social support avoidant coping strategy, which account for 60.96% of the variance.

In our study, internal consistency for the subscale of social support coping corrected (7,8,13,17) was an alpha of 0.70 for active coping subscale corrected (1,6,9,12) alpha was of 0.75 and avoidant coping subscale corrected (2,3,4,5,14) was 0.77.

Social and emotional loneliness. The short version of the Social and Emotional Loneliness Scale for Adults (SELSA-S) was used to measure both types of loneliness [45]. In fact, SELSA-S consists of three subscales labelled (a) social loneliness, (b) family-emotional loneliness and (c) romantic-emotional loneliness. Participants rated 15 items, 5 of every subscale. Items were rated on a 7-point Likert-type scale that ranged from 1 (strongly disagree) to 7 (strongly agree). The total score of every subscale was obtained by summing up the items, with possible scores ranging from 7 to 35. There is no total score for loneliness because this measure comes from a multidimensional perspective of loneliness. In this study Cronbach's alpha was 0.83 for family-emotional, 0.77 for social and 0.74 for romantic-emotional.

Sexual satisfaction. The subscale of sexual satisfaction of the Multidimensional Sexual Self-Concept Questionnaire (MSSCQ) was used to measure this aspect [7]. A total 5 of 5 items were scored on a 7-point Likert-type scale (expanding upon the original 5-point Likert-type scale) ranging from 1 (not at all characteristic of me) to 7 (very characteristic of me) comparable to a SELSA scale. Alpha was 0.96 and 0.95 in this study.

2.3.2. Moderator Variable

Gender was recorded as 0 for transgender women and 1 for transgender men.

2.3.3. Outcome Variables

The Anxiety and Depression subscales of The Symptom Checklist of Derogatis (SCL-90-R) were used to assess anxiety and depression [62]. Twenty-three items were scored, ten items for anxiety and thirteen for depression. For each item the person was asked to rate severity of depression experienced over the past week. Responses were scored on a five-point scale ranging from (1) not at all to (5) extremely. Cronbach's alpha was 0.92 for anxiety and 0.94 for depression,

For all the scales and subscales, a total score was obtained by adding up the individual scores and dividing them by the number of items answered.

2.4. Analysis Strategy

As the method of obtaining data was the interview method, no missing data was obtained; all of the participants answered every question. After data curation, statistical techniques were used to process the data using descriptive, Pearson correlations and hierarchical regression analysis with the IBM SPSS 22 package (IBM, Armonk, NY, USA). Firstly, pertinent analyses were carried out to verify the reliability, normality, independence and homoscedasticity assumptions using Cronbach's alpha, Kolmogorov-Smirnov test and Q-Q plots, the collinearity statistics (tolerance index and variance inflated factor—VIF and the Breusch-Pagan test respectively. Secondly, independent samples t-test were used to assess the statistical significance of gender differences. Thirdly, Pearson bivariate correlations were used to explore the associations between men's and women's mental health and stressors. Fourthly, hierarchical multiple linear regression analysis was used to study the moderating effect of gender on the criterion variables (anxiety and depression). Before computing these, the assumptions of the presence of normality, linearity and homoscedasticity, along with the absence of multicollinearity were tested. Predictors were entered into the first step (main effects) and interactions between gender and predictors were entered in the second step (interactions between gender and those predictor variables that showed a different association seem to have responded in a different way in relation to the gender of the participants). When an interaction is significant, two separate regression models for each level of the moderator were conducted. Alpha level of 0.05 was used. Finally, power analysis was obtained using the G*Power program [63] and heteroscedasticity between the predictor and the criterion variable was run through the macro Heteroskedasticity SPSS [64].

3. Results

The Cronbach's alpha showed a good reliability and the residual variance was constant with normality distribution.

All the predictors showed a linear relationship with anxiety and depression as it was observed in the scatterplot of the standardized residuals with the standardized predicted values. Q-Q plots and the level of significance obtained when applying the Kolmogorov-Smirnov test (up to 0.05) showed a good normality. When testing multicollinearity, the tolerance index values for the studied variables were up to 0.78 for anxiety and 0.69 for depression, which indicated the independence of the contributions of the predictor variables, producing variance inflated factor (VIF) scores lower than 10 for all the predictors. Finally, heteroscedasticity was an accomplished assumption because Breusch-Pagan (LM = 9.87; p = 0.20 for anxiety and LM = 3.05; p = 0.96 for depression) test was not found significant.

3.1. Gender Differences in Proximal and Mental Health Variables

Descriptive statistics of predictor and outcome variables are displayed in Table 1 for transgender men and women respectively. To examine whether there are mean differences based on the study variables, t-tests for independent samples were conducted. Differences in anxiety, body image, social loneliness and sexual satisfaction were found. Transgender women showed higher levels of anxiety, social loneliness and sexual satisfaction and a poorer body image.

Table 1. Descriptive statistics for men and women in predictor and outcome variables.

N = 120	Answer Range	Mean		SD		t	p
		Tr. Men	Tr. Women	Tr. Men	Tr. Women		
Anxiety	1–5	1.13	1.43	0.78	0.84	1.92	<0.05
Depression	1–5	1.65	1.89	0.94	0.98		
Body Image	1–5	2.81	3.09	0.58	0.72	2.35	<0.05
Self-esteem	1–5	3.42	3.44	0.54	0.53		
Active coping	1–4	2.74	2.79	0.48	0.48		
Soc. support coping	1–4	2.59	2.52	0.58	0.72		
Avoidant coping	1–4	2.17	2.25	0.46	0.50		
Social loneliness	1–7	3.30	3.54	1.39	1.45		
Family loneliness	1–7	3.78	3.54	1.67	1.77		
Romantic loneliness	1–7	3.82	4.39	1.55	1.39	2.13	<0.05
Sexual satisfaction	1–5	2.53	2.91	0.99	1.10	2.01	<0.05

3.2. Proximal Aspects and Mental Health for Transgender Men and Women

Bivariate correlations of interpersonal variables with anxiety and depression for both men and women, are shown in Table 2. All the stressors were associated with anxiety and depression except for the case of active and social support coping strategies which were not significantly correlated with anxiety. Similarly, high correlations were observed between anxiety and depression.

Table 2. Bivariate correlations for all the sample (men and women together).

	1.	2.	3.	4.	5.	6.	7.	8.	9.	10.	11.
1. Anxiety		0.75 *	−0.29 **	−0.22 *	−0.09	−0.06	0.29 **	0.40 **	0.48 **	0.19 *	−0.19 *
2. Depression			−0.53 **	−0.45 **	−0.26 **	−0.25 **	0.58 **	0.50 **	0.59 **	0.23 **	−0.41 **
3. Body image				0.41 **	0.18 *	0.20 *	−0.46 **	−0.43 **	−0.35 **	−0.17	0.51 **
4. Self esteem					0.51 **	0.25 **	−0.36 **	−0.57 **	−0.54 **	−0.23 **	0.33 **
5. Active cop.						0.32 **	−0.33 **	−0.35 **	−0.43 **	−0.10	0.24 **
6. Soc. supp. cop.							−0.24 **	−0.18 *	−0.27 **	0.02	−0.03
7. Avoidant cop.								0.33 **	0.39 **	0.17	−0.33 **
8. Fam. lonel.									0.69 **	0.12	−0.19 *
9. Soc. lonel.										0.31 **	−0.26 **
10. Rom. lonel.											−0.38 **
11. Sex. satisfact.											

* $p < 0.05$; ** $p < 0.01$.

To identify whether associations of stressors with anxiety and depression varied by gender, two separate bivariate correlational analyses were conducted for transgender men and women (see Table 3). Regarding the correlation between the stressors and anxiety, men showed higher associations for family loneliness, whereas women showed higher associations for body image and social loneliness. With respect to the correlations between stressors and depression, men showed higher correlations for family and social loneliness, whereas women presented higher correlations for body image and avoidant coping strategies, interestingly not showing significant correlations with loneliness. Some correlations differ for men and women: anxiety and self-esteem, body image, avoidant coping strategy and romantic loneliness, depression and active coping strategy, social support coping strategy and romantic loneliness. These variables would be entered in the regression models as interactions with gender (see Table 3).

Table 3. Bivariate correlations for men and women separately (transgender men above the diagonal and transgender women below the diagonal).

	1.	2.	3.	4.	5.	6.	7.	8.	9.	10.	11.
1. Anxiety	1	0.73 **	−0.22	−0.26 *	−0.01	−0.08	0.23	0.47 **	0.52	0.29 *	−0.22
2. Depression	0.77 **	1	−0.51 **	−0.56 **	−0.20	−0.28 *	0.52 **	0.61 **	0.69 **	0.40 **	−0.47 **
3. Body image	−0.44 **	−0.63 **	1	0.34 **	0.04	0.15	−0.33 **	−0.31 *	−0.21	−0.24	0.57 **
4. Self esteem	−0.19	−0.36 **	0.48 **	1	0.49 **	0.22	−0.36 **	−0.62 **	−0.65 **	−0.32 *	0.36 **
5. Active cop.	−0.17	−0.33**	0.29 *	0.53 **	1	0.35 **	−0.25	−0.37 **	−0.44 **	−0.01	0.12
6. Soc. supp. cop.	−0.03	−0.21	0.26 *	0.28 *	0.29 *	1	−0.31 *	−0.18	−0.19	−0.01	0.02
7. Avoidant cop.	0.34 **	0.63 **	−0.60 **	−0.37 **	−0.42 **	−0.18	1	0.24	0.40 **	0.36 **	−0.44 **
8. Fam. lonel.	0.38 **	0.43 **	−0.51 **	−0.52 **	−0.33 **	−0.20	0.43 **	1	0.71 **	0.16	−0.17
9. Soc. lonel.	0.44 **	0.49 **	−0.51 **	−0.44 **	−0.43 **	−0.32 *	0.38 **	0.69 **	1	0.41 **	−0.35 **
10. Rom. lonel.	0.03	0.01	0.20	−0.15	−0.23	0.08	−0.05	0.11	0.19	1	−0.47 **
11. Sex. satisfact.	−0.24	−0.43 **	0.44 **	0.32 *	0.36 **	−0.06	−0.26 *	−0.19	−0.23	−0.39 **	1

* $p < 0.05$; ** $p < 0.01$.

3.3. Proximal Stressors as Predictors of Mental Health (Anxiety and Depression)

To test the effects of all predictor variables on symptoms of anxiety and depression, taking into account the role of gender variable in those relationships (moderating effect), two hierarchical multiple regression analysis were conducted using the two-step model with two steps of independent variables.

Taking into account anxiety as a criterion variable, the main effects model was significant ($F (1, 118) = 36.87$, $p < 0.001$). This model accounted for 23% of the variance of anxiety. In order to the study the moderating effect of gender, the interaction of each predictor with gender was also included in a second step (i.e., self-esteem, body image, avoidant coping strategy and romantic loneliness). The interactions model produced an increment of 4% variance and romantic loneliness × gender interaction was found to be significant. Hence, the interaction effects model was selected to explain anxiety ($F (1, 117) = 7.79$, $p < 0.01$) and its observed power was 0.85. In this sense, the predictor found to be significant for both genders was social loneliness and the predictor found only for men was romantic loneliness. Therefore, higher scores in social loneliness were associated with higher levels of anxiety for transgender men and women and higher scores in romantic loneliness were associated with higher levels of anxiety only for transgender men ($F (1, 58) = 32.77$, $B = -0.78$, $p < 0.001$) (see Table 4 and Figure 1).

Regarding the regression analysis conducted to explain depression, the main effects model was also significant ($F (1, 116) = 12.15$, $p < 0.001$). This model accounted for 53% of the variance of depression. The interaction of each predictor with gender was also included in a second step (i.e., active coping strategy, social support strategy and romantic loneliness) to study the moderating effect of gender. The interactions model produced an increment of 5% variance and romantic loneliness × gender interaction was found to be significant. Hence, the interaction effects model was selected to explain depression ($F (1, 115) = 10.84$, $p < 0.001$) and its observed power was 0.99. In this sense, the predictor found to be significant for both genders was social loneliness, avoidant coping strategy and body image and the predictor found only for men was romantic loneliness. Therefore, higher scores in social loneliness, avoidant coping strategy and a poor body image was associated with higher levels of depression for transgender men and women, and higher scores in romantic loneliness explained higher levels of depression for transgender men ($F (1, 55) = 6.31$, $B = -0.49$, $p < 0.05$) (see Table 4 and Figure 1).

Table 4. Hierarchical multiple regression analysis with anxiety and depression as dependent variables.

	Anxiety							Depression					
	Model 1			Model 2				Model 1			Model 2		
Predictor Variables	(B)	SE B		(B)	SE B	95% CI (LL, UL)	Predictor Variables	(B)	SE B		(B)	SE B	95% CI (LL, UL)
Step 1: Proximal Stressors:							**Step 1: Proximal Stressors:**						
Self-esteem	0.06	0.09		0.04	0.07	(−0.05, 0.33)	Self-esteem	0.05	−0.18		−0.05	−0.03	(−0.25, 0.14)
Body image	−0.14	−0.11		−0.22	−0.19	(−0.19, 0.04)	Body image	−0.25 ***	−0.35		−0.31 ***	−0.23	(−0.24, −0.05)
Avoidant coping	0.12	0.10		0.13	0.10	(−0.36, 0.62)	Active coping	0.07	−0.02		0.01	0.02	(−0.24, 1.23)
Family loneliness	0.13	0.09		0.17	0.13	(−0.12, 0.32)	Soc. support coping	−0.03	−0.10		−0.02	−0.05	(−0.97, 0.31)
Social loneliness	0.56 ***	0.50		0.51 ***	0.45	(0.33, 0.68)	Avoidant coping	0.32 ***	0.40		0.33 ***	0.30	(0.63, 1.77)
Rom. loneliness	0.04	0.04		−0.01	−0.01	(−0.29, 0.10)	Family loneliness	0.13	0.16		0.06	0.07	(−0.14, 0.40)
Sex. satisfaction	−0.06	−0.07		−0.12	−0.13	(−0.47, 0.12)	Social loneliness	0.37 ***	0.60		0.26 ***	0.27	(0.21, 0.71)
							Rom. loneliness	0.02	0.05		−0.06	−0.12	(−0.34, 0.13)
							Sex. satisfaction	−0.11	−0.28		−0.13	−0.15	(−0.67, −0.03)
Moderator							**Moderator**						
Gender	−0.14	−0.13		0.49	0.51	(−5.80, −0.31)	Gender	−0.14	−0.07		0.39	0.33	(−6.09, −0.65)
Step 2: Interaction model:							**Step 2: Interaction model:**						
Self-esteem × Gend.				0.48	0.50	(−0.26, 0.25)	Active cop. × Gend.				0.10	0.14	(−1.9, 1.35)
Body image × Gend.				0.19	0.21	(−0.11, 0.20)	Soc. sup. cop. × Gend.				−0.20	−0.24	(−1.80, 0.68)
Avoidant cop. × Gend.				0.34	0.35	(−0.84, 1.11)	Rom. lonel × Gend.				−0.58 ***	−0.58	(−0.95, −0.20)
Rom. lonel. × Gend.				−0.46 ***	−0.22	(−0.26, −0.04)							
R^2	0.24			0.29			R^2	0.54			0.58		
ΔR^2	0.24 ***			0.05 **			ΔR^2	0.05 ***			0.04 ***		

** $p < 0.01$; *** $p < 0.001$/LL = Lower Level; UL = Upper Level.

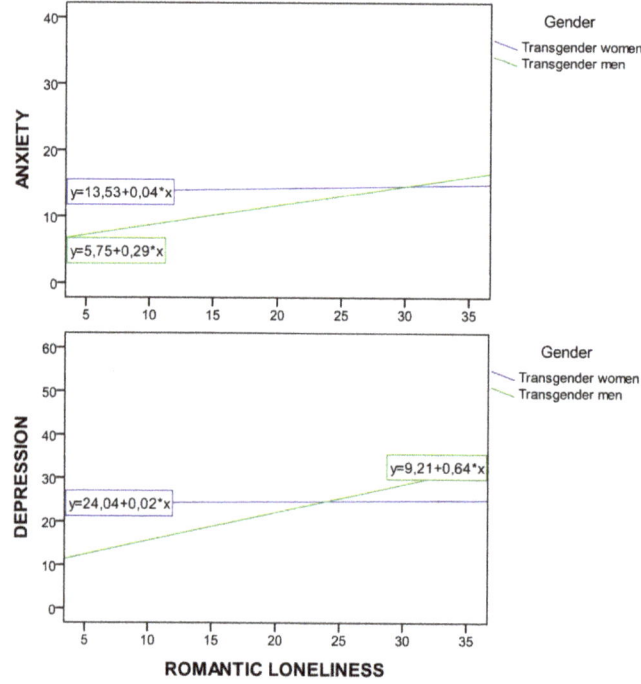

Figure 1. Romantic loneliness × gender interaction effect on mental health: (**a**) Depression; (**b**) Anxiety.

4. Discussion

The study aimed to investigate the situation and the relationship between proximal stressors and mental health capacity among transgender adults in Spain. Several significant differences were found in some stressors and in the mental health of both men and women. Specifically, transgender women were found to have higher levels of anxiety, poorer body image, higher social loneliness and higher sexual satisfaction, similar to the results found in previous literature [65,66]. Women have been particularly stigmatized because by transitioning from male to female and deviating from their expected gender role, prior social status is lost [1,67]. Perhaps women show greater sexual satisfaction due to the fact that their sexual life is a private sphere, one that is not publicly visible and, unlike other contexts such as social relationships, it is a realm in which they can experience more freedom. There is no literature on this subject but it has become a topic of special interest for future research.

On the subject of mental health, anxiety and depression typically occur simultaneously [68], a fact which holds true for transgender people as well [69], although they are commonly accepted as separate concepts [70]. Considering the association between proximal stressors and mental health, this study investigated the effects of proximal personal (self-esteem, body image and coping skills) and proximal interpersonal (social, family and romantic loneliness and sexual satisfaction) stressors on transgender men's and women's psychological health (anxiety and depression). Identifying which are the most important predictors and how to minimize them would be a useful tool for the design of future clinical and research interventions. The findings are consistent with previous research in that several proximal stressors were found to be associated with poor mental health among transgender people [8,46,71].

With respect to the ways in which these stressors are associated with poor mental health, social loneliness accounts for anxiety in both men and women, whereas romantic loneliness only accounts for it in men. Additionally, depression is accounted for by the level of social loneliness, body image and the use of avoidant coping skills in both men and women, though it is only accounted for by romantic loneliness, again, in in the case of men. Gender differences, therefore, are only significant in the case of romantic loneliness. These results substantiate previous findings regarding these variables and that of psychological health in different populations. In fact, there is empirical evidence regarding the fact that loneliness anticipates anxiety and depression [44,72–75]. There are no previous studies, however, concerning the role of gender in regard to romantic loneliness.

On the other hand, coping skills also play a role in one's mental health. The use of ineffective coping skills can either hinder or promote anxiety and depression [33]. The coping strategy of avoidance, which has shown to be ineffective in resolving complex life circumstances, causes people to experience significant levels of distress [76]. Discomfort with body and high desire of reassignment between the participants (at different levels) is common among members of our sample, related with a poor mental health [27].

For the results of our study to be accurately interpreted, certain limitations must be considered. First, the measures used in the study were all self-reported, a factor that may be associated to higher levels of response bias. Nevertheless, self-reported measures are an effective method in which to assess mental health [77]. Second, the study used a cross-sectional design which does not allow for understanding causal pathways. Nevertheless, the study contributes to our understanding of the significant association between proximal stressors and mental health, taking into account the moderating effect of gender. Third, the use of convenience sampling limits the generalizability of the findings, although it allowed us to access people in different situations. Fourth, the bidirectionality of the relationship between some of the stressors and the mental health can be considered a limitation. This issue is partially ameliorated by the fact that the outcome variables had a timeframe that was more proximal to the reporting period, whereas the independent variables had more distal timeframes, meaning that a larger body of literature exists in which proximal stressors foresee issues related to mental health. Finally, no other situations of disadvantage linked to mental health (socioeconomic status, culture, ethnicity, etc.), that could potentially have affected what was found in the analysis have been studied. Thus, in addition to transgender experience, gender was included as an important variable to be considered.

Future research should delve deeper, including looking into distal stressors and other mental health indicators. It could be interesting as well to separate those who have long-term mental health issues and those who do not. In this way, data collection and research projects are possible not only in the short-term but long-term as well, which would then allow for a more developmental perspective. Finally, qualitative research would allow for better understanding of subjective experiences in relation to stressors and mental health. All these research suggestions could be useful for a better understanding of the transgender experience.

Finally, notwithstanding the mentioned limitations and future research suggestions, the current study contributes to the literature on the subject by (1) exploring proximal personal and proximal interpersonal stressors and mental health in the transgender population, as well as differentiating between men and women; (2) highlighting the relationship between proximal stressors and mental health in this population; and (3) emphasizing the role of gender as a moderator of the relationship between stressors, specifically romantic loneliness and mental health. These contributions could lead to professional intervention which would promote the mental health of transgender people. Based on our results, interventions looking to reduce social loneliness, avoidant coping strategies, poor body image and romantic loneliness (among men) would be compelling, as would the impact each has on transgender individuals' mental health. Practitioners should to be aware the importance of relationships and the impact of loneliness on in transgender's mental health. Promoting a good relational network, both friendships and romantic partners, has always to be considered in any intervention with this population. In fact, working on social meaningful connections would buffer other feelings of loneliness, such as romantic loneliness. In this case, this seems to be especially important for transgender men in the context of romantic relationships.

Additionally, it is known that this population lives in stressful an environment due to different situations such as stigma, transphobia, and/or violence [1]. All these circumstances may promote the utilization of avoidant coping strategies in order to protect themselves from distress. However, as we have observed in this study, the use of these strategies may individuals be more prone to depression.

Finally, practitioners should focus on individuals' body image. This is an important aspect in order to prevent depression. Developing an accurate evaluation and intervention and also working on individuals' context to prevent from discrimination due to body image are important elements to be considered.

Author Contributions: Conceptualization, N.F.-R., F.L. and R.J.C.; Methodology, N.F.-R., R.J.C. and B.O.; Software, N.F.-R. and R.J.C.; Validation, N.F.-R. and R.J.C.; Formal analysis, N.F.-R., R.J.C. and B.O.; Investigation, N.F.-R.; Resources, N.F.-R. and R.J.C.; Data curation, N.F.-R.; Writing—original draft preparation, N.F.-R., R.J.C., F.L. and B.O.; writing—review and editing, N.F.-R., R.J.C., F.L. and B.O.; visualization, N.F.-R. and R.J.C.; supervision, N.F.-R.; Project administration, N.F.-R.

Conflicts of Interest: The authors declare no conflict of interest.

References

1. Fernández-Rouco, N.; Carcedo, R.J.; Yeadon-Lee, T. Transgender Identities, Pressures and Social Policy: A Study Carried Out in Spain. *J. Homosex.* **2018**, 1–19. [CrossRef]
2. Meyer, I.H. Prejudice, social stress and mental health in lesbian, gay and bisexual populations: Conceptual issues and research evidence. *Psychol. Bull.* **2003**, *129*, 674. [CrossRef]
3. Hendricks, M.L.; Testa, R.J. A conceptual framework for clinical work with transgender and gender nonconforming clients: An adaptation of the Minority Stress Model. *Prof. Psychol. Res. Pract.* **2012**, *43*, 460. [CrossRef]
4. Marone, P.; Iacoella, S.; Cecchini, M.; Rabean, A. An Experimental Study of Body Image and Perception in Gender Identity Disorders. *Int. J. Transgend.* **1998**, *2*. Available online: http://www.symposion.com/ijt/ijtvo06no01_03.htm (accessed on 15 December 2018).
5. Diener, E.; Suh, E.; Oishi, S. Recent findings on subjective Wellbeing. *Indian J. Clin. Psychol.* **1997**, *24*, 25–41.
6. Van Tilburg, T.; Havens, B.; de Jong Gierveld, J. Loneliness among older adults in the Netherlands, Italy and Canada: A multifaceted comparison. *Can. J. Aging.* **2004**, *23*, 169–180. [CrossRef] [PubMed]
7. Snell, W.E. The Multidimensional Sexual Self-Concept Questionnaire. In *Handbook of Sexuality Related Measures*; Davis, C.M., Yarber, W.L., Bauserman, R., Schreer, G., Davis, S.L., Eds.; Sage Publications: Thousand Oaks, CA, USA, 1995; pp. 521–527.
8. Budge, S.L.; Adelson, J.L.; Howard, K.A. Anxiety and depression in transgender individuals: The roles of transition status, loss, social support and coping. *J. Consult. Clin. Psychol.* **2013**, *81*, 545. [CrossRef] [PubMed]
9. Stavrakaki, C.; Vargo, B. The relationship of anxiety and depression: A review of the literature. *Br. J. Psychiatry* **1986**, *149*, 7–16. [CrossRef] [PubMed]
10. Gorman, J.M. Comorbid depression and anxiety spectrum disorders. *Depress. Anxiety* **1996**, *4*, 160–168. [CrossRef]
11. Tanaka, E.; Sakamoto, S.; Kijima, N.; Kitamura, T. Different personalities between depression and anxiety. *J. Clin. Psychol.* **1998**, *54*, 1043–1051. [CrossRef]
12. Oliver, M.I.; Pearson, N.; Coe, N.; Gunnell, D. Help-seeking behaviour in men and women with common mental health problems: Cross-sectional study. *Br. J. Psychiatry* **2005**, *186*, 297–301. [CrossRef]
13. Dell'Osso, B.; Glick, I.D.; Baldwin, D.S.; Altamura, A.C. Can long-term outcomes be improved by shortening the duration of untreated illness in psychiatric disorders: A conceptual framework. *Psychopathology* **2013**, *14*, 14–21. [CrossRef] [PubMed]
14. Link, B.; Phelan, J.C. Conceptualizing stigma. *Am. Rev. Sociol.* **2001**, *27*, 363–385. [CrossRef]
15. Clement, S.; Schauman, O.; Graham, T.; Maggioni, F.; Evans-Lacko, S.; Bezborodovs, N.; Morgan, C.; Rüsch, N.; Brown, J.S.; Thornicroft, G. What is the impact of mental health-related stigma on help-seeking? A systematic review of quantitative and qualitative studies. *Psychol. Med.* **2015**, *45*, 11–27. [CrossRef] [PubMed]
16. Hughto, J.M.W.; Reisner, S.L.; Pachankis, J.E. Transgender stigma and health: A critical review of stigma determinants, mechanisms and interventions. *Sol. Sci. Med.* **2015**, *147*, 222–231. [CrossRef]

17. Arcelus, J. Non-Suicidal Self Injury in Transsexualism: Associations with Psychological Symptoms, Victimization, Interpersonal Functioning and Perceived Social Support. *J. Sex. Med.* **2015**, *12*, 168–179.
18. Mustanski, B.; Andrews, R.; Puckett, J.A. The effects of cumulative victimization on mental health among lesbian, gay, bisexual and transgender adolescents and young adults. *Am. J. Public Health Res.* **2016**, *106*, 527–533. [CrossRef]
19. Roberts, A.L.; Rosario, M.; Slopen, N.; Calzo, J.P.; Austin, S.B. Childhood gender nonconformity, bullying victimization and depressive symptoms across adolescence and early adulthood: An 11-year longitudinal study. *J. Am. Acad. Child Adolesc. Psychiatry* **2013**, *52*, 143–152. [CrossRef]
20. Kessler, R.C. The epidemiology of depression among women. In *Women and Depression*; Keyes, C.L.M., Goodman, S.H., Eds.; Cambridge University Press: New York, NY, USA, 2006; pp. 22–37.
21. Spitzer, R.L.; Kroenke, K.; Williams, J.B.; Löwe, B. A brief measure for assessing generalized anxiety disorder: The GAD-7. *Arch. Intern. Med.* **2006**, *166*, 1092–1097. [CrossRef]
22. Clements-Nolle, C.; Marx, R.; Guzman, R.; Katz, M. HIV prevalence, risk behaviors, health care use and mental health status of transgender persons: Implications for public health intervention. *Am. J. Public Health* **2001**, *91*, 915–921.
23. Nemoto, T.; Bodeker, B.; Iwamoto, M. Social support, exposure to violence and transphobia: Correlates of depression among male-to female transgender women with a history of sex work. *Am. J. Public Health* **2011**, *101*, 1980–1988. [CrossRef]
24. Bockting, W.; Coleman, E.; Deutsch, M.B.; Guillamon, A.; Meyer, I.; Meyer, W., III; Reisner, S.; Sevelius, J.; Ettner, R. Adult development and quality of life of transgender and gender nonconforming people. *Curr. Opin. Endocrinol. Diabetes Obes.* **2016**, *23*, 188. [CrossRef] [PubMed]
25. Koken, J.A.; Bimbi, D.S.; Parsons, J.T. Experiences of familial acceptance–rejection among transwomen of color. *J. Fam. Psychol.* **2009**, *23*, 853. [CrossRef] [PubMed]
26. Erich, S.; Tittsworth, J.; Kerstein, A.S. An examination and comparison of transsexuals of color and their white counterparts regarding personal well-being and support networks. *J. GLBT Fam. Stud.* **2010**, *6*, 25–39. [CrossRef]
27. Pruzinski, T. Psychopatology of body experience: Expanded perspectives. In *Body Images: Development, Deviance and Change*; Cash, T.F., Pruzinski, T., Eds.; The Guilford Press: New York City, NY, USA, 1990; pp. 170–189.
28. White, J.M.; Reisner, S.L. A systematic review of the effects of hormone therapy on psychological functioning and quality of life in transgender individuals. *Transgend. Health* **2016**, *1*, 21–31. [CrossRef] [PubMed]
29. McClelland, S.I. Intimate justice: A critical analysis of sexual satisfaction. *Soc. Personal. Psychol. Compass* **2010**, *4*, 663–680. [CrossRef]
30. Devor, H. *FTM: Female-to-Male Transsexuals in Society*; Indiana University Press: Bloomington, IN, USA, 1997.
31. Bowlby, J. *Attachment and Loss*; Basic Books: New York, NY, USA, 1969.
32. Leary, M.R.; Tambor, E.S.; Terdal, S.K.; Downs, D.L. Self-esteem as an interpersonal monitor: The sociometer hypothesis. *J. Personal. Soc. Psychol.* **1995**, *68*, 518–530. [CrossRef]
33. Antonovsky, A. *Unraveling the Mystery of Health. How People Manage Stress and Stay Well*; Jossey-Bass: San Francisco, CA, USA, 1988.
34. McCubbin, M.A.; McCubbin, H.I. Theoretical orientations to family stress and coping. In *Treating Stress in Families*; Brunner/Mazel: Philadelphia, PA, USA, 1989; pp. 3–43.
35. Orth, U.; Robins, R.W.; Meier, L.L. Disentangling the effects of low self-esteem and stressful events on depression: Findings from three longitudinal studies. *J. Personal. Soc. Psychol.* **2009**, *97*, 307–321. [CrossRef]
36. Crocker, J.; Park, L.E. The costly pursuit of self-esteem. *Psychol. Bull.* **2004**, *130*, 392–414. [CrossRef] [PubMed]
37. Bouman, W.P.; Claes, L.; Brewin, N.; Crawford, J.R.; Millet, N.; Fernandez-Aranda, F.; Arcelus, J. Transgender and anxiety: A comparative study between transgender people and the general population. *Int. J. Transgend.* **2017**, *18*, 16–26. [CrossRef]
38. Witcomb, G.L.; Bouman, W.P.; Claes, L.; Brewin, N.; Crawford, J.R.; Arcelus, J. Levels of depression in transgender people and its predictors: Results of a large matched control study with transgender people accessing clinical services. *J. Affect. Disord.* **2018**, *235*, 308–315. [CrossRef] [PubMed]
39. Pruzinsky, T.; Cash, T.F. Integrative themes in body-image development, deviance and change. In *Body Images: Development, Deviance and Change*; Cash, T.F., Pruzinski, T., Eds.; Guilford Press: New York City, NY, USA, 1990; pp. 337–349.

40. Beiter, R.; Nash, R.; McCrady, M.; Rhoades, D.; Linscomb, M.; Clarahan, M.; Sammut, S. The prevalence and correlates of depression, anxiety and stress in a sample of college students. *J. Affect. Disord.* **2015**, *173*, 90–96. [CrossRef] [PubMed]
41. Röder, M.; Barkmann, C.; Richter-Appelt, H.; Schulte-Markwort, M.; Ravens-Sieberer, U.; Becker, I. Health-related quality of life in transgender adolescents: Associations with body image and emotional and behavioral problems. *Int. J. Transgend.* **2018**, *19*, 78–91. [CrossRef]
42. Martinsen, K.D.; Kendall, P.C.; Stark, K.; Neumer, S.P. Prevention of anxiety and depression in children: Acceptability and feasibility of the transdiagnostic EMOTION program. *Cogn. Behav. Pract.* **2016**, *23*, 1–13. [CrossRef]
43. Grossman, A.H.; D'augelli, A.R.; Frank, J.A. Aspects of psychological resilience among transgender youth. *J. LGBT Youth* **2011**, *8*, 103–115. [CrossRef]
44. Hawkley, L.C.; Burleson, M.H.; Berntson, G.G.; Cacioppo, J.T. Loneliness in everyday life: Cardiovascular activity, psychosocial context and health behaviors. *J. Personal. Soc. Psychol.* **2003**, *85*, 105–120. [CrossRef]
45. DiTommaso, E.; Brannen, C.; Best, L.A. Measurement and validity characteristics of the short version of the social and emotional loneliness scale for adults. *Educ. Psychol. Meas.* **2004**, *64*, 99–119. [CrossRef]
46. Klein, A.; Golub, S.A. Family rejection as a predictor of suicide attempts and substance misuse among transgender and gender nonconforming adults. *LGBT Health* **2016**, *3*, 193–199. [CrossRef]
47. López, F. Necesidades en la infancia y en la adolescencia. In *Respuesta Familiar, Escolar y Social*; Pirámide: Madrid, Spain, 2008.
48. Zimmer, D. Does marital therapy enhance the effectiveness of treatment for sexual dysfunction? *J. Sex Marital Ther.* **1987**, *13*, 193–209. [CrossRef]
49. Carcedo, R.J.; Perlman, D.; López, F.; Orgaz, M.B.; Toth, K.; Fernández-Rouco, N. Men and women in the same prison: Interpersonal needs and psychological health of prison inmates. *Int. J. Offender Ther. Comp. Criminol.* **2008**, *52*, 641–657. [CrossRef] [PubMed]
50. Carcedo, R.J.; Perlman, D.; Orgaz, M.B.; López, F.; Fernández-Rouco, N.; Faldowski, R.A. Heterosexual romantic relationships inside of prison: Partner status as predictor of loneliness, sexual satisfaction and quality of life. *Int. J. Offender Ther. Comp. Criminol.* **2011**, *55*, 898–924. [CrossRef] [PubMed]
51. Carcedo, R.J.; Perlman, D.; López, F.; Orgaz, M.B. Heterosexual romantic relationships, interpersonal needs and quality of life in prison. *Span. J. Psychol.* **2012**, *15*, 187–198. [CrossRef] [PubMed]
52. Carcedo, R.J.; Perlman, D.; López, F.; Orgaz, M.B.; Fernández-Rouco, N. The relationship between sexual satisfaction and psychological health of prison inmates. *Prison J.* **2015**, *95*, 43–65. [CrossRef]
53. Davis, S.A.; Meier, S. Effects of testosterone treatment and chest reconstruction surgery on mental health and sexuality in female-to-male transgender people. *Int. J. Sex Health* **2014**, *26*, 113–128. [CrossRef]
54. Timmins, L.; Rimes, K.A.; Rahman, Q. Minority stressors and psychological distress in transgender individuals. *Psychol. Sex. Orientat. Gend. Divers.* **2017**, *4*, 328. [CrossRef]
55. Goodman, L.A. Snowball sampling. *Ann. Math. Stat.* **1961**, *32*, 148–170. [CrossRef]
56. CSIC. Código de Buenas Prácticas Científicas del CSIC. Comité de Ética del CSIC. Madrid: Consejo Superior de Investigaciones Científicas. 2011. Available online: https://www.cnb.csic.es/documents/CBP_CSIC.pdf (accessed on 1 February 2019).
57. Fitts, W.; Warren, W. *Tennessee Self-Concept Scale (2ª Ed.)*; Western Psychological Services: Los Angeles, CA, USA, 1996.
58. Fitts, W.H. *The Tennessee Self-Concept Scale, Mind Over Matter*; Dept. of Mental Health: Nashivlle, TN, USA, 1964.
59. Lindgren, T.; Pauly, I. A body image scale for evaluating transsexuals. *Arch. Sex. Behav.* **1975**, *4*, 639–656. [CrossRef] [PubMed]
60. Basabe, N.; Valdoseda, M.; Páez, D. Memoria afectiva, salud, formas de afrontamiento y soporte social. In *Salud, Expresión y Represión Social de las Emociones*; Páez, D., Ed.; Promolibro: Valencia, Spain, 1993; pp. 339–377.
61. Lazarus, R.; Folkman, S. *Estrés y Procesos Cognitivos*; Martínez Roca: Barcelona, Spain, 1986.
62. Derogatis, L.R.; Lipman, R.S.; Covi, L. SCL-90: An outpatient psychiatric rating scale—Preliminary report. *Psychopharmacol. Bull.* **1973**, *9*, 13–28. [PubMed]
63. Erdfelder, E.; Faul, F.; Buchner, A. GPOWER: A general power analysis program. *Behav. Res. Methods Instrum. Comput.* **1996**, *28*, 1–11. [CrossRef]

64. Daryanto, A. Heteroskedasticity Test for SPSS (2nd Version). 2018. Available online: https://sites.google.com/site/ahmaddaryanto/scripts/Heterogeneity-test (accessed on 28 January 2018).
65. Hoffman, B.R. The interaction of drug use, sex work and HIV among transgender women. *Subst. Use Misuse* **2014**, *49*, 1049–1053. [CrossRef]
66. Sevelius, J.M.; Reznick, O.G.; Hart, S.L.; Schwarcz, S. Informing interventions: The importance of contextual factors in the prediction of sexual risk behaviors among transgender women. *AIDS Educ. Prev.* **2009**, *21*, 113–127. [CrossRef]
67. Sirin, S.R.; McCreary, D.R.; Mahalik, J.R. Differential reactions to men and women's gender role transgressions: Perceptions of social status, sexual orientation and value dissimilarity. *J. Mens. Stud.* **2004**, *12*, 119–132. [CrossRef]
68. Maser, J.D.; Cloninger, C.R. Comorbidity of anxiety and mood disorders: Introduction and overview. In *Comorbidity of Mood and Anxiety Disorders*; American Psychiatric Press: Washington, DC, USA, 1990; pp. 3–12.
69. Endler, N.S.; Macrodimitris, S.D.; Kocovski, N.L. Anxiety and Depression: Congruent, Separate or Both? *J. Appl. Biobehav. Res.* **2003**, *8*, 42–60. [CrossRef]
70. Endler, N.S.; Cox, B.J.; Parker, J.D.; Bagby, R.M. Self-reports of depression and state-trait anxiety: Evidence for differential assessment. *J. Pers. Soc. Psychol.* **1992**, *63*, 832. [CrossRef] [PubMed]
71. Meyer, I.H. Minority stress and mental health in gay men. *J. Health Soc. Behav.* **1995**, *36*, 38–56. [CrossRef] [PubMed]
72. DiTommaso, E.; Spinner, B. Social and emotional loneliness: A re-examination of Weiss' typology of loneliness. *Personal. Individ. Differ.* **1997**, *22*, 417–427. [CrossRef]
73. Nangle, D.W.; Erdley, C.A.; Newman, J.E.; Mason, C.A.; Carpenter, E.M. Popularity, friendship quantity and friendship quality: Interactive influences on children's loneliness and depression. *J. Clin. Child. Adolesc. Psychol.* **2003**, *32*, 546–555. [CrossRef]
74. Prince, M.J.; Harwood, R.H.; Blizard, R.A.; Thomas, A.; Mann, A.H. Social support deficits, loneliness and life events as risk factors for depression in old age. The Gospel Oak Project VI. *Psychol. Med.* **1997**, *27*, 323–332. [CrossRef] [PubMed]
75. Segrin, C.; Powell, H.L.; Givertz, M.; Brackin, A. Symptoms of depression, relational quality and loneliness in dating relationships. *Pers. Relatsh.* **2003**, *10*, 25–36. [CrossRef]
76. Dear, G.E.; Thomson, D.M.; Hall, G.J.; Hall, K. Self-inflicted injury and coping behaviours in prison. In *Suicide Prevention: The Global Context*; Kosky, R.J., Eshkevarky, S., Hassan, R., Goldney, R., Eds.; Plenum Press: New York, NY, USA, 1998; pp. 198–199.
77. Mustanski, B.S.; Garofalo, R.; Emerson, E.M. Mental health disorders, psychological distress and suicidality in a diverse sample of lesbian, gay, bisexual and transgender youths. *Am. J. Public Health* **2010**, *100*, 2426–2432. [CrossRef] [PubMed]

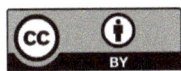

© 2019 by the authors. Licensee MDPI, Basel, Switzerland. This article is an open access article distributed under the terms and conditions of the Creative Commons Attribution (CC BY) license (http://creativecommons.org/licenses/by/4.0/).

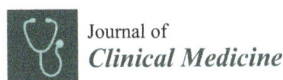

Article

Couple Relationship and Parent-Child Relationship Quality: Factors Relevant to Parent-Child Communication on Sexuality in Romania

Meda Veronica Pop * and Alina Simona Rusu *

School of Psychology and Education Sciences, Babes-Bolyai University, 400029 Cluj-Napoca, Romania
* Correspondence: medavpop@gmail.com (M.V.P.); alina.rusu@ubbcluj.ro (A.S.R.)

Received: 5 February 2019; Accepted: 14 March 2019; Published: 19 March 2019

Abstract: This study of parents in Romania explores how perceptions of their couple relationship quality and of factors associated with it (such as sexual communication anxiety and sexual perfectionism) were related to their perception of aspects describing parenting dimensions relevant to the sexual education and sexual health of their children. The hypotheses tested in this study were supported by the data collected from 106 participants (aged 25 to 51 years), parents of 1 to 3 children: (1) sexual communication anxiety with one's partner (but not sexual perfectionism) is a significant predictor for parents' self-efficacy, outcome expectancy and communication and parenting behavior related to sexuality education; (2) parents' self-efficacy and outcome expectancy about parent-child communication on sexual topics (including involvement in risky sexual behaviors) predict the level of parenting behavior in this respect; (3) parents' sexual communication anxiety (but not their sexual perfectionism) together with their self-efficacy and outcome expectancy regarding parent-child communication about sexuality predict the level of parental sexuality-communication-and-education behavior.

Keywords: sexual communication anxiety; sexual perfectionism; parent-child communication; risky sexual behavior

1. Introduction

Available data from most parts of world indicate that young people are often lacking competencies and are erroneously or partially informed about sexuality, sexual health and sexual risk behavior, and that they are the population that is at the highest risk of negative outcomes associated with sexual health, but the literature also indicates that many of these aspects could be overcome through effective sexuality education programs and interventions [1–3]. Thus, improving or optimizing sexual health in young people should and oftentimes does constitute a priority for families and care-givers, local communities, states and global society.

There is a considerable need expressed and identified for successful sexuality education programs and interventions, both formal and informal, for young people and for parents, given the costs and consequences of a lack of competencies and of risky sexual behavior in young people [4]. In line with this, identifying psychosocial factors relevant to the quality of the parent-child relationship and thus for the sexuality education and sexuality communication behavior between parents and their children is a promising line of research [5–7].

The quality of a couple's relationship and their perception of it could influence a number of aspects of the parent-child relationship [8] and vice versa [9,10]. Kouros and colleagues [11] found a positive association between daily evaluations of the emotional quality of a parent's intimate/couple relationship and that of the parent-child relationship after controlling for relationship satisfaction and conflict and for parenting levels [11]. This *spillover effect* [10–12], that is the transfer of a person's (particularly negative) affect, mood and behavior from one context to another or from one interaction to another, could be bidirectional [10,11]. The *compensation hypothesis* proposes that a compensation of negative aspects of the couple relationship might translate into a person investing parenting resources (time, attention, knowledge) and positive affect into their parent-child relationship [13]. The two models should not necessarily be mutually exclusive [11]. Studies investigating the influence that the quality of parent-child relationship might have on the parents' couple relationship or the bi-directionality of these influences have found support for both hypotheses [9,10,14].

Empirical evidence exists highlighting the (primary and secondary) effect that some parenting interventions might have on childrens' behavior, on the parent-child relationship and also on the couple relationship [9]. Also, it appears that mothers might be less vulnerable than fathers to the spillover effect from the couple relationship into the parent-child relationship [14].

Parents' concern over their communication with their children on sexuality topics is an aspect commonly addressed by parental programs and interventions (as a means or a goal) due to communication's intrinsic role in parent-child relationships [15,16]. Studies investigating parental *connectedness* [17] with its component parent-child (sexual) communication, found communication (and connectedness) to be playing a protective role against certain sexual risk behavior in which young people might engage [18,19].

Communication on sexual topics between adolescents and parents predicted adolescents' sexual communication with their partners on similar topics and for the sexually active ones it predicted the use of protection during sex (such as condoms) [20]. Although some parents express fear of the possibility that communication about sexuality might cause adolescents and young people to start their sex lives earlier or increase the chances of them engaging in particular sexual behavior, data generally does not support this association [15,19,21,22].

The majority of parents report they wish to communicate "openly" with their children on this subject [23], although data indicates that many of the adolescents perceive their communication on various sexuality issues with their parents to be less than satisfactory [22]. Generally, mothers tend to communicate more (frequently and diversely) than fathers about sexuality and more with their daughters than with their sons [24]. Also, there is a similar discrepancy with regard to parent-child sexuality communication related outcomes (e.g., sexually protective behavior) in favor of girls/daughters [15]. Widman and colleagues [15] suggest that besides other factors associated with the parent-child relationship, the quality of the parents' couple relationship might interact with the parent-child communication and with its effects on children and young people's sexual behavior [15].

The perceived self-efficacy and outcome expectancies (both in parents and in young people) about certain sexuality and sexuality education behaviors and outcomes were identified as good predictors for the level of sexually protective behavior in which young people engage and for their intentions in that sense [25–27]. Perceived self-efficacy is a person's beliefs and expectations of their capacity to successfully follow a certain behavior while outcome expectancy is the person's beliefs regarding the likelihood of a particular behavior to produce a certain outcome [28].

The sexuality (education) and sexual health of young people with intellectual or developmental disabilities has not been the subject of many research efforts thus far [29]. Significantly fewer aspects of the association between couple relationship factors and parent-child relationship factors in parents and their children with developmental problems or difficulties have been investigated. In comparison to others, these parents experience higher levels of stress and lower levels of couple relationship satisfaction [30,31].

Although the literature on the subject is not extensive, it is known that young LGBT people and their parents face various additional and specific challenges regarding sexuality education, sexual health and general well-being [32]. Research efforts in the health promotion and prevention of risk behavior in sexual and gender minorities revealed that positive parenting practices, acceptance and support from families, and communication between parents and LGBT youth were found to have protective roles for young people's health and well-being [32].

There is very little research in the area of sexual risk behavior and sexuality education with participants, young or otherwise, from Romania. Romania does not have sexuality education in the national curriculum; currently, it lacks a national strategy and has had inconsistent or partially successful public policies regarding sexual and reproductive health. Data provided by reports from various international health promotion organizations have, in recent years, placed Romania in undesired leading positions among European countries with respect to various sexual and reproductive health outcomes [33].

This study aims to explore the ways in which, for parents in Romania, the perception of their couple-relationship quality and of several factors associated with it (such as sexual communication anxiety and sexual perfectionism) is related to the perception of factors describing parenting dimensions relevant for the sexuality education of children and young people. The perception of the quality of the couple relationship was previously, in studies [34] of adult participants from Romania, associated with their perception of the quality of their sexual relationship, with their anxiety to talk about sexual issues with their partners, and with aspects of their sexual perfectionism. Sexual communication anxiety is the anxiety or fear associated with a real or anticipated communication with one's sexual partner about sexuality [35]. Perfectionism is defined as a person's constant striving to avoid mistakes (*flawlessness*), their establishing extremely high standards of performance, accompanied by a tendency to make excessively critical self-evaluations and to be preoccupied with others' negative evaluations of them [36]. Sexual perfectionism refers to the perfectionistic beliefs, standards and expectations people have for sexual performance and relationships, i.e., perfectionism related to the sexual aspects of a relationship [37,38].

Thus, the following hypotheses were tested: (1) Sexual communication anxiety and sexual perfectionism are significant predictors (individually and together) for parents' self-efficacy, outcome expectancy and communication-and-parenting behavior regarding sexuality education; (2) Parents' self-efficacy and outcome expectancy about parent-child communication on sexual topics are predictors (separately and together) of the level of parenting behavior in this respect; and (3) Parents' sexual perfectionism and sexual communication anxiety together with their self-efficacy and outcome expectancy regarding parent-child communication about sexuality predict the level of parental sexuality-communication-and-education behavior.

2. Experimental Section

The research design was non-experimental, correlational and predictive (with an exploratory component), with five variables: (1) sexual communication anxiety (SCA), (2) multidimensional sexual perfectionism (MSP), (3) parental self-efficacy about communicating with children about sexuality (SESC), (4) parental sexuality-education-and-communication behavior (SECB) and (5) parental outcome expectancy about communicating with children about sexuality (OECS).

2.1. Participants and Procedure

Data were collected online from a convenience sample ("chain" selection, [39]) of N = 106 participants from various regions in Romania between April and June 2017. The participants were aged between 25 and 51 years (M = 37.83 years, SD = 5.99). A percentage of 92.5% of them were women; 76.4% of the participants were married, 16% divorced, 5.7% were unmarried but in a relationship and 1.9% were single at that time. For participants in a relationship at that time (98.1%), the mean duration of that relationship was M = 13.48 years (SD = 7.07). The mean duration of the participants' longest relationship was 13.64 years (SD = 6.94). The mean number of participants' sexual/romantic partners up to the study time was M = 4.86 (SD = 5.11). 96.4% of the participants had university degrees. 46 (43.4%) participants were raising 1 child, 56 (52.8%) were raising 2 children and 4 participants (3.8%) were parents to 3 children. The mean age of the 170 children raised by the study participants was M = 8.34 years (SD = 5.54).

The selection was based on a single criterion: participants had to be parents (legal guardians) of at least one child (younger than 18 years) at the moment of the study. The survey was completed anonymously online on the www.esurveycreator.com platform. General research ethics prescriptions were followed, as well as the regulations on Research Ethics of Babes-Bolyai University (informed consent, confidentiality and anonymity of the data).

2.2. Instruments

(1) Multidimensional Sexual Perfectionism Questionnaire (MSPQ) [37,38] for MSP, (2) Sexual Communication Apprehension Items (SCAI) [35] for SCA; (3) Parenting and Child Sexuality Questionnaire (PCSQ) [40] for SESC and SECB; (4) and Parenting Outcome Expectancy Scale (POES) [41] for OECS. All measures were previously indicated by the literature to have had good psychometric qualities. Socio-demographic items were created for the purpose of this study (e.g., gender, educational background, professional status, relationship status, relationship lengths, number of lifetime partners, number of children, self-rated religiosity level).

Data analyses were performed with the Statistical Package for the Social Sciences (SPSS 17.0) program. Normality of score-frequency-distribution tests, correlation analyses and simple and multiple (hierarchical) linear regression analyses were conducted.

3. Results

The results (Spearman rho coefficients) of the correlation analyses on subscale scores of study measures can be seen in Table 1.

Table 1 shows significant Spearman rho correlation coefficients ($p < 0.01$, 2-tailed) of adequate values, describing the relation between global scores on OECS and PCSQ ($r_{est} = 0.628$, $p < 0.01$), on OECS and SCAI ($r_s = -0.564$, $p < 0.01$) and on PCSQ and SCAI ($r_s = -0.516$, $p < 0.01$). MSPQ global scores had no statistically significant relation with global scores on other measures in the study, although the Spearman rho correlation coefficient's value for the MSPQ and SCAI global scores almost reached statistical significance ($p = 0.06$, 2-tailed). Of particular interest are PCSQ subscales 1 and 2, which assess two different variables of the study: the OECS scores significantly positively correlate with the PCSQ1-SE scores ($r_{est} = 0.657$, $p < 0.01$) and with the PCSQ2-B scores ($r_s = 0.478$, $p < 0.01$); the SCAI global scores significantly negatively correlate with the PCSQ1-SE scores ($r_s = -0.526$, $p < 0.01$) and with the PCSQ2-B scores ($r_s = -0.391$, $p < 0.01$) (see Table 1).

Regarding sexual perfectionism and its dimensions' correlations with other variables of the study, the only statistically significant ones were between scores on: MSPQ2-PS and PCSQ1-SE ($r_{est} = -0.330$, $p < 0.01$); MSPQ3-DP and PCSQ1-SE ($r_s = -0.215$, $p < 0.05$); MSPQ5-PSD and OECS ($r_s = -0.245$, $p < 0.05$), MSPQ5-PSD and PCSQ1-SE ($r_s = -0.392$, $p < 0.01$); MSPQ5-PSD and SCAI ($r_s = 0.301$, $p < 0.01$); and MSPQ global scores and PCSQ1-SE ($r_s = -0.300$, $p < 0.01$) (see Table 1).

Simple linear regression analyses were carried out to test the predictor quality of some study variables as posited by hypotheses 1 and 2. Simple linear regression equations (df = 1 and residual df = 104) indicated that the following significant predictors were found: (1) the MSPQ5-PSD scores predicted the PCSQ1-SE scores (F = 12.557, $p < 0.01$; $R^2 = 0.108$) and SCAI global scores (F = 11.384, $p < 0.01$ $R^2 = 0.099$); (2) the SCAI global scores predicted the PCSQ1-SE scores (F = 39.982, $p < 0.01$, $R^2 = 0.278$), PCSQ2-B scores (F = 22.244, $p < 0.01$, $R^2 = 0.176$) and POES scores (F = 47.265, $p < 0.01$, $R^2 = 0.312$); (3) the POES scores predicted the PCSQ1-SE scores (F = 81.050, $p < 0.01$, $R^2 = 0.438$) and PCSQ2-B scores (F = 32.401, $p < 0.01$, $R^2 = 0.238$) and (4) the PCSQ1-SE scores predicted the PCSQ2-B scores (F = 74.308, $p < 0.01$, $R^2 = 0.417$) and POES global scores (F = 81.050, $p < 0.01$, $R^2 = 0.438$).

Table 1. Spearman bivariate correlation coefficients for study variables (and dimensions) and significance levels.

	1	2	3	4	5	6	7	8	9	10	11	12	13	14	15
1 POES total															
2 PCSQ1-SE	0.657 ** 0.000														
3 PCSQ2-B	0.478 ** 0.000	0.654 ** 0.000													
4 PCSQ3-E	0.273 ** 0.005	0.289 ** 0.003	0.389 ** 0.000												
5 PCSQ total	0.628 ** 0.000	0.925 ** 0.000	0.848 ** 0.000	0.498 ** 0.000											
6 MSPQ1-SO	0.072 0.462	−0.080 0.414	0.059 0.545	0.154 0.115	−0.019 0.849										
7 MSPQ2-SP	−0.149 0.128	−0.330 ** 0.001	−0.068 0.489	0.060 0.540	−0.217 * 0.025	0.517 ** 0.000									
8 MSPQ3-PD	−0.106 0.280	−0.215 * 0.027	−0.005 0.958	0.138 0.159	−0.117 0.231	0.713 ** 0.000	0.468 ** 0.000								
9 MSPQ4-PSO	−0.013 0.894	−0.234 * 0.016	−0.039 0.690	0.156 0.109	−0.120 0.219	0.556 ** 0.000	0.443 ** 0.000	0.568 ** 0.000							
10 MSPQ5-PSD	−0.245 * 0.011	−0.392 ** 0.000	−0.119 0.225	0.062 0.528	−0.279 ** 0.004	0.510 ** 0.000	0.596 ** 0.000	0.704 ** 0.000	0.627 ** 0.000						
11 MSPQ total	−0.103 0.291	−0.300 ** 0.002	−0.013 0.896	0.162 0.098	−0.170 0.081	0.793 ** 0.000	0.716 ** 0.000	0.852 ** 0.000	0.775 ** 0.000	0.854 ** 0.000					
12 SCAII-G	−0.547 ** 0.000	−0.509 ** 0.000	−0.402 ** 0.000	−0.277 ** 0.004	−0.507 ** 0.000	0.029 0.769	0.180 0.065	0.146 0.135	0.059 0.550	0.283 ** 0.003	0.174 0.074				

Table 1. Cont.

	1	2	3	4	5	6	7	8	9	10	11	12	13	14	15
13 SCAI2-SS	−0.437 ** 0.000	−0.475 ** 0.000	−0.287 ** 0.003	−0.219 * 0.024	−0.441 ** 0.000	0.091 0.352	0.187 0.055	0.196 * 0.045	0.141 0.150	0.341 ** 0.000	0.230 * 0.017	0.709 ** 0.000			
14 SCAI3-ND	−0.536 ** 0.000	−0.495 ** 0.000	−0.359 ** 0.000	−0.231 * 0.017	−0.483 ** 0.000	−0.058 0.553	0.173 0.077	0.089 0.367	0.001 0.996	0.249 * 0.010	0.112 0.252	0.829 ** 0.000	0.691 ** 0.000		
15 SCAI total	−0.564 ** 0.000	−0.526 ** 0.000	−0.391 ** 0.000	−0.283 ** 0.003	−0.516 ** 0.000	0.024 0.810	0.182 0.062	0.154 0.116	0.065 0.507	0.301 ** 0.002	0.183 0.060	0.983 ** 0.000	0.797 ** 0.000	0.869 ** 0.000	

** = level of significance $p < 0.01$ (2-tailed); * = level of significance $p < 0.05$ (2-tailed). Note: PCSQ subscales: PCSQ1-SE = Confidence and Comfort; PCSQ2-B = Parenting Behavior; PCSQ3-E = Sexuality Education; MSPQ subscales: MSPQ1-SO = Self-oriented sexual perfectionism; MSPQ2-SP = Socially prescribed sexual perfectionism; MSPQ3-PD = Partner-directed sexual perfectionism; MSPQ4-PSO = Partner's self-oriented sexual perfectionism; MSPQ5-PSD = Partner's self(respondent)-directed sexual perfectionism; SCAI subscales: SCAI1-G = General sexual communication anxiety; SCAI2-SS = Safer sex communication anxiety SCAI3-ND = Negative disclosure anxiety. Bolded characters indicate the category of statistical significant results.

Simple linear regression analyses were followed (when the case) by a multiple linear regression. For all regression models proposed, the data satisfactorily verified all the assumptions of a multiple regression analysis [39,42,43].

The regression equation found for the "predictors SCA and MSP-PSD and criterion SESC" model was significant: $F(2,103) = 22.821$, $p < 0.000$, with $R^2 = 0.307$. The SESC predicted level was 220.912–0.658 (SCA) −1.280 (MSP-PSD), where 220.912 was the constant's regression coefficient's value. Only SCA predicted SESC significantly at a $p < 0.01$ level, but at $p < 0.05$ both predictors were significant.

The regression equation found for the "predictors OECS and SESC and criterion SECB" model was significant: $F(2,103) = 37.782$, $p < 0.000$, with $R^2 = 0.423$. The SECB predicted level was −0.500 + 0.210 (SESC) + 0.151 (OECS), where −0.500 was the constant's regression coefficient's value. Only SESC was a significant predictor for SECB. The regression equation found for the "predictors OECS and SCA and criterion SESC" model was significant: $F(2,103) = 46.381$, $p < 0.000$, with $R^2 = 0.474$. The SESC predicted level was 1.247–0.320 (SCA) + 2.062 (OECS), where 1.247 was the constant's regression coefficient's value. Both SCA and OECS were significant predictors for SESC.

The regression equation found for the "predictors SCA and SESC and criterion SECB" model was significant: $F(2,103) = 38.144$, $p < 0.000$, cu $R^2 = 0.426$. The SECB predicted level was 15.114–0.056 (SCA) + 0.215 (SESC), where 15.114 was the constant's regression coefficient's value. Only SESC was a significant predictor for SECB.

A two-step hierarchical regression analysis was carried out to test the third hypothesis of this study. One of the distal predictors (i.e., MSP) for the SECB criterion was excluded from the analysis due to the fact that previous analyses revealed that it was not a good predictor for the dependent variable of the model. As such, the first predictor block included only SCA as an independent variable while the second regression predictor block contained SESC and OECS (see Figure 1). Tests of the model data revealed that it met the assumptions of a multiple regression analysis.

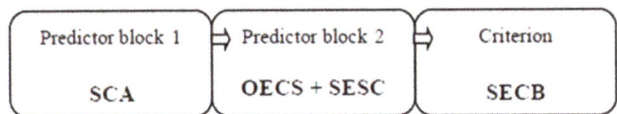

Figure 1. Hierarchical multiple regression model (Hypothesis 3 of study).

The linear hierarchical (2-step) regression analysis returned significant ($p < 0.001$) regression equations for both models (steps): *model 1* (only predictor block 1) and *model 2* (predictor blocks 1 and 2) (see Table 2).

Table 2. Parameters of the hierarchical regression models (model 1 and model 2).

Regression Model	Model Parameters					Change Parameters		
	R	R^2	R^2 Adjust.	F	p	R^2 Change	F Change	p_{Fch}
1	0.420 a	0.176	0.168	22.244	0.000 [a]	0.176	22.244	0.000
2	0.654 b	0.428	0.411	25.465	0.000 [b]	0.252	22.481	0.000

R = correlation coefficient; R^2 = determination coefficient; R^2 adjust. = adjusted determination coefficient; F = global significance of predictor; p = level of significance; [a] Predictors: (Constant), SCA; [b] Predictors: (Constant), SCA, OECS, SESC; Criterion: SECB.

For *model 1*, the regression equation was $F(1,104) = 22.244$, $p < 0.000$, with $R^2 = 0.176$. The level of the predicted SECB was 59.470–0.215 (SCA), where 59.470 was the constant's regression coefficient value. For *model 2*, the regression equation was $F(2,102) = 25.465$, $p < 0.000$, with $R^2 = 0.428$. The level of the predicted SECB was 7.573 - 0.045 (SCA) + 0.104 (OECS) + 0.201 (SESC), where 7.573 was the constant's regression coefficient value (see Table 3). Both models contributed significantly (F value is significant, $p < 0.000$) to the capacity of predicting the criterion in comparison to models with estimated population parameters [44].

Table 3. Hierarchical regression coefficients (hypothesis 3 of the study).

Regression Model		Unstandard. Coeff.		Standard. Coeff.	t	p	95% Confidence Interval for B		Correlations		
		B	SE	β			Lower Limit	Upper Limit	Zero-Order	Partial	Semi-Partial
1	(Constant)	59.470	2.655		22.399	0.000	54.205	64.735			
	SCAI total	−0.215	0.046	−0.420	−4.716	0.000	−0.305	−0.124	−0.420	−0.420	−0.420
2	(Constant)	7.573	12.881		0.588	0.558	−17.976	33.123			
	SCAI total	−0.045	0.048	−0.089	−0.950	0.344	−0.140	0.049	−0.420	−0.094	−0.071
	POES total	0.104	0.149	0.074	0.698	0.487	−0.192	0.400	0.487	0.069	0.052
	PCSQ1-SE	0.201	0.038	0.550	5.328	0.000	0.126	0.276	0.646	0.467	0.399

B = regression coefficient/slope value; SE = coefficient standard error; β = standardized coefficient value; t = significance of coefficient test statistic; p = probability significance level.

Both models explained a significant variance at the criterion level (see Table 2). *Model 1* indicated that SCA significantly ($p < 0.000$) predicted the criterion SECB, i.e., 17.6% of its variance. *Model 2* indicated that together the three predictors (SCA, OECS and SESC) significantly ($p < 0.000$) predicted the criterion SECB, i.e., 42.8% of its variance. Thus, adding the two predictors (in block 2) to the hierarchical regression brought a significant ($p < 0.000$) improvement to the prediction model ($R^2_{change} = 0.252$) of SECB. Adding OECS and SESC as predictors increased the percentage of criterion-variance prediction by 25.2% [44].

The values of the adjusted coefficient of determination (R^2 *adjust.*) for both models of the hierarchical regression analysis were very similar to those of the coefficient of determination R^2 (see Table 2), which indicates that if they were to be derived from the population and not from the study sample the two models of the hierarchical regression would explain approximately similar levels of the criterion variance. It could be thus said that the two models have a high generalizability level (Field, 2013).

Table 3 indicated that when SCA was the only independent variable in the model, it was a significant predictor for SECB ($t = -4.716$, $p < 0.000$), but once the other two predictors (OECS and SESC) were introduced in the regression analysis, SCA did not remain significant as a predictor of SECB ($t = -0.950$, $p = 0.344$). Also, OECS proved not to be a significant predictor for SECB when considered together with the other two predictors ($t = 0.698$, $p = 0.487$). In this model (i.e., 2) the only predictor that remained significant for the criterion variance was SESC ($t = 5.328$, $p < 0.000$). Thus, although the three predictors had, separately, a significant direct influence on the criterion (as shown by the results of simple regression analyses), when their interaction was taken into consideration (controlling for levels of any two of them), the only one retaining a significant direct influence on SECB in this model was SESC. SCA and OECS lost their influence in this model as direct predictors of SECB and only showed an indirect influence [44].

Based on these results a mediation model was proposed with SESC mediating the relation/path between the predictors SCA and OECS with SECB. Figure 2 describes this model. The validity of this model needs further testing in future studies.

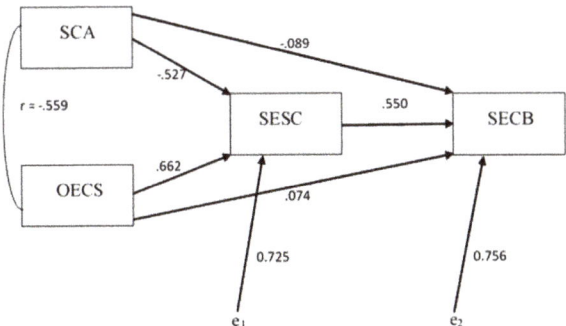

Figure 2. Mediation model of the relation between the predictors SCA, OECS and the criterion SECB by the predictor SESC.

The information offered by the parents in Romania participating in the study based on their answers to the socio-demographic data questionnaire revealed that a percentage of 94.3% (N = 100) did not consider their children to have ever been in a sexual risk situation. Only 31.13% (N = 33) of them were able to describe what in their opinion could constitute such a situation (e.g., exposure to online pornography, unprotected sex or being approached for sex by strangers, adults or older children/young people). 23.6% (n = 25) of the 106 participants reported that they had never used any type of resources to help them with the communication about sexuality and sexuality education they provided to their children; the majority of the participants, 64.2% (n = 68), mentioned books as a source of information, while 56.6% (n = 60) of them mentioned online resources and 40.6% (n = 43) of them mentioned talking to friends. Only 17.9% (n = 19) had talked to professionals while 11.3% (n = 12) had attended a specific course/training. During the 6 months prior to the study, 35 (33%) participants did not use any type of resource, 27 (25.5%) participants used them rarely, another 27 participants used them moderately frequently, while only 14 (13.2%) used them quite frequently and 3 (2.8%) used them very frequently. 17.9% (n = 19) of participants had not communicated to their children about sexuality in the 6 months prior to the study, 27.4% (n = 29) had only communicated rarely, 32.1% (n = 34) had communicated moderately frequently, 21.7% (n = 23) quite often, and 0.9% (n = 1) reported communicating very often.

Participants' self-rated level of religiosity was not a good predictor for any of the variables of the study. The number of sexual partners that participants estimated they had had by that time ($M = 4.86$, $SD = 5.109$) proved to be a moderate predictor for their level of self-efficacy regarding communication with children on sexuality topics and for their level of sexuality education parenting behavior. The majority of participants responded to the three optional open-ended questions in PCSQ [40] regarding communication about sexuality and sexuality education programs, i.e., all of the participants responded to the question "Please describe how you communicate with your child about sexuality?", more than 99% of them responded to "What would make it easier for you to talk to your child about sexuality?" and 95% responded to "What additional information or topics would you like to see included in a parenting program to help parents develop skills to support children's developing sexuality?".

The responses to the first of these questions were very diverse, although participants predominantly answered that they communicated "openly" and in a "relaxed" way, and that they had "positive" and "natural" conversations on the topic with their children, many using, as expected, the verbal approach to communication. Only seven participants stated they didn't communicate with their children about sexuality, citing mainly the child's "inappropriate" age as a reason for it. Some parents (around 25%) used the only-answer-when-asked approach, while others (also approximately 25%) mentioned they initiated conversations. Many of them stressed the anatomic and physiological aspects of development in their conversations with their children and expressed beliefs about the "age-appropriateness" of the conversations' content. One parent said "With honesty, trust and responsibility and without thinking my children are too young to know the truth. I tell them what they need to know at their age based on their cognitive development phase. I answer their questions about sexuality. We do not hide our bodies, we use the appropriate names for genitalia" while another said, "I haven't talked to my children about this subject. I don't feel prepared for such conversations. I don't have the necessary courage to talk to them."

To the second question, 13 participants responded with "I don't know", while 18 parents (17%) said schools (and also sometimes pre-schools) should provide sexuality education classes for children. Participants mostly mentioned the following means of facilitating communication with children about sexuality: being properly informed and trained; having access to various types of resources and support; changed societal and individual (their own) attitudes regarding sexuality; their children's age and perceived interest for the topic. Almost a fifth of the participants considered that the communication with their children about sexuality was good and it couldn't be improved. One parent said that "Sexuality education in schools using accurate scientific resources and leaving aside any unnecessary self-consciousness would help", while another participant responded that "It would be helpful to involve parents in having all the necessary knowledge to approach all the aspects of sexuality in a competent and relaxed way".

To the third open-ended question, approximately one third of the participants responded by saying they wouldn't add anything to a sexuality education parenting program besides the topics already mentioned in the previous item of PCSQ. Almost a quarter of the respondents considered that the parent-child relationship and communication about sexuality should be part of a parental sexuality education program, and a similar number of parents thought that such a program should include information on how to access accurate information sources for both parents and children and also information about children's and adolescents' development and about age-appropriate communication. Approximately 10% of the parents considered that information about negative consequences of sexual activity, sexually transmitted infections, protection, pregnancy and contraception, sexual orientation and gender identity, morality, religion and their relation to sexuality, should be added. A few parents mentioned that a sexuality education parenting program should also be about romantic relationships, consent, abuse, media influence and pornography. One participant said that "If we want a healthier generation, adopting older generations' models will only bring negative consequences; as such, sexuality education should be provided by professionals and with minimum involvement from dilettantes in the subject, be they well-intended parents" and another noted, "How to communicate so that we don't push them away from us and that they come and ask for advice when they need it, even in this sensitive domain. Children rarely talk to their parents about this subject".

4. Discussion

The results of the investigation on parents from Romania support the fact that participants' level of sexual communication (with their partner) anxiety predicted their level of parental outcome expectancy and self-efficacy regarding communication with children about sexuality, as well as the level of communication-with-children-about-sexuality behavior they engaged in.

With regard to the sexual perfectionism dimensions, partners' self-directed (towards respondent) sexual perfectionism was found to be a significant predictor for respondents' level of sexual communication anxiety and for their level of parental self-efficacy about discussing sexuality. Moreover, this dimension of sexual perfectionism proved to be significantly correlated with the majority of the study's variables and their dimensions, with the exception of parental communication-about-sexuality-and-sexuality-education behavior. As a result of that, sexual perfectionism was replaced by this dimension (partners' self-directed sexual perfectionism) throughout the following analyses of the study. Sexual communication anxiety and partners' self-directed sexual perfectionism together significantly predicted the level of parental self-efficacy of communication with children about sexuality, sexual communication anxiety being a mediator in their relation.

Other multiple prediction models were not tested due to the fact that partners' self-directed sexual perfectionism was not a significant predictor for the other variables. Since no prior results on this subject (hypothesis 1) were found in literature, a comparison could not be made, but theoretical models and other connected results encouraged such a hypothesis being formulated and the attempt made in this direction by this study indicated promising results.

Regarding the second hypothesis of the study, the data analysis revealed that parental self-efficacy and outcome expectancy about communicating with children on topics of sexuality were significant predictors (both separately and together) for the parental level of communication about sexuality and sexual education with the children. Parents' communication self-efficacy appeared to mediate the relation of the other two variables.

Both self-efficacy and outcome expectancy were good predictors for each other. When taking into account their interaction, only self-efficacy about communicating with children on sexuality topics remained significant in predicting the level of communication behavior between parents and children about sexuality. These results confirmed, on the one hand, the predictions of Bandura's theory of self-efficacy regarding the role that self-efficacy and outcome expectancy played in predicting the performance and intention to perform certain behaviors. On the other hand, they partially contradicted Bandura's view [28] of these processes, offering alongside other results [45] valuable insights about the possibility of a bi-causal relation existing between parental self-efficacy and outcome expectancy with regard to their communication with children on sexuality topics.

The third hypothesis of the study tested a two-step multiple prediction model for the level of parental communication-with-children-about-sexuality behavior. Sexual communication anxiety was a predictor in the first block of predictors and parental outcome expectancy and self-efficacy regarding communication with children about sexuality were in the second prediction block. The results of the model testing pointed out that only parental self-efficacy about communication with children on sexuality topics remained a significant predictor for their levels of parenting behavior in that respect. The other two predictors had only an indirect effect over the parental communication with children about sexuality. A path model describing these relations was built. These findings are among the very few results proposing a model that describes the relations between these variables (i.e., characterizing parents' perceptions of their couple relationship and of their parental relationship and parenting aspects) with an explanatory value for the variance in the levels of parents' communication-with-children-about-sexuality behavior and with implications both at a theoretical and a practical level.

From a practical point of view, these results have a potential applicability in the configuration of new or in the adjustment of already-existing family counselling interventions, as well as in educational approaches such as sexuality education programs addressed to young people and/or to their parents. Based on the explored model of prediction and mediation from this study, these interventions could target the perception of a couple's sexual relationship or of the parent-child relationship with the projected outcome of changing the sexuality-communication behavior between parents and children while also bringing other secondary benefits in the parent-child relationship and also in the couple relationship. Specifically, these benefits refer to lowering the levels of anxiety about communication on sexual topics with one's partner or the levels of one's sexual perfectionism, which in turn could contribute to the quality of one's intimate relationships. Understandably, these results, especially the ones obtained by testing exploratory hypotheses, need further investigation in future studies with the purpose of better comprehending this research area and the associations between individual characteristics, family dynamics and processes which influence the sexual health outcomes in young people.

There are some possible limitations to the conclusions drawn from the results of this study. Among them might be the characteristics of the study sample (e.g., mostly women, mostly married or in a long-term relationship, mostly holding a university degree), while others relate to the study procedure and the assessment instruments (e.g., access restricted to online participation, some of instruments translated but not validated), and others relate to the data sample. Our opinion is that these possible limitations affecting the generalizability of our conclusions could be seen as an opportunity and a basis for future studies, where their influence on the results could be additionally investigated and understood.

In conclusion, the study successfully explored and investigated how factors characterizing parents-from-Romania's perceptions of their (sexual) couple relationships and of their parent-child relationships were both relevant for their communication with their children on sexual topics. The more anxious participating parents were about communicating about sexual issues with their partner and the less confident they were about their capacity to communicate with their children about sexuality or about the effects of such a communication, the less likely they were to talk with their children about sexuality.

Author Contributions: For the elaboration of this study, the two authors contributed as follows: conceptualization, M.V.P. and A.S.R.; data collection and analysis: M.V.P., data interpretation: M.V.P. and A.S.R., supervision of the study: A.S.R., manuscript writing: M.V.P. and A.S.R.

Funding: This research received no external funding.

Conflicts of Interest: The authors declare no conflict of interest.

References

1. Hirst, J. Developing sexual competence? Exploring strategies for the provision of effective sexualities and relationships education. *Sex Educ.* **2008**, *8*, 399–413. [CrossRef]
2. United Nations Educational, Scientific and Cultural Organization (UNESCO). The Rationale for Sexuality Education. In *International Technical Guidance on Sexuality Education: An Evidence-Informed Approach for Schools, Teachers and Health Educators*; United Nations Educational, Scientific and Cultural Organization: Paris, France, 2009; Volume 1.
3. Bourke, A.; Boduszek, D.; Kelleher, C.; McBride, O.; Morgan, K. Sex education, first sex and sexual health outcomes in adulthood: Findings from a nationally representative sexual health survey. *Sex Educ.* **2014**, *14*, 299–309. [CrossRef]
4. Kirby, D. *Sex Education: Access and Impact on Sexual Behaviour of Young People*; Department of Economic and Social Affairs, United Nations Secretariat: New York, NY, USA, 2011.
5. de Graaf, H.; Vanwesenbeeck, I.; Woertman, L.; Meeus, W. Parenting and adolescents' sexual development in western societies: A literature review. *Eur. Psychol.* **2011**, *16*, 21. [CrossRef]
6. Kelleher, C.; Boduszek, D.; Bourke, A.; McBride, O.; Morgan, K. Parental involvement in sexuality education: Advancing understanding through an analysis of findings from the 2010 Irish Contraception and Crisis Pregnancy Study. *Sex Educ.* **2013**, *13*, 459–469. [CrossRef]
7. Stone, N.; Ingham, R.; Gibbins, K. 'Where do babies come from?' Barriers to early sexuality communication between parents and young children. *Sex Educ.* **2013**, *13*, 228–240. [CrossRef]
8. Morrill, M.I.; Hawrilenko, M.; Córdova, J.V. A longitudinal examination of positive parenting following an acceptance-based couple intervention. *J. Fam. Psychol.* **2016**, *30*, 104–113. [CrossRef]
9. Zemp, M.; Milek, A.; Davies, P.T.; Bodenmann, G. Improved child problem behavior enhances the parents' relationship quality: A randomized trial. *J. Fam. Psychol.* **2016**, *30*, 896–906. [CrossRef]
10. Sears, M.S.; Repetti, R.L.; Reynolds, B.M.; Robles, T.F.; Krull, J.L. Spillover in the home: The effects of family conflict on parents' behavior. *J. Marriage Fam.* **2016**, *78*, 127–141. [CrossRef]
11. Kouros, C.D.; Papp, L.M.; Goeke-Morey, M.C.; Cummings, E.M. Spillover between marital quality and parent–child relationship quality: Parental depressive symptoms as moderators. *J. Fam. Psychol.* **2014**, *28*, 315–325. [CrossRef]
12. Stroud, C.B.; Meyers, K.M.; Wilson, S.; Durbin, C.E. Marital quality spillover and young children's adjustment: Evidence for dyadic and triadic parenting as mechanisms. *J. Clin. Child Adolesc. Psychol.* **2015**, *44*, 800–813. [CrossRef]
13. Nelson, J.A.; O'Brien, M.; Blankson, A.N.; Calkins, S.D.; Keane, S.P. Family stress and parental responses to children's negative emotions: Tests of the spillover, crossover, and compensatory hypotheses. *J. Fam. Psychol.* **2009**, *23*, 671–679. [CrossRef]
14. Khajehei, M. Parenting challenges and parents' intimate relationships. *J. Hum. Behav. Soc. Environ.* **2015**, *26*, 447–451. [CrossRef]

15. Widman, L.; Choukas-Bradley, S.; Noar, S.M.; Nesi, J.; Garrett, K. Parent-adolescent sexual communication and adolescent safer sex behavior: A meta-analysis. *JAMA Pediatr.* **2016**, *170*, 52–61. [CrossRef]
16. Wight, D.; Fullerton, D. A review of interventions with parents to promote the sexual health of their children. *J. Adolesc. Health* **2013**, *52*, 4–27. [CrossRef]
17. Vidourek, R.A.; Bernard, A.L.; King, K.A. Effective parent connectedness components in sexuality education interventions for African American youth: A review of the literature. *Am. J. Sex. Educ.* **2009**, *4*, 225–247. [CrossRef]
18. Markham, C.M.; Lormand, D.; Gloppen, K.M.; Peskin, M.F.; Flores, B.; Low, B.; House, L.D. Connectedness as a predictor of sexual and reproductive health outcomes for youth. *J. Adolesc. Health* **2010**, *46*, S23–S41. [CrossRef]
19. De Looze, M.; Constantine, N.A.; Jerman, P.; Vermeulen-Smit, E.; ter Bogt, T. Parent–adolescent sexual communication and its association with adolescent sexual behaviors: A nationally representative analysis in the Netherlands. *J. Sex Res.* **2015**, *52*, 257–268. [CrossRef]
20. Widman, L.; Choukas-Bradley, S.; Helms, S.W.; Golin, C.E.; Prinstein, M.J. Sexual communication between early adolescents and their dating partners, parents, and best friends. *J. Sex Res.* **2014**, *51*, 731–741. [CrossRef]
21. Zamboni, B.D.; Silver, R. Family sex communication and the sexual desire, attitudes, and behavior of late adolescents. *Am. J. Sex. Educ.* **2009**, *4*, 58–78. [CrossRef]
22. Angera, J.J.; Brookins-Fisher, J.; Inungu, J.N. An investigation of parent/child communication about sexuality. *Am. J. Sex. Educ.* **2008**, *3*, 165–181. [CrossRef]
23. Kirkman, M.; Rosenthal, D.A.; Shirley Feldman, S. Being open with your mouth shut: The meaning of 'openness' in family communication about sexuality. *Sex Educ.* **2005**, *5*, 49–66. [CrossRef]
24. Sneed, C.D.; Somoza, C.G.; Jones, T.; Alfaro, S. Topics discussed with mothers and fathers for parent–child sex communication among African-American adolescents. *Sex Educ.* **2013**, *13*, 450–458. [CrossRef]
25. DiIorio, C.; Dudley, W.N.; Kelly, M.; Soet, J.E.; Mbwara, J.; Potter, J.S. Social cognitive correlates of sexual experience and condom use among 13-through 15-year-old adolescents. *J. Adolesc. Health* **2001**, *29*, 208–216. [CrossRef]
26. DiIorio, C.; McCarty, F.; Denzmore, P. An exploration of social cognitive theory mediators of father–son communication about sex. *J. Pediatric Psychol.* **2006**, *31*, 917–927. [CrossRef]
27. Lehr, S.T.; Demi, A.S.; DiIorio, C.; Facteau, J. Predictors of father-son communication about sexuality. *J. Sex Res.* **2005**, *42*, 119–129. [CrossRef] [PubMed]
28. Bandura, A. Self-efficacy: Toward a unifying theory of behavioral change. *Psychol. Rev.* **1977**, *84*, 191–215. [CrossRef]
29. Sinclair, J.; Unruh, D.; Lindstrom, L.; Scanlon, D. Barriers to sexuality for individuals with intellectual and developmental disabilities: A literature review. *Educ. Train. Autism Dev. Disabil.* **2015**, *50*, 3–16.
30. Kersh, J.; Hedvat, T.T.; Hauser-Cram, P.; Warfield, M.E. The contribution of marital quality to the well-being of parents of children with developmental disabilities. *J. Intellect. Disabil. Res.* **2006**, *50*, 883–893. [CrossRef] [PubMed]
31. Miodrag, N.; Hodapp, R.M. Chronic stress and health among parents of children with intellectual and developmental disabilities. *Curr. Opin. Psychiatry* **2010**, *23*, 407–411. [CrossRef]
32. Bouris, A.; Guilamo-Ramos, V.; Pickard, A.; Shiu, C.; Loosier, P.S.; Dittus, P.; Gloppen, K.; Waldmiller, J.M. A systematic review of parental influences on the health and well-being of lesbian, gay, and bisexual youth: Time for a new public health research and practice agenda. *J. Prim. Prev.* **2010**, *31*, 273–309. [CrossRef]
33. Pop, M.V.; Rusu, A.S. Developing a sexuality education program for parents in Romania–preliminary analysis. *J. Psychol. Educ. Res.* **2017**, *25*, 57–73.
34. Pop, M.V.; Rusu, A.S. Satisfaction and communication in couples of parents and potential parents—psychological predictors and implications for sexuality education of children. *Procedia-Soc. Behav. Sci.* **2015**, *209*, 402–410. [CrossRef]
35. Babin, E.A. An examination of predictors of nonverbal and verbal communication of pleasure during sex and sexual satisfaction. *J. Soc. Pers. Relationsh.* **2012**, 1–23. [CrossRef]
36. Hewitt, P.L.; Flett, G.L. Perfectionism in the self and social contexts: Conceptualization, assessment, and association with psychopathology. *J. Personal. Soc. Psychol.* **1991**, *60*, 456–470. [CrossRef]
37. Snell, W.E., Jr. (Ed.) Chapter 16: Sexual perfectionism among single sexually experienced females. In *New Directions in the Psychology of Human Sexuality*; Snell Publications: Cape Girardeau, MO, USA, 2001.

38. Snell, W.E., Jr.; Rigdon, K.L. Chapter 15: The Multidimensional Sexual Perfectionism Questionnaire: Preliminary evidence for reliability and validity. In *New Directions in the Psychology of Human Sexuality*; Snell, W.E., Jr., Ed.; Snell Publications: Cape Girardeau, MO, USA, 2001.
39. Clark-Carter, D. *Quantitative Psychological Research: The Complete Student's Companion*, 3rd ed.; Psychology Press, Taylor & Francis Group: Hove, UK; New York, NY, USA, 2010.
40. Morawska, A.; Walsh, A.; Grabski, M.; Fletcher, R. Parental confidence and preferences for communicating with their child about sexuality. *Sex Educ.* **2015**, *15*, 235–248. [CrossRef]
41. DiIorio, C.; Dudley, W.N.; Wang, D.T.; Wasserman, J.; Eichler, M.; Belcher, L.; West-Edwards, C. Measurement of parenting self-efficacy and outcome expectancy related to discussions about sex. *J. Nurs. Meas.* **2001**, *9*, 135–149. [CrossRef]
42. Howitt, D.; Cramer, D. *Understanding Statistics in Psychology with SPSS*; Pearson: London, UK, 2017.
43. Tabachnick, B.G.; Fidell, L.S. *Using Multivariate Statistics*, 6th ed.; Pearson: Boston, MA, USA, 2013.
44. Field, A. *Discovering Statistics Using IBM SPSS Statistics*; Sage: London, UK, 2013.
45. Williams, D.M. Outcome expectancy and self-efficacy: Theoretical implications of an unresolved contradiction. *Personal. Soc. Psychol. Rev.* **2010**, *14*, 417–425. [CrossRef]

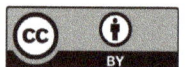

© 2019 by the authors. Licensee MDPI, Basel, Switzerland. This article is an open access article distributed under the terms and conditions of the Creative Commons Attribution (CC BY) license (http://creativecommons.org/licenses/by/4.0/).

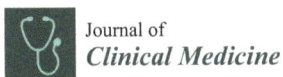

Article

Sexual Dysfunction and Quality of Life in Chronic Heroin-Dependent Individuals on Methadone Maintenance Treatment

Carlos Llanes [1,*], Ana I. Álvarez [2], M. Teresa Pastor [3], M. Ángeles Garzón [2], Nerea González-García [4] and Ángel L. Montejo [5]

1   Department of Psychiatry, Complejo Asistencial de Zamora, Zamora 49022, Spain
2   Department of Psychiatry, Hospital Clínico Universitario de Salamanca, Salamanca 37007, Spain; aialvarez@saludcastillayleon.es (A.T.Á.); magarzon@saludcastillayleon.es (M.Á.G.)
3   Castilla y León Health Authority, Complejo Asistencial de Zamora, Zamora 49022, Spain; mtpastor@saludcastillayleon.es
4   Department of Statistics, University of Salamanca, Institute of Biomedical Research of Salamanca IBSAL, Salamanca 37007, Spain; nerea_gonzalez_garcia@usal.es
5   Psychiatry, University of Salamanca, Institute of Biomedical Research of Salamanca IBSAL, Salamanca 37007, Spain; amontejo@usal.es
*   Correspondence: cllanes@saludcastillayleon.es; Tel.: +34-980-548-820 (ext. 48200)

Received: 31 January 2019; Accepted: 1 March 2019; Published: 7 March 2019

Abstract: This study examined whether methadone (hereinafter referred to as MTD) maintenance treatment (MMT) is correlated with sexual dysfunction (SD) in heroin-dependent men. This was conducted to determine the prevalence of sexual dysfunction and if there is a relationship between duration and dose among men on MMT and its impact on the quality of life. The study combined a retrospective and a cross-sectional survey based on the Kinsey Scale, TECVASP, and PRSexDQ-SALSEX clinical interviews of 85 patients who are currently engaged in MMT. Sexual dysfunction in all five PRSexDQ-SALSEX domains (lack of libido, delay in orgasm, inability to orgasm, erectile dysfunction, and tolerance or acceptance of changes in sexual function) was associated with dose and long-term use of heroin. All dimensions of SD were affected by the MTD intake. From the analysis of our sample, we may conclude that dose of MTD and overall score of SD were directly associated. However, no evidence was found to prove that treatment duration and severity of SD were linked. It is notable that only one tenth of the patients spontaneously reported their symptoms of the sexual sphere, but up to a third considered leaving the MMT for this reason.

Keywords: opioid-related disorders; methadone; adverse effects; erectile dysfunction; medication adherence

1. Introduction

Opioid dependence is a rising drug use disorder with a substantial contribution to the global disease burden. The absolute number (age standardized prevalence) of people with opioid dependence worldwide increased from 10.4 million (0.20%) in 1990 to 15.5 million (0.22%) in 2010, and the disability adjusted years of life lost attributable to opioid dependence rose from 5.3 million (0.21% of global disease burden) in 1990 to 9.2 million (0.37%) in 2010 [1]. Opioid substitution treatment, either with methadone or buprenorphine, has been shown to be safe and effective in suppressing illicit opioid use, improving physical and mental wellbeing, and reducing all cause and overdose mortality [2]. However, methadone is more commonly used for maintenance treatment [3]. Methadone maintenance treatment (MMT) is a comprehensive treatment program that involves the long-term prescribing of methadone as a substitution therapy for opioid dependence. Despite the effectiveness of the methadone maintenance treatment [4], previous studies have found that sexual dysfunction, including hypoactive sexual desire disorder, erectile dysfunction, and orgasmic dysfunction, is common in heroin users and individuals being treated for heroin addiction [5]. In a recent meta-analysis, the meta-analytical pooled prevalence for sexual dysfunction among methadone users was 52% (95% confidence interval, 0.39–0.65). Hypoactive sexual desire disorder and low libido were the most prevalent sexual dysfunctions, accounting for 51% of cases [6]. Several hypotheses have been suggested to explain the correlation between methadone use and sexual dysfunction. One well-known hypothesis is that methadone exerts neuroendocrinological effects on the tubero-infundibular and hypothalamic-pituitary-gonadal axes. The chronic stimulation of the μ-opioid receptors by methadone alters the function of the tubero-infundibular axis and the dopaminergic control of prolactin, with a consequential impact on sexual functioning [7]. A high level of circulating prolactin causes the inhibition of the gonadotropin-releasing hormone, which lowers the levels of sex hormones, especially testosterone. Men with low testosterone levels may exhibit a decrease in sexual interest [8]. A recent qualitative study has found that some MMT subjects who experienced sexual dysfunction chose to withdraw from interactions with their partners, which led to conflicts. Such conflicts negatively impacted the rehabilitation. Furthermore, inappropriate reactions to the sexual problems included premature treatment discontinuation under pressure from partners, methadone dose reduction, and the use of other illicit drugs to enhance sexual performance [9]. The measurement of the health-related quality of life construct (HRQoL) is widely used in the field of health. This represents individual responses to the physical, mental, and social effects that a health alteration produces on daily life. In drug addiction, this construct has been used for a relatively short time [10].

Although sexual dysfunction is not life threatening, it may often result in withdrawal from sexual intimacy, thereby reducing quality of life [11]. Therefore, we conducted this study to investigate sexual dysfunction in men and women on MMT. We also investigated the correlation and association between sexual dysfunction and quality of life in this group of patients.

2. Experimental Section

Methods and study design: this cross-sectional study was conducted in the drug detoxification unit in Complejo Asistencial de Salamanca Hospital in Salamanca, Spain, which is the Castilla y León regional reference unit for the treatment of addictions in hospitalization. The research period was from May 2017 to October 2018.

Participants: all participants were recruited on admission to the drug detoxification unit to voluntarily withdraw or reduce methadone. Subjects were eligible for this study if: (1) They were men or women over 18 years old; (2) they had been engaged in MMT; (3) they had a diagnosis of mental and behavioral disorders due to the use of opioids (F11.3 ICD-10); (4) their urine was found to be negative in drug use in the weekly analytical control for the six months prior to admission; and (5) they were not under treatment with any psychodrugs except benzodiazepines.

Interviews and measures: an original form was developed to record the information of the participants. The questionnaire included items on demographic characteristics (sex and age) and methadone treatment status (such as the time of receiving MMT and methadone dose). It also include if they were being treated with benzodiazepines or not and if they were, the equivalent dose in diazepam.

The Kinsey scale [12], also called the Heterosexual–Homosexual Rating Scale, is used to describe a person's sexual orientation based on their experience or response at a given time. It consists of nine items that explore the importance of sexual life for the patient and the degree of satisfaction with it, the identification of the patient with the different groups of sexual orientations, and the frequency of sexual intercourse of the patient. The first seven items are answered on a scale of 1 to 5 and the last two are of a dichotomous nature. The scale is self-applied and typically ranges from "0", Exclusively heterosexual to "1", Predominantly heterosexual, only incidentally homosexual; "2", Predominantly heterosexual, but more than incidentally homosexual; "3", Equally heterosexual and homosexual; "4", Predominantly homosexual, but more than incidentally heterosexual; "5", Predominantly homosexual, only incidentally heterosexual; and "6", Exclusively homosexual. In both the male and female volumes of the Kinsey Reports, an additional grade, listed as "X", indicated no socio-sexual contacts or reactions.

PRSexDQ-SALSEX is a brief and clinician-administered questionnaire that includes seven questions in total [12]. The presence of sexual function impairment in patients with psychiatric disorders is very common and could be an effect of the medication (mainly antidepressants and neuroleptics) [13]. Questions A and B are screening items used to assess whether the patient had noticed changes in sexual function since pharmacotherapy or during the last four weeks and reported it spontaneously. Items 3–7 are questions evaluating five dimensions of SD on a scale of 0–3: loss of libido, delayed orgasm or ejaculation, lack of orgasm or ejaculation, erectile dysfunction in men/vaginal lubrication dysfunction in women, and patient's tolerance. The total score of PRSexDQ-SALSEX ranges from 0 to 15 [14].

For the measurement of the health-related quality of life (HRQoL), the test specifically designed for the drug-dependent population TECVASP [15] was used. TECVASP (acronym in Spanish of Test for the Evaluation of the Quality of Life in Addicts to Psychoactive Substances) consists of 22 items (18 positive and four negative [items 15, 19, 20, and 21]), with a graduated response format of five alternatives. The response alternatives are coded with the following scores: (a) in the positive items: nothing (5 points), little (4 points), sometimes (3 points), enough (2 points), and a lot (1 point); (b) in the negative items: nothing (1 point), little (2 points), sometimes (3 points), enough (4 points), and a lot (5 points). In this way, for each item, a higher score represents a more positive assessment of the content, and in the test, a higher score represents a better HRQoL.

Statistical Analysis: Kolmogorov-Smirnov was one sample test used to examine the quantitative variables' distribution. Normally distributed variables were described as mean ± standard deviation; otherwise, their information was summarized by median ± interquartile range. Categorical response features were measured through absolute or relative frequencies and percentages. Differences between two independent groups were tested by the Student's t-test (for normal distribution data) or Mann-Whitney U test. Comparisons of more than two independent groups were studied by ANOVA (for data with parametric distribution) or the Kruskal-Wallis test (for non-normal distributions). The Chi-Square test, Fisher's exact test, and tau de Kendall measure were used to evaluate the association in qualitative variables.

Patients were classified based on the categorization of SALSEX total score into four different groups: no Sexual Dysfunction (SD) (a score of 0 points), mild SD (a score of 1–5 points, where no items scored ≥ 2), moderate SD (a score of 6–10 points or an item scoring 2 and no items scoring 3), or severe SD (a score of 11–15, or any items scoring 3 points). In addition, based on the cut-off points of the first and third quartiles, the dose of methadone (MTD) consumed was categorized as <30 mg, 30–60 mg, and >60 mg. Subsequently, Correspondence Factor Analysis (CFA) was used to analyze the relationship between methadone consumption and sexual problems, taking into account tolerance, dose, and time of methadone treatment. CFA is a statistical technique that produces a graphical representation of a contingency table, facilitating the interpretation of the association between two categorical variables. The categories of these variables are represented by points on a plane. For a correct interpretation of a CFA representation, it should be taken into account that two close points in the graph refer to positive associated categories.

Finally, relationships between sexual activity and quality of life of patients based on SD severity groups were studied. Differences in questions with five Likert response options were evaluated by means of an ANOVA or Kruskal-Wallis test, since this treatment is admitted when the number of Likert alternatives is greater than four. The global quality of life score was computed by the sum of the 22 items' scores of the TECVASP scale. Here, it is important to note that: (i) there were 18 inverse items and four direct questions; (ii) scores' range vary from 22 to 110 points; and (iii) the higher the score in the test, the worse the quality of life of patients.

3. Results

3.1. Clinical and Sociodemographic Characteristics of Patients

Patients' characteristics are shown in Table 1. The sample consisted of 85 patients, mainly men ($n = 72$, 84.7%), with a mean age of 43.1 ± 7.7 years, with 23 years being the youngest patient and 58 years the oldest. The mean dose of methadone consumed by patients was 49.01 ± 29.87 mg, with a mean treatment time of 7.21 ± 6.95 years. Differentiating by sexes, the mean age of men was 42.76 ± 7.79 years, and the mean duration of treatment and mean dose were 6.34 ± 6.74 years and 45.33 ± 25.29 mg, respectively. For women, the mean age was 44.85 ± 7.2 and they consumed a mean dose of 69.38 ± 43.92 mg, during 9.85 ± 7.78 years of treatment.

Table 1. Clinical and sociodemographic characteristics.

Characteristic	N = 85
Age (years)	43.1 ± 7.7
<30 years, n (%)	6 (7.1)
30–40, n (%)	22 (25.9)
40–50, n (%)	45 (52.9)
>50, n (%)	12 (14.1)
Sex (males), n (%)	72 (84.7)
Treatment time (years)	7.21 ± 6.95
MTD[1] dose	49.01 ± 29.87
MTD[1] tolerance	
Good tolerance, n (%)	37 (43.5)
Middle tolerance, n (%)	44 (51.8)
Poor tolerance, n (%)	4 (4.7)
Personality disorder, n (%)	49 (57.6)
Consumption of self-administered benzodiazepines, n (%)	27 (31.8)
Dose (mg)	95.19 ± 98.45
Consumption of medicated benzodiazepines, n (%)	22 (25.9%)
Dose (mg)	36.36 ± 32.74

[1] MTD, Methadone.

About half of the patients from the sample suffered from a personality disorder ($n = 49$, 57.6%). One-third of the patients consumed self-administered benzodiazepines (31.8%; mean dose 95.2 ± 98.5 mg), while one quarter took benzodiazepines by medical prescription (25.9%; mean dose 36.4 ± 32.7 mg). There was a significant statistical difference between the doses of self-administered and medicated doses of benzodiacepines ($p = 0.001$), with the self-administered benzodiazepines being the greater dose. None of the patients taking self-administered benzodiazepines had received medical advice to get them.

Differences between Sexes in Clinical and Sociodemographic Characteristics

Table 2 contains features of patients according to their sex. During their treatment time, which was significantly different in men and women ($p = 0.01$), men received a lower dose of MTD. Tolerance toward MTD was significantly better in men than women, who presented low percentages of good tolerance. Although the doses of both self-administered and medically prescribed benzodiazepines were lower in women, no statistically significant differences were observed by sex. No age difference was found between sexes.

Table 2. Comparison of sexes in clinical and sociodemographic characteristics.

Characteristic	Men (n = 72)	Women (n = 13)	p-Value
Age (years)	42.76 ± 7.79	46 ± 15.5	0.49
Treatment time (years)	6.74 ± 6.74	9 ± 17.5	0.01
MTD' dose (mg)	45.33 ± 25.29	60 ± 23.5	0.20
MTD's tolerance	-	-	0.01
Good tolerance, n (%)	35 (48.6)	2 (15.4)	
Middle tolerance, n (%)	35 (48.6)	9 (69.2)	
Poor tolerance, n (%)	2 (2.8)	2 (15.4)	
Personality disorder, n (%)	41 (56.9)	8 (61.5)	0.77
Dose of self-administered benzodiazepines (mg)	96.46 ± 103.78	85 ± 44.44	0.74
Dose of medicated benzodiazepines (mg)	40 ± 36.52	20 ± 40.0	0.59

3.2. Sexual Activity, Frequency of SD and Group Differences in SALSEX Scores

83.5% of the participants described themselves as heterosexual, 35.3% had an exclusively monogamous sexual relationship, and 23.5% had non-monogamous sexual relations. Furthermore, 15.3% had sexual intercourse in the last semester to get money or cover a material need, or paid for sexual intercourse (24.7%). Kinsey results showed that a high percentage of the sample gave importance to sex (71.7%), but only 24.7% were satisfied with their sexual activity.

At the same time, a total of 85.9% of the patients in this investigation suffered from SD. Among them, 24.7% showed mild SD, 21.2% suffered from moderate SD, and 40% had severe SD. There was a highly significant difference between men and women in terms of the PRSexDQ-SALSEX total score (p = 0.000; Figure A1), being more serious in female patients. 76.5% felt alteration in their sexual activity after the beginning of methadone treatment, but only 11.8% reported it to the doctor without being questioned. In addition, 76.9% of patients were disturbed by SD and 32.7% of them considered interrupting the MTD treatment.

Dysfunction groups showed a statistically different behaviour in items 5 (p = 0.037), 6 (p = 0.003), and 7 (p = 0.005) of the Modified Kinsey scale. Patients without sexual dysfunction had sex more frequently than patients with SD (Figure 1, median values of items 5 and 6), with the patients having severe sexual dysfunction having the lowest score.

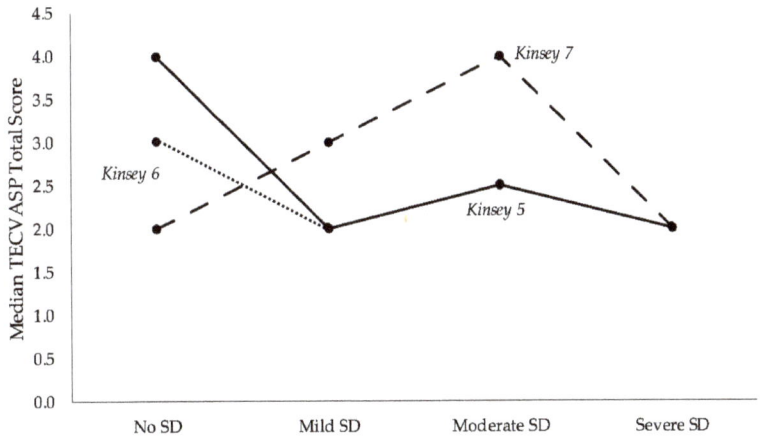

Figure 1. Differences in Kinsey questionnaire items, distinguished by the four SD classes of SALSEX.

Impact of Treatment Duration, Methadone Dose Consumed, Tolerance toward Methadone, and Effect of Using Benzodiazepines on Sexual Dysfunction

Generally, correlation analysis allowed us to conclude that the dose of MTD and overall score of SD were directly associated (Pearson correlation coefficient 0.332; $p = 0.002$). However, no evidence was found that treatment duration and severity of SD were linked (Pearson correlation coefficient 0.183; $p = 0.094$).

The frequency of SD problems by dose and tolerance toward MTD are summarized in Tables 3 and 4. Differences (Kruskal-Wallis analysis) between the four SD groups of patients (no SD, mild SD, moderate SD, severe SD) showed statistically significant dissimilarities on MTD's dose ($p = 0.005$) and MTD's tolerance ($p = 0.000$). Patients with severe sexual dysfunction were those who took higher doses of MTD, as well as those who showed the worst tolerance towards the opiate. All cases with poor tolerance toward MTD presented severe sexual dysfunction.

Table 3. Comparison of clinical characteristics between patients with no SD and patients with SD, distinguishing those with mild, moderate, and severe SD.

Characteristic	No SD Patients ($n = 12$)	SD Patients ($n = 73$)			p-Value
		Mild ($n = 21$)	Moderate ($n = 18$)	Severe ($n = 34$)	
Age (years)	44 ± 9.75	43 ± 11	45.5 ± 10	42.5 ± 10.5	0.871
MTD's dose (mg)	32.5 ± 13.75	40 ± 28	39 ± 18.75	53 ± 40.75	0.005
MTD's tolerance					
Good tolerance, n (%)	9 (75)	13 (61.9)	10 (55.6)	5 (14.7)	
Medium tolerance, n (%)	3 (25)	8 (38.1)	8 (44.4)	25 (73.5)	0.000
Poor tolerance, n (%)	-	-	-	4 (11.8)	
Personality disorder, n (%)	8 (66.7)	11 (52.4)	10 (55.6)	20 (58.8)	0.947

Table 4. Effect of MTD dose and tolerance on the frequency (%) of sexual dysfunction problems.

Characteristic	No SD Patients ($n = 12$)	Mild SD Patients ($n = 21$)				Moderate/Severe SD Patients ($n = 52$)			
		DL	DEO	A	ELP	DL	DEO	A	ELP
MTD dose									
<30 mg	0	87.5	75	12.5	50	100	72.7	54.5	81.8
30–60 mg	0	72.7	72.7	18.2	27.3	95.8	79.2	83.3	83.3
>60 mg	-	0	100	50	0	94.1	94.1	88.2	94.1
MTD tolerance									
Poor	-	-	-	-	-	100	100	100	100
Medium	0	62.5	75	0	12.5	93.9	87.9	87.9	87.9
Good	0	76.9	76.9	30.8	46.2	93.3	66.6	53.3	80

Decreased libido (DL); Delay in ejaculation/orgasm (DEO); Anorgasmia (A); Erection/lubrication problem (ELP).

In Table 4, the percentage of patients suffering from some libido, eyaculation/orgasm, anorgasmia, or erection/lubrication problem are summarized, regardless of whether the symptoms were mild. Patients who did not suffer from SD, did not present problems in any of the evaluated dimensions (decreased libido (DL), delay in eyaculation/orgasm (DEO), anorgasmia (A), and erection/lubrication problem (ELP)). However, all dimensions of SD were affected by the MTD intake in those with mild, moderate, or severe SD. Patients treated with a lower amount of MTD suffered from less problems of delay in ejaculation/orgasm or in the inability to ejaculate/have orgasm during intercourse. The same occurred with those patients with a better tolerance to this opiate. The dose associated with the highest erection/lubrication problem (94.1%) was more than 60 mg of MTD.

As seen in the CFA graphical representation (Figure 2a) and remembering that the proximity between points can be understood as a direct association between categories, it was observed that:

- Patients which had no SD or their SD was not severe showed good tolerance to MTD;
- Patients with moderate SD were those that had good or medium tolerance;

- Severe SD was associated with poor MTD tolerance.

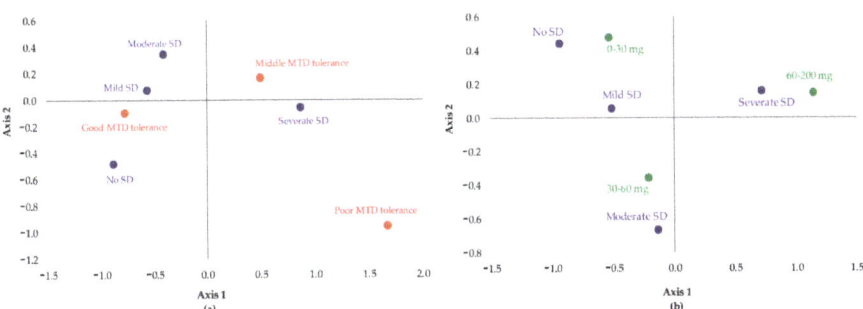

Figure 2. CFA graphical representations of the categories of two qualitative variables: (**a**) Tolerance to MTD (red) vs severity of SD (blue); (**b**) dose of MTD (green) vs severity of SD (blue).

After examining the influence of mg of dose with the grade of dysfunction (Figure 2b), it could be concluded that:

- Patients which had no SD or their SD was mild were those who took a dose between 0 and 30 mg;
- Patients with moderate SD took 30–60 mg of MTD;
- Severe SD was associated with the highest doses: 60–200 mg.

Finally, 57.6% of the patients also used benzodiazepines (both self-administered and medically prescribed). Due to this last characteristic, the presence of DS was then examined depending on whether the patients used methadone alone or methadone combined with benzodiazepines. Firstly, SALSEX scores difference analysis between both groups presented non-significant differences ($p = 0.242$). In other words, no significant evidence was found to corroborate that the use of benzodiazepines combined with methadone influences the presence and/or severity of DS. Secondly, CFA graphical representation (Figure A2) shows the differences in the association between DS and doses of MTD and DS and tolerance to MTD in patients who only consume MTD (panels a and c) and patients who consume both methadone and benzodiazepines (panels b and d). In the case of patients who only take MTD the association between not suffering from SD or mild SD and having a good tolerance to MTD is very strong (panel a), while those who consume MTD and benzodiazepines suffer from moderate SD, although they have a good tolerance to MTD (panel b). Regarding the dose consumed, patients taking a dose of 0–30 mg of MTD and also benzodiazepines (panel d) are associated with mild SD, while patients who only take MTD (dose of 0–30 mg) are associated with a diagnosis of no presence of DS (panel c).

3.3. Quality of Life in Presence of Sexual Dysfunction Problems

The mean score of the quality of life test TECVASP was 58.12 ± 13.74 points. Statistically significant differences were found for SALSEX classes in questions 4 ($p = 0.006$), 10 ($p = 0.019$), 14 ($p = 0.034$), 16 ($p = 0.019$), and 22 ($p = 0.005$).

Figure A3 contains the global quality of life score test for patients that had no SD versus patients which suffered from SD of any grade. The median score of the SD group was higher than the median score of patients without dysfunction problems, mirroring the results of worse quality of life in those patients. A comparison of four classes of SD reported a significant difference ($p = 0.011$, Figure A2b), where patients with severe sexual dysfunction suffered from the worst quality of life and patients with mild sexual dysfunction had the best quality of life.

4. Discussion

The Kinsey scale results showed that a high percentage of the sample gave importance to sex (71.7%), but only 24.7% were satisfied with their sexual activity. Patients in MMT had problems with sexual function in one or more of the five PRSexDQ-SALSEX domains (loss of libido, delayed orgasm or ejaculation, lack of orgasm or ejaculation, erectile dysfunction in men/vaginal lubrication dysfunction in women, and patient's tolerance.). The research literature has noted high rates of sexual dysfunction in heroin users and MMT patient populations [14]. Our study found that 85.9% of participants in MMT had sexual dysfunction (40% of them severe dysfunction), which is perhaps higher than reported in other studies [15,16], although the results found varied greatly [17,18].

Older age, for example, was highly hypothesized to be correlated with increased sexual dysfunction in patients receiving methadone [19]. In our sample, we did not find statistically significant differences between the presence of sexual dysfunction and age ($p = 0.871$). There are also significant differences ($p = 0.005$) in the methadone dose among patients who presented mild, moderate, or severe sexual dysfunction. This finding agrees with what was found by others [11], who showed that patients on higher methadone doses had more sexual dysfunction, and differed slightly from others [14].

Although it is commonly accepted that sexual dysfunction is a direct pharmacological effect of opioids, recent studies have revealed that the etiology of sexual dysfunction in methadone-maintained patients is rather complex [20,21]. Some research has suggested that heroin, amphetamine, alcohol, tobacco, and marijuana can cause sexual dysfunction by a number of mechanisms, including effects on the male reproductive system at the level of the hypothalamus, the pituitary gland, and the testes [22,23]. Additionally, because of this, those patients who had positive toxic control in the six months prior to our study were excluded from the sample. Other factors commonly pointed out are psychological factors (i.e., psychiatric symptoms). To avoid this, we have excluded all those patients who had a psychiatric diagnosis, apart from a substance use disorder (except for personality disorder). The diagnosis of personality disorder appears in 57.6% of the sample, which in itself is linked to sexual dysfunction [24,25], however, and as a limitation of this research, we did not consider physical health and biological factors (i.e., sex hormone), which also significantly contribute to it [26].

There were several limitations to our study. Firstly, we found that a proportion of the participants in MMT used benzodiazepines (both self-administered and medically prescribed) during methadone treatment. This was the only admitted psychopharmacological treatment, and although its presence may interfere with the results [27] (benzodiazepines are psychotropic drugs with some adverse sexual effects) [28], it is not easy to find patients on methadone treatment in monotherapy. Secondly, another limitation of the study is bias due to its retrospective design (instead of prospective one); however, the relatively high mean duration of methadone treatment (6.34 ± 6.74 and 9.85 ± 7.78 years of treatment for men and women, respectively) avoids bias in the recalling symptoms of sexual dysfunction prior to initiating MMT, which would influence the result of this study. We emphasize that they did not take antidepressants or antipsychotics, which have been shown in the literature to cause many sexual dysfunctions [29].

Sexual functioning is critical for improving the quality of life in patients enrolled in an opioid rehabilitation program. The methadone treatment programs should be progressively oriented to the person, valuing their opinions, encouraging their active participation in the process, and improving their quality of life levels, so that the approach to their problems is similar to that of any another health issue.

Clinical implications: clinicians may consider asking about sexual dysfunction while treating heroin dependents, as only 11.8% of the patients in our sample reported it without being questioned about it; however, 32.7% of them considered interrupting the treatment for this reason. As the results of our study showed high rates of sexual dysfunction secondary to methadone treatment (not spontaneously reported), we think it is very important to use scales like these, including brief and relatively nonintrusive questionnaires that ease the exploration and detection of these symptoms and avoid discontinuation of the treatment

5. Conclusions

A high prevalence of sexual life dissatisfaction was found in our sample. It suggests that the sexual dysfunction of MMT patients deserves special attention from specialists of addiction treatment settings.

Author Contributions: Conceptualization, C.L.; Data curation, A.I.Á., M.Á.G., and N.G.-G.; Formal analysis, N.G.-G.; Methodology, Á.L.M.; Project administration, C.L., A.I.Á., and Á.L.M.; Supervision, M.T.P.; Writing—original draft, C.L.

Acknowledgments: The authors wish to acknowledge the patients and staff of the drug detoxification unit in Complejo Asistencial de Salamanca for their participation in this study.

Conflicts of Interest: The authors declare no conflict of interest. The funders had no role in the design of the study; in the collection, analyses, or interpretation of data; in the writing of the manuscript, or in the decision to publish the results.

Appendix A

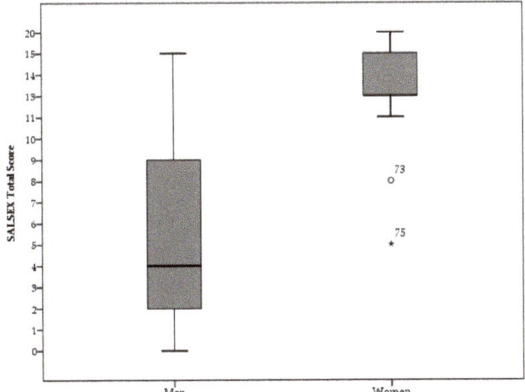

Figure A1. Difference between men and women in SALSEX total score. The ° symbol represents an outlier and the * symbol corresponds to extreme value.

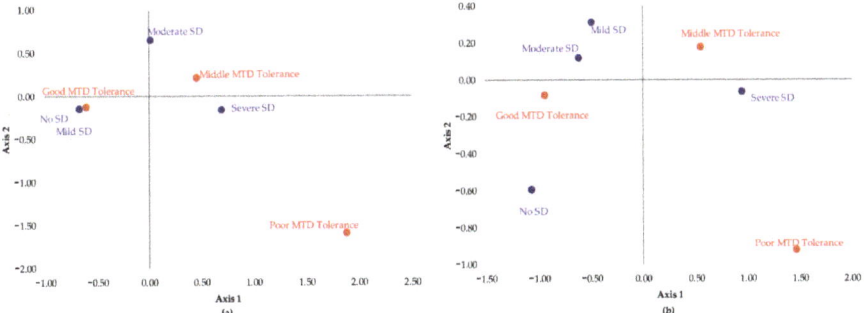

Figure A2. *Cont.*

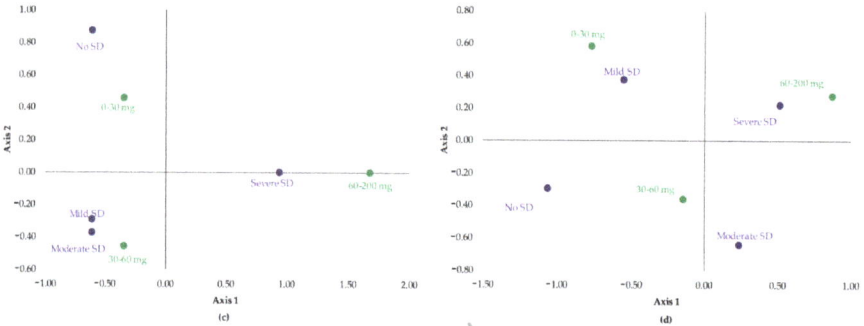

Figure A2. CFA graphical representations of the categories of two qualitative variables: (**a**) Tolerance to MTD (red) vs severity of SD (blue) of patients that only use MTD; (**b**) tolerance to MTD (red) vs severity of SD (blue) of patients that use MTD and benzodiazepines; (**c**) dose of MTD (green) vs severity of SD (blue) of patients that only use MTD; (**d**) dose of MTD (green) vs severity of SD (blue) that use MTD and benzodiazepines.

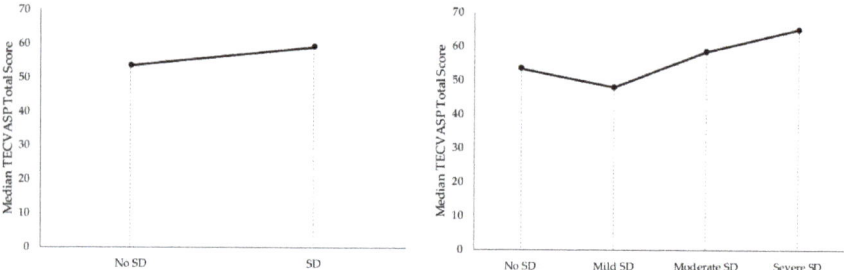

Figure A3. Quality of life based on SALSEX classes (no SD, mild SD, moderate SD, and severe SD).

References

1. Degenhardt, L.; Charlson, F.; Mathers, B.; Hall, W.D.; Flaxman, A.D.; Johns, N.; Vos, T. The global epidemiology and burden of opioid dependence: Results from the global burden of disease 2010 study. *Addiction* **2014**, *109*, 1320–1333. [CrossRef] [PubMed]
2. Mattick, R.P.; Breen, C.; Kimber, J.; Davoli, M. Methadone maintenance therapy versus no opioid replacement therapy for opioid dependence. *Cochrane Database Syst. Rev.* **2009**, *3*, CD002209. [CrossRef] [PubMed]
3. Mattick, R.P.; Breen, C.; Kimber, J.; Davoli, M. Buprenorphine maintenance versus placebo or methadone maintenance for opioid dependence. *Cochrane Database Syst. Rev.* **2014**, *2*, CD002207. [CrossRef] [PubMed]
4. Degenhardt, L.; Randall, D.; Hall, W.; Law, M.; Butler, T.; Burns, L. Mortality among clients of a state-wide opioid pharmacotherapy program over 20 years: Risk factors and lives saved. *Drug Alcohol Depend.* **2009**, *105*, 9–15. [CrossRef] [PubMed]
5. Hallinan, R.; Byrne, A.; Agho, K.; McMahon, C.; Tynan, P.; Attia, J. Erectile dysfunction in men receiving methadone and buprenorphine maintenance treatment. *J. Sex. Med.* **2008**, *5*, 684–692. [CrossRef] [PubMed]
6. Yee, A.; Loh, H.S.; Ng, C.G. The prevalence of sexual dysfunction among male patients on methadone and buprenorphine treatments: A meta-analysis study. *J. Sex. Med.* **2014**, *11*, 22–32. [CrossRef] [PubMed]
7. Matuszewich, L.; Ormsby, J.L.; Moses, J.; Lorrain, D.S.; Hull, E.M. Effects of morphiceptin in the medial preoptic area on male sexual behavior. *Psychopharmacology* **1995**, *122*, 330–335. [CrossRef] [PubMed]
8. Argiolas, A.; Melis, M.R. Neuropeptides and central control of sexual behaviour from the past to the present: A review. *Prog Neurobiol.* **2013**, *108*, 80–107. [CrossRef] [PubMed]

9. Xia, Y.; Zhang, D.; Li, X.; Chen, W.; He, Q.; Jahn, H.J.; Li, X.; Chen, J.; Hu, P.; Ling, L. Sexual dysfunction during methadone maintenance treatment and its influence on patient's life and treatment: A qualitative study in South China. *Psychol. Health Med.* **2013**, *18*, 321–329. [CrossRef] [PubMed]
10. Reno, R.R.; Aiken, L.S. Life activities and life quality of heroin addicts in and out of methadone treatment. *Int. J. Addict.* **1993**, *28*, 211–232. [CrossRef] [PubMed]
11. Brown, R.; Balousek, S.; Mundt, M.; Fleming, M. Methadone maintenance and male sexual dysfunction. *J. Addict. Dis.* **2005**, *24*, 91–106. [CrossRef] [PubMed]
12. Kinsey, A.C.; Pomeroy, W.R.; Martin, C.E. Sexual Behavior in the Human Male. *Am. J. Public Health* **2003**, *93*, 894–898. [CrossRef] [PubMed]
13. Montejo, A.L.; Llorca, G.; Izquierdo, J.A.; Rico-Villademoros, F. Incidence of sexual dysfunction associated with antidepressant agents: A prospective multicenter study of 1022 outpatients. Spanish Working Group for the Study of Psychotropic-Related Sexual Dysfunction. *J. Clin. Psychiatry* **2001**, *62* (Suppl. 3), 10–21. [PubMed]
14. Montejo, A.L.; Rico-Villademoros, F. Psychometric properties of the Psychotropic-Related Sexual Dysfunction Questionnaire (PRSexDQ-SALSEX) in patients with schizophrenia and other psychotic disorders. *J. Sex Marital Ther.* **2008**, *34*, 227–239. [CrossRef] [PubMed]
15. Lozano Rojas, O.M.; Rojas Tejada, A.J.; Pérez Meléndez, C. Development of a specific health-related quality of life test in drug abusers using the Rasch rating scale model. *Eur. Addict. Res.* **2009**, *15*, 63–70. [CrossRef] [PubMed]
16. Zhang, M.; Zhang, H.; Shi, C.X.; McGoogan, J.M.; Zhang, B.; Zhao, L.; Zhang, M.; Rou, K.; Wu, Z. Sexual dysfunction improved in heroin-dependent men after methadone maintenance treatment in Tianjin, China. *PLoS ONE* **2014**, *9*, e88289. [CrossRef] [PubMed]
17. Quaglio, G.; Lugoboni, F.; Pattaro, C.; Melara, B.; Mezzelani, P.; Des Jarlais, D.C. Erectile dysfunction in male heroin users, receiving methadone and buprenorphine maintenance treatment. *Drug Alcohol Depend.* **2008**, *94*, 12–18. [CrossRef] [PubMed]
18. Grover, S.; Mattoo, S.K.; Pendharkar, S.; Kandappan, V. Sexual dysfunction in patients with alcohol and opioid dependence. *Indian J. Psychol. Med.* **2014**, *36*, 355–365. [CrossRef] [PubMed]
19. Yee, A.; Loh, H.S.; Ng, C.G.; Sulaiman, A.H. Sexual Desire in Opiate-Dependent Men Receiving Methadone-Assisted Treatment. *Am. J. Mens Health* **2018**, *12*, 1016–1022. [CrossRef] [PubMed]
20. Hanbury, R.; Cohen, M.; Stimmel, B. Adequacy of sexual performance in men maintained on methadone. *Am. J. Drug Alcohol Abuse* **1977**, *4*, 13–20. [CrossRef] [PubMed]
21. Jaafar, N.R.N.; Mislan, N.; Aziz, S.A.; Baharudin, A.; Ibrahim, N.; Midin, M.; Das, S.; Sidi, H. Risk Factors of Erectile Dysfunction in Patients Receiving Methadone Maintenance Therapy. *J. Sex. Med.* **2013**, *10*, 2069–2076. [CrossRef] [PubMed]
22. Gerra, G.; Manfredini, M.; Somaini, L.; Maremmani, I.; Leonardi, C.; Donnini, C. Sexual Dysfunction in Men Receiving Methadone Maintenance Treatment: Clinical History and Psychobiological Correlates. *Eur. Addict. Res.* **2016**, *22*, 163–175. [CrossRef] [PubMed]
23. Trajanovska, A.S.; Vujovic, V.; Ignjatova, L.; Janicevic-Ivanovska, D.; Cibisev, A. Sexual dysfunction as a side effect of hyperprolactinemia in methadone maintenance therapy. *Med. Arch Sarajevo Bosnia Herzeg* **2013**, *67*, 48–50. [CrossRef]
24. Quinta Gomes, A.L.; Nobre, P. Personality traits and psychopathology on male sexual dysfunction: An empirical study. *J. Sex. Med.* **2011**, *8*, 461–469. [CrossRef] [PubMed]
25. Crisp, C.C.; Vaccaro, C.M.; Pancholy, A.; Kleeman, S.; Fellner, A.N.; Pauls, R. Is female sexual dysfunction related to personality and coping? An exploratory study. *Sex. Med.* **2013**, *1*, 69–75. [CrossRef] [PubMed]
26. Zhong, B.-L.; Xu, Y.-M.; Zhu, J.-H.; Li, H.-J. Sexual life satisfaction of methadone-maintained Chinese patients: Individuals with pain are dissatisfied with their sex lives. *J. Pain Res.* **2018**, *11*, 1789–1794. [CrossRef] [PubMed]
27. Uhde, T.W.; Tancer, M.E.; Shea, C.A. Sexual dysfunction related to alprazolam treatment of social phobia. *Am, J. Psychiatry. abril de* **1988**, *145*, 531–532.

28. Mazzilli, R.; Angeletti, G.; Olana, S.; Delfino, M.; Zamponi, V.; Rapinesi, C.; Del Casale, A.; Kotzalidis, G.D.; Elia, J.; Callovini, G.; et al. Erectile dysfunction in patients taking psychotropic drugs and treated with phosphodiesterase-5 inhibitors. *Arch. Ital. Urol. Androl.* **2018**, *90*, 44–48. [CrossRef] [PubMed]
29. Montejo-González, A.L.; Llorca, G.; Izquierdo, J.A.; Ledesma, A.; Bousoño, M.; Calcedo, A.; Carrasco, J.L.; Ciudad, J.; Daniel, E.; De la Gandara, J. SSRI-induced sexual dysfunction: Fluoxetine, paroxetine, sertraline, and fluvoxamine in a prospective, multicenter, and descriptive clinical study of 344 patients. *J. Sex Marital Ther.* **1997**, *23*, 176–194. [CrossRef] [PubMed]

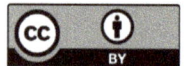

© 2019 by the authors. Licensee MDPI, Basel, Switzerland. This article is an open access article distributed under the terms and conditions of the Creative Commons Attribution (CC BY) license (http://creativecommons.org/licenses/by/4.0/).

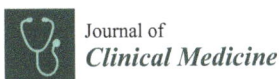

Article

Same Same but Different: A Clinical Characterization of Men with Hypersexual Disorder in the Sex@Brain Study

Jannis Engel [1,*], Maria Veit [1], Christopher Sinke [1], Ivo Heitland [1], Jonas Kneer [1], Thomas Hillemacher [1,2], Uwe Hartmann [1] and Tillmann H.C. Kruger [1]

1. Department of Psychiatry, Social Psychiatry and Psychotherapy, Hannover Medical School, Carl-Neuberg-Str. 1, 30625 Hannover, Germany; veit.maria@mh-hannover.de (M.V.); sinke.christoph@mh-hannover.de (C.S.); heitland.ivo-aleksander@mh-hannover.de (I.H.); kneer.jonas@mh-hannover.de (J.K.); thomas.hillemacher@klinikum-nuernberg.de (T.H.); hartmann.uwe@mh-hannover.de (U.H.); krueger.tillmann@mh-hannover.de (T.H.C.K.)
2. Department for Psychiatry and Psychotherapy, Paracelsus University Hospital Nuremberg, Prof. Ernst-Nathan-Str. 1, 90419 Nürnberg, Germany
* Correspondence: engel.jannis@mh-hannover.de; Tel.: +49-511-532-2631

Received: 19 December 2018; Accepted: 28 January 2019; Published: 30 January 2019

Abstract: Problems arising from hypersexual behavior are often seen in clinical settings. We aimed to extend the knowledge about the clinical characteristics of individuals with hypersexual disorder (HD). A group of people who fulfilled the proposed diagnostic criteria for HD (men with HD, $n = 50$) was compared to a group of healthy controls ($n = 40$). We investigated differences in sociodemographic, neurodevelopmental, and family factors based on self-report questionnaires and clinical interviews. Men with HD reported elevated rates of sexual activity, paraphilias, consumption of child abusive images, and sexual coercive behavior compared to healthy controls. Moreover, rates of affective disorders, attachment difficulties, impulsivity, and dysfunctional emotion regulation strategies were higher in men with HD. Men with HD seem to have experienced various forms of adverse childhood experiences, but there were no further differences in sociodemographic, neurodevelopmental factors, and family factors. Regression analyses indicated that attachment-related avoidance and early onset of masturbation differentiated between men with HD and healthy controls. In conclusion, men with HD appear to have the same neurodevelopment, intelligence levels, sociodemographic background, and family factors compared to healthy controls, but they report different and adverse experiences in childhood, problematic sexual behavior, and psychological difficulties.

Keywords: hypersexuality; sexual addiction; sexual compulsivity; phenomenology; comorbidities

1. Introduction

Hypersexual disorder (HD) is characterized by intense, repetitive sexual fantasies, urges, and behaviors that lead to clinically significant psychological impairment [1–3]. Kafka [3] proposed that hypersexual disorder should be included as a category in the Diagnostic and Statistical Manual of Mental Disorders, 5th edition (DSM-5) [4], but the proposal was ultimately rejected. One of the reasons given was the lack of experimental research on hypersexual disorder [5,6]. In the forthcoming version of the International Classification of Diseases, ICD-11, hypersexual disorder will be classified as compulsive sexual behavior disorder [7].

Alarming numbers are shown by a recent representative study of men ($n = 1151$) and women ($n = 1174$) in the United States that found 10.3% of men and 7% of women showed clinically relevant levels of distress and/or impairment due to difficulties in controlling sexual urges, feelings, and behaviors [8]. Manifestations of hypersexual behavior can include both real-world sexual contacts and online sexual activities. Online use of sexual content in combination with masturbation is the most common behavior that leads to men being diagnosed with hypersexual disorder according to the Kafka criteria [3,9].

Cooper [10] pointed out that the triad of access, affordability, and anonymity enables people to access whatever content they like anonymously, regardless of economic and social constraints. Of course, internet usage patterns vary greatly between individuals with some engaging excessively in online sexual activities [11] whereas others use dating platforms to find partners for sexual encounters [12]. The main driving forces for excessive online sexual activity may be the anticipated and experienced gratification associated with sexual arousal and the accessibility of virtually all types of sexual stimulus [13].

Little is known about the clinical characteristics of people with HD. Data from a study without a control group suggest that most subjects with men with HD are in intimate relationships, educated, and employed [14]; however, many also report intimacy deficits due to disengagement from family and a history of sexual, physical, and/or emotional abuse [15]. Intensive use of pornography [16,17] and hypersexual behavior in general [18] have been linked to risky sexual behaviors. Studies indicate that psychiatric comorbidities, particularly mood disorders, are prevalent in HD with rates ranging from 72%–90% in the case of mood disorders [14,19–21], and 42% in the case of substance use disorders [22]. Findings on the relationship between hypersexual disorder and impulsivity are mixed. Two studies [23,24] of treatment-seeking individuals fulfilling the proposed criteria for hypersexual disorder [3] found that between 48% and 53.3% displayed elevated impulsivity in self-report measures. Reid, Berlin, and Kingston [25] suggested that a context-specific form of sexual impulsivity, but not general impulsivity, might be prevalent in hypersexual disorder. Hypersexual behavior has been shown to be associated with neuropsychological impairments and alterations in attentional bias [26] and executive control [27,28].

From a biological perspective, the testosterone system plays a crucial role for the development and maintenance of sexual behavior [29]. As a marker of prenatal androgen exposure, the ratio of the lengths of the second and fourth digits (2D:4D) can be used, and there is some evidence that a lowered 2D:4D ratio might be connected to hypersexual behavior [30], although mixed findings have been reported. Some studies of the general population have demonstrated that a lower 2D:4D ratio (a more masculine pattern) is linked to having a higher number of sexual partners and more offspring [30–32], whereas others have shown that a high 2D:4D ratio is linked to promiscuity in men [33].

The aim of this study was to investigate the clinical and some specific (neuro-)developmental characteristics of men with hypersexual disorder in a large sample of people who fulfill the proposed diagnostic criteria [3] and compare them with healthy controls. Furthermore, detailed analyses should identify potential risk factors contributing to hypersexual behavior, such as biographical factors, i.e., adverse childhood events and attachment difficulties [34], as well as early age of sexual interest [35]. We present data on parameters not previously measured in comparable samples and we discuss the results in the light of the current understanding of hypersexuality.

2. Experimental Section

2.1. Recruitment

2.1.1. Hypersexual Disorder Group

Men with HD were recruited between December 2016 and August 2017 through a press release by the Section of Clinical Psychology and Sexual Medicine, Department of Psychiatry, Social Psychiatry, and Psychotherapy at Hannover Medical School, Germany. The press release was taken up by local newspapers and social media (e.g., www.facebook.com, www.instagram.com) and resulted in 539 self-identified men with HD expressing an interest in participating in the study (see Figure 1). Two-hundred-and-sixty men responded to an email asking for a telephone number. Fifty-nine of the 260 individuals who provided a telephone number could not be reached by telephone, but the remaining 201 were screened for hypersexual disorder in a semi-standardized telephone interview of about 45 minutes carried out by a trained psychologist using Kafka's [3] proposed criteria. Individuals were eligible for the study if they fulfilled Kafka's [3] proposed criteria for hypersexual disorder. The questionnaires used in this study were sent by mail to eligible participants. Three participants whose scores did not reach the cut-off (53) of Hypersexual Behavior Inventory 19 [36] were excluded post hoc. Kafka's [3] criteria for hypersexual disorder consist of clinically significant symptoms that arise from sexual urges, fantasies or behaviors, and recur over a period of 6 months that individuals struggle to control and are not due to the direct physiological effect of an exogenous substance. Seventy-three of the 201 individuals who were screened met these criteria and were deemed eligible for the study; 50 decided to participate and they formed the hypersexual disorder group (HD group, see Figure 1 chart).

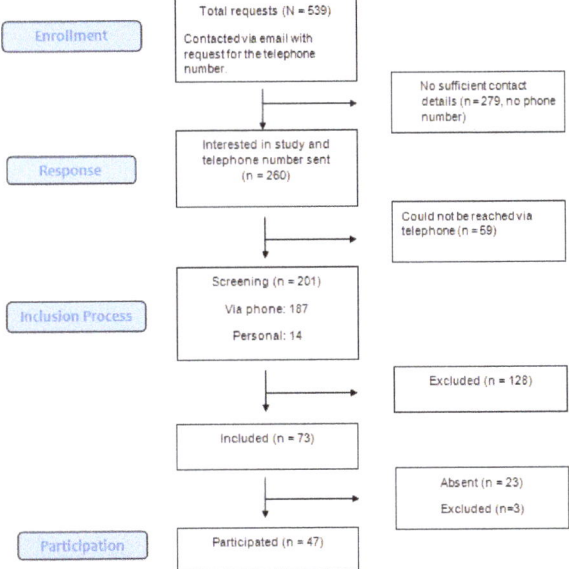

Figure 1. Recruitment of the hypersexual disorder group.

2.1.2. Healthy Controls

Healthy controls were recruited via advertisements on the Hannover Medical School, Germany, intranet homepage. Eighty-five individuals responded to the advertisements (see Figure 2) of whom 56 responded to an email asking for a telephone number. Twenty-nine of these 56 could not be reached via telephone for screening. The controls were matched for age ($p = 0.587$) and education ($p = 0.503$) with HD group. Data from two healthy controls were subsequently excluded from analysis (one reported a severe head injury prior to study participation, one reported a homosexual orientation, and one control participant did not show up to assessment).

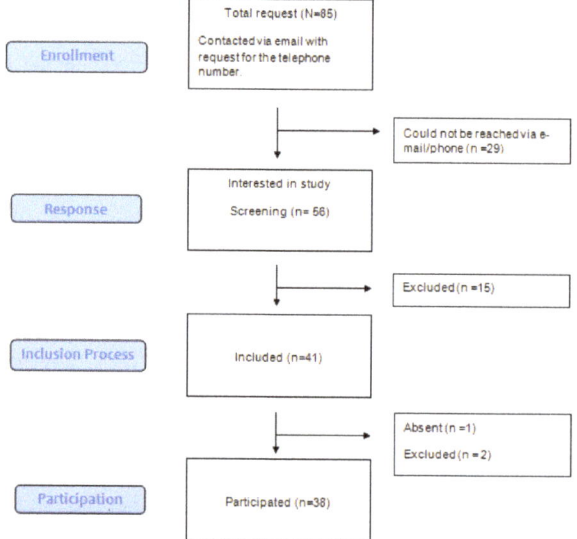

Figure 2. Recruitment of healthy controls.

2.1.3. Exclusion Criteria

Exclusion criteria for all participants were: intellectual disability (as measured by Wechsler Adult Intelligent Scale-IV), a psychotic disorder (assessed with Structured Clinical Interview for DSM-IV Axis 1 disorders, SCID-I), severe head injury, homosexual orientation on the Kinsey scale, and pedophilic sexual preference (assessed in a semi-structured interview). In our Sex@brain project we focused on heterosexual participants due to the heterosexual nature of the stimuli in the upcoming experiments. All participants declared that their primary sexual interest was in women although some reported a history of same-sex sexual contact.

All participants provided written, informed consent before participating and received monetary compensation for participation. They were informed that they could withdraw from the study at any time. The study was conducted in accordance with the Declaration of Helsinki and was approved by the ethics commission of the Hannover Medical School, Germany. The results reported here were obtained as part of a larger assessment that included a neuropsychological test battery and functional magnetic resonance imaging.

2.2. Measures

The variables were classified into three categories: (1) sociodemographic, neurodevelopmental, and family factors, (2) sexual characteristics, and (3) psychological characteristics including psychiatric comorbidities. For an exact description of items please see the notes to Tables 1–4.

2.2.1. Sociodemographic, Neurodevelopmental, and Family Factors

A questionnaire was used to collect sociodemographic data, namely age, highest educational qualification, employment status, lifetime criminal history, and relationship status. There were also questions about neurodevelopmental perturbations, sibling position, parental health at birth, and maternal and paternal age at birth. Aversive childhood experiences were assessed with the Childhood Trauma Questionnaire (CTQ) [37]. The developmental and neurodevelopmental perturbations investigated were birth complications, prolonged bedwetting, delayed walking, delayed speech development, and childhood accidents leading to unconsciousness. Handedness was determined using a 10-item adaptation of the Edinburgh Handedness Inventory [38] and 2D:4D ratio was estimated using images obtained from a portable scanner. The lengths of digits of the right hand were estimated independently by two research assistants (inter-rater reliability: $r = 0.83$) and calculations were based on the means of the two ratings.

Intelligence was estimated from the four subtests of the fourth edition of the Wechsler Adult Intelligent Scale (WAIS-IV) [39] that are most highly correlated with full scale IQ as measured by the German WAIS-IV. These four subtests are Vocabulary (verbal comprehension; $r = 0.7$), Block Design (perceptual reasoning; $r = 0.65$), Arithmetic (working memory; $r = 0.73$), and Coding (processing speed; $r = 0.5$).

2.2.2. Sexual Characteristics

Sexual development and behavior were assessed via a semi-structured interview and a set of questionnaires. We collected data on age at first ejaculation, masturbation in the week prior to assessment (duration and frequency), intercourse in the week prior to assessment, and lifetime total of sexual partners. Moreover, we assessed duration and frequency of pornography consumption, number of affairs, paraphilias, sexual coercive behavior, consumption of child abuse images, and sexual dysfunctions. Specific instruments were used to measure sexual excitation and inhibition proneness (Sexual Excitation Scale, SES and Sexual Inhibition Scale, SIS) [40], symptoms of hypersexual disorder (Hypersexual Behavior Inventory-19, HBI-19) [36], symptoms of cybersex addiction (Internet Addiction Test for online sexual activities—short version, sIATsex; [41] and sexual addiction (Sexual Addiction Screening Test-Revised, SAST-R) [42].

2.2.3. Psychological Characteristics and Comorbidities

Psychiatric comorbidities were diagnosed using the German version of the SCID-I [43]. Additional questionnaires were used to assess impulsivity (Barrat Impulsiveness Scale-11, BIS-11) [44], substance abuse (Fagerström Test for Nicotine Dependence, FTND) [45], hazardous and harmful patterns of alcohol consumption (The Alcohol Use Disorder Identification Test, AUDIT) [46], depressive symptoms (Beck Depression Inventory-II, BDI-II) [47], bonding (Experiences in Close Relationships-Revised, ECR-R) [48], alexithymia (Toronto Alexithymia Scale, TAS-26) [49], and emotion regulation (ERQ, Emotion Regulation Questionnaire [50]; Fragebogen zur Erhebung der Emotionsregulation, FEEL-E) [51].

Attention deficit hyperactivity disorder (ADHD) was diagnosed on the basis of scores ≥ 15 on both the Wender Utah Rating Scale (WURS-K) [52] and ADHD self-assessment scale (ADHS-SB) [53].

2.2.4. Logistic Regression Analysis

To identify possible predictive factors for hypersexual disorder we carried out a binary logistic regression analysis with group classification as dichotomous dependent variables. Our aim was to identify factors that differentiated between men with HD and healthy controls. The number of independent variables was chosen on recommendations by Agresti [54] (p. 138).

2.3. Data Analysis

All analyses were executed with SPSS Statistics Version 24 (IBM® Corporation, Amonk, NY, USA). Analyses were carried out using independent t-tests, Mann–Whitney U tests or Fisher's exact tests for dichotomous variables. Fisher tests for tables larger than 2×2 were also used, as all polytomous categorical variables had at least one expected cell frequency of less than 5. As this was one of the first extensive phenomenological studies that included both men with hypersexual disorder and healthy controls in the search for group differences regarding the theoretically derived set of clinical variables tested here, we opted for an exploratory approach and report two-tailed significance levels without correction for multiple comparisons (all analyses $p < 0.05$). However, for interested readers we also included Bonferroni corrected significance in Tables 1–4. Effect sizes for parametric tests were expressed as Cohen's d, with $d = 0.2$ indicating a small effect, $d = 0.5$ a medium effect, and $d = 0.8$ a large effect [55]. There are variations in group sizes on the various tests because questionnaires with missing data were excluded from analysis. To control for the effects of psychiatric disorders other than hypersexual disorder, all group comparisons were also computed after excluding participants with a history of any SCID-I diagnosis; this procedure yielded an N of 45 (HD = 21; HC = 22). The results of these analyses are presented in the Supplementary Materials.

3. Results

3.1. Sociodemographic, Neurodevelopmental, and Family Factors

As intended by subject matching there were no group differences in the sociodemographic variables regarding age ($t(83) = 0.55$, $p = 0.587$) and highest educational qualification (Fisher's exact test ($N = 85$), $p = 0.503$; see Table 1). Also, employment status (Fisher's exact test ($N = 85$), $p = 0.458$), lifetime criminal history (Fisher's exact test ($N = 85$), $p = 0.368$), and relationship status (Fisher's exact test ($N = 85$), $p = 0.128$) were not different between groups. There were also no differences in scores on the four WAIS-IV subscales used including the subtests vocabulary ($t(82) = -1.28$, $p = 0.204$), block design ($t(82) = 0.92$, $p = 0.359$), arithmetic ($t(82) = 0.112$, $p = 0.911$), and coding ($t(82) = 1.66$, $p = 0.100$), indicating similar intelligence levels among groups.

Indicators of neurodevelopmental perturbations were similar in men with HD and healthy controls including general developmental factors during childhood (Fisher's exact test ($N = 82$), $p = 1$) distribution of handedness (Fisher's exact test ($N = 85$), $p = 0.645$) and 2D:4D finger length ratio ($t(77) = 0.34$, $p = 0.738$).

Our data show that men with HD and healthy controls grew up in families with similar structural family factors such as number of children in the household in which the participant grew up ($t(78) = 0.01$, $p = 0.995$); position in the birth order ($w(78) = 718$, $z = -0.402$, $p = 0.687$); position among children in the household ($w(78) = 750$, $z = -0.464$, $p = 0.642$); maternal age at birth ($t(79) = 0.88$, $p = 0.384$); and paternal age at birth ($t(73) = 0.09$, $p = 0.93$). Men with HD reported more frequently maternal psychiatric problems (Fisher's exact test ($N = 62$), $p = 0.001$), but not paternal psychiatric problems (Fisher's exact test ($N = 68$), $p = 0.307$) than healthy controls. Furthermore, the aversive childhood memories of men with HD differed substantially from healthy controls. Men with HD reported elevated rates of overall adverse childhood experiences (CTQ; $t(68) = 2.71$, $p = 0.009$, $d = 0.57$), in particular emotional abuse ($t(73) = 3.53$, $p < 0.001$, $d = 0.73$), emotional neglect ($t(81) = 2.46$, $p = 0.016$, $d = 0.54$), and sexual abuse ($t(45) = 2.49$, $p = 0.017$, $d = 0.49$) compared to healthy controls. However, physical abuse ($t(80) = 1.60$, $p = 0.113$) and physical neglect ($t(83) = 1.49$, $p = 0.141$) did not reach statistical significance.

Table 1. Sociodemographic, neurodevelopmental, and family factors.

	Hypersexual Disorder Group ($n = 47$)		Healthy Volunteers ($n = 38$)		p-Value	d
Sociodemographic Variables	%	M (SD)	%	M (SD)		
Age		36.51 (11.47)		37.92 (12.33)	0.587 [a]	
Highest educational qualification [b]						
no school-leaving qualification	2		0			
secondary school leaving certificate of 4 years secondary education	4		3			
secondary school leaving certificate (5 years)	11		5		0.503 [c]	
completed apprenticeship	28		26			
secondary school leaving certificate (8 years)	21		40			
university degree	34		26			
Employment status [d]						
unemployed	9		14			
in training	27		30		0.458 [c]	
retired	4		8			
employed	66		48			
Lifetime criminal history (yes) [e]	19		11		0.368 [c]	
Current intimate relationship (yes)	43		61		0.128 [c]	

Table 1. Cont.

	Hypersexual Disorder Group ($n = 47$)	Healthy Volunteers ($n = 38$)	p-Value	d
Neurodevelopmental Factors				
Developmental perturbations (yes) [f]	43	42	1 [c]	
Handedness [g]				
right	83	79		
left	4	10.5	0.645 [c]	
ambidextrous	13	10.5		
2D:4D finger length ratio [h]	0.97 (.33)	0.96 (0.29)	0.738 [a]	
Family Factors				
Number of siblings	1.51 (1.42)	1.51 (0.93)	0.995 [a]	
Position in the birth order [i]	1.67 (0.95)	1.72 (0.82)	0.687 [j]	
Position among children in the household [k]	1.57 (0.94)	1.72 (0.82)	0.642 [j]	
Age at participants birth				
Paternal	30.02 (8.41)	29.88 (4.57)	0.930 [a]	
Maternal	27.64 (7.77)	26.35 (4.79)	0.384 [a]	
Childhood Trauma Questionnaire (CTQ) [l,m]	57.42 (16.06)	49.97 (8.38)	0.009 [a,*]	0.57
Emotional abuse	10.13 (4.76)	7.29 (2.51)	0.001 [a,†,*]	0.73
Physical abuse	7.32 (3.67)	6.26 (2.38)	0.113 [a]	
Sexual abuse	6.28 (2.38)	5.03 (3.42)	0.017 [a,*]	0.49
Emotional neglect	11.74 (4.86)	9.24 (3.5)	0.016 [a,*]	0.54
Physical neglect	7.34 (3.02)	6.53 (1.67)	0.141 [a]	
Psychiatric problems [n]				
Father (yes)	20	3	0.307 [c]	
Mother (yes)	39	9	0.001 [c,†,*]	
Intelligence [WAIS-IV] [o]				
Vocabulary	46.26 (7.40)	43.97 (8.97)	0.204 [a]	
Block-design-test	48.91 (9.68)	50.79 (8.77)	0.359 [a]	
Arithmetic	17.15 (3.10)	17.24 (3.84)	0.911 [a]	
Coding	66.67 (15.73)	71.92 (12.62)	0.1 [a]	

Note. [a] Statistical analysis: t-test. [b] 0 = no school-leaving qualification; 1 = secondary school leaving certificate of secondary education (4 years); 2 = secondary school leaving certificate (5 years); 3 = completed apprenticeship 4 = secondary school leaving certificate (8 years); 5 = university degree. [c] Statistical analysis: Fishers exact test. [d] 0 = unemployed; 1 = in training; 2 = retired; 3 = employed. [e] Criminal status was assessed with a semi-structured interview (voluntary disclosure of confidential information) in which we asked participants to disclose all incidents of criminal behavior regardless of whether they had resulted in conviction. Lifetime history of any criminal behavior was coded 1; absence of criminal behavior was coded 0. [f] Assessed with a semi-structured questionnaire. Coded 1 if any of the following problems had occurred, otherwise coded 0: Complications at birth, problems with toilet training, problems with development of speech, problems with development of walking, head injuries, cranio-cerebral trauma, unconsciousness, childhood diseases (e.g., measles, mumps, rubella, diphtheria, chickenpox, poliomyelitis, meningitis, cerebral abscess, encephalitis and other illnesses resulting in a long stay in hospital). [g] Handedness was assessed using a 10-item adaptation of the German version of the Edinburgh Handedness Inventory [38]. [h] The participants' right hands were photocopied to measure individual finger lengths. This was done by laying the surface of the palm of the right hand onto a photocopier, the photocopied image was then used to estimate the ratio. The basal crease where the finger joins the palm and the distal point of the fingertip were used as landmarks to assess length. 2D:4D ratio was calculated by two independent raters, by dividing the length of the second digit by the length of the fourth digit. The computed means of the two raters were used. [i] Position in birth order with regard to mother's other children. (What position are you in the birth order of your full siblings and the half-siblings on your mother's side?). [j] Statistical analysis: Wilcoxon–Mann–Whitney Test. [k] Position with regard to children growing up in the same household. (What position are you with regard to the siblings you grew up with?). [l] Five dimensions of childhood trauma were assessed via retrospective self-reports using the German version of the Childhood Trauma Questionnaire [37]. [m] Higher values indicate more problems. [n] Participants were asked about maternal and paternal psychiatric problems in a semi-structured interview. Presence was coded 1, absence 0. [o] Sum scores in the German version of the Wechsler Adult Intelligence Scale WAIS—Fourth Edition [39]. * p-values < 0.05 were considered significant. † significant after Bonferroni α-correction. In this section p-values < 0.002 (0.05/22) were considered as significant.

3.2. Sexual Characteristics

The sexual history from men with HD differed substantially from healthy controls (see Table 2). First of all, men with HD had earlier sexual experiences than control group. Men with HD reported that they were over a year younger when they started masturbating ($t(79) = 3.59, p < 0.001, d = 0.80$) and about a year younger when they first ejaculated ($t(77) = 2.79, p = 0.007, d = 0.63$). But they did not differ in age of first intercourse ($t(83) = 1.868, p = 0.065$). Men with HD and healthy controls reported similar duration of last/current relationship in months ($t(42) = 0.14, p = 0.886$), and number of children ($w(75) = 728$, $z = -0.081, p = 0.936$). However, men with HD differed in their sexual relationships from healthy controls. On average men with HD reported about eighty more female sexual partners ($w(79) = 470.5$, $p = 0.001$) and female coital partners ($w(81) = 443$, $p < 0.000$) than healthy controls. Moreover, despite their predominant heterosexual orientation, men with HD reported sexual activities with men with more male sexual partners ($w(83) = 567.5$, $p < 0.000$) and male coital partners ($w(83) = 664$, $p = 0.002$), whereas healthy controls reported almost no sexual activities with men. Moreover, men with HD were more likely to report that they had an affair during their last or current relationship (Fisher's exact test ($N = 81$), $p < 0.001$), with 67% reporting an affair compared to only 19% in healthy controls. Furthermore, men with HD report more received problems through online sexual activities than healthy controls indicated by a group difference in sIATsex score ($t(80) = -11.70$, $p < 0.001$, $d = 2.45$). Accordingly, they reported that they consumed pornography more often in the week before the assessment (Fisher's exact test ($N = 84$), $p < 0.001$), about 85% of men with HD reported at least three times of pornography consumption per week, compared to about 40% in healthy controls. Moreover, men with HD watched on average about seventy minutes more of pornography ($t(47) = -3.61$, $p = 0.001$, $d = 0.73$) than healthy controls. Duration of pornography consumption varied greatly between groups, with more than half of men with HD watching over an hour per week, compared to only 9% in healthy controls. Relating to sexual excitation and inhibition, men with HD reported more pronounced sexual excitation (SES: $t(83) = 5.01$, $p < 0.001$, $d = 1.09$), a lower sexual inhibition due to threat of performance consequences (SIS2: $t(83) = -3.75$, $p < 0.001$, $d = 0.82$). However, men with HD showed a higher score for perceived threat of performance failure (SIS1; $t(80) = 2.30$, $p = 0.024$, $d = 0.48$). Interestingly, the prevalence of reported sexual dysfunction was similar in men with HD and healthy controls (Fisher's exact test ($N = 85$), $p = 0.765$), specifically there were no differences in erectile disorder, hypoactive desire disorder, premature and delayed ejaculation.

Table 2. Sexual characteristics.

	Hypersexual Disorder Group ($n = 47$)		Healthy Volunteers ($n = 38$)		p-Value	d
Sexual History and Development	%	M (SD)	%	M (SD)		
Onset of masturbation		11.16 (2.41)		12.97 (2.06)	<0.001 [a,†,*]	0.8
Age at first ejaculation		11.91 (1.67)		12.81 (1.06)	0.007 [a,*]	0.628
Age at first intercourse		16.57 (3.08)		17.71 (2.37)	0.065 [a]	
Number of sexual partners [b]						
Male		75.32 (376.12)		0.03 (0.16)	<0.001 [c,†,*]	
Female		99.10 (211.10)		19.24 (22.00)	0.001 [c,†,*]	
Number of coital partners [d]						
Male		16.90 (76.52)		0.03 (0.16)	0.002 [c,*]	
Female		86.71 (204.43)		15.00 (19.65)	<0.001 [c,†,*]	
Number of relationships		4.81 (3.51)		5.35 (3.82)	0.506 [a]	
Duration of last/current relationship [in month] [e]		66.90 (99.24)		70.67 (73.48)	0.886 [a]	
Number of children		0.74 (1.06)		0.77 (1.03)	0.936 [c]	
Affairs in last/current relationship (yes)	67		19		<0.001 [f,†,*]	
Consumption of pornography in the last week [g]						
5	35.5		0			
4	17.8		10.8			
3	31.1		27		<0.001 [f,†,*]	
2	6.7		21.6			
1	8.9		40.5			
Duration (minutes)		87.53 (125.50)		18.93 (19.82)	0.001 [c,†,*]	0.73
Hypersexual Behavior Inventory (HBI-19) [h,y]		72.37 (10.31)		30.26 (10.09)	<0.001 [a,†,*]	4.123
Sexual Addiction Screening Test (SAST-R) [i,y]		13.04 (3.20)		2.61 (2.71)	<0.001 [a,†,*]	3.49
Short Internet Addiction Test—modified for cybersex (sIATsex) [j,y]		39.62 (10.59)		17.11 (7.07)	<0.001 [a,†,*]	2.45
Sexual excitation (SES) [k,y]		60.92 (9.79)		50.41 (9.39)	<0.001 [a,†,*]	1.093
Sexual inhibition [k,y] (SIS1/Threat of performance failure)		35.79 (8.18)		32.39 (5.39)	0.024 [a,*]	0.481
Sexual inhibition [k,y] (SIS2/Threat of performance consequences)		25.66 (4.90)		29.45 (4.26)	<0.001 [a,†,*]	0.819
Sexual dysfunctions (yes) [l]	17		13		0.765 [f]	

Note. [a] Statistical analysis: t-test. [b] Number of partners with whom the participant engaged in sexual behavior of any kind (including petting). [c] Statistical analysis: Wilcoxon–Mann–Whitney U Test. [d] Number of partners with whom the participant in vaginal or anal intercourse. [e] Participants were asked: How long has your current relationship lasted? or How long did your last relationship last? [d] Positive responses to the question Have you had/did you have sex with others in your current/last relationship? were coded 1; negative responses were coded 0.

^{f} Statistical analysis: Fisher's exact test. ^{g} Frequency of pornography consumption was classified as follows: 5 = Several times a day, 4 = once a day, 3 = several times a week, 2 = once a week, 1 = less than that. ^{h} Hypersexual behavior was assessed using the Hypersexual Behavior Inventory-19, for which the suggested cut-off score is 53 [36]. ^{i} Sexual addiction was assessed using the first 20 Items of the Sexual Addiction Screening Test-Revised [42]. ^{j} Cybersex addiction was assessed using an adaption of an Internet Addiction Test [41]. ^{k} Propensity to sexual excitation and inhibition was assessed using German versions of the Sexual Inhibition and Sexual Excitation Scales. Sexual inhibition was assessed using two independent subscales "Threat of performance consequences" and "Threat of performance failure" [40]. ^{l} All data given in this section based on the ICD-10 criteria for sexual dysfunctions. ^{y} Higher values indicate greater problems. * p-values < 0.05 were considered significant. † significant after Bonferroni α-correction. In this section p-values < 0.002 (0.05/22) were considered as significant.

Paraphilias like exhibitionism, voyeurism, masochism, sadism, fetishism, frotteurism or transvestism were more prevalent in men with HD (Fisher's exact test ($N = 85$), $p < 0.001$) (see Table 3). Men with HD were also more likely to report sexually coercive behavior (Fisher's exact test ($N = 85$), $p < 0.001$) and a higher rate of having consumed images of child abuse at least once in their lives (Fisher's exact test ($N = 82$), $p = 0.009$); none of the healthy controls reported having consumed child abuse images.

Table 3. Sexual characteristics.

	Hypersexual Disorder Group ($n = 47$)		Healthy Volunteers ($n = 38$)		p-Value
	n	%	n	%	
Paraphilias (yes) ^{a}	22	47	1	3	<0.001 †,*
Exhibitionism (yes)	3	6	0	0	0.25
Voyeurism (yes)	5	11	0	0	0.062
Masochism (yes)	7	15	0	0	0.015 *
Sadism (yes)	5	11	0	0	0.062
Fetishism (yes)	16	34	1	3	<0.001 †,*
Frotteurism (yes)	4	8	0	0	0.125
Transvestism (yes)	1	2	0	0	1
Sexual coercive behavior (yes) ^{b}	33	70	8	21	<0.001 †,*
Lifetime consumption of images of child abuse (yes) ^{c}	38	81	0	0	0.009 *

Note. Statistical Analysis: Fisher's exact tests. ^{a} All data given in this section are based on the ICD-10 criteria for paraphilias. ^{b} Sexual violence was assessed using a four-item questionnaire asking about verbal assault, non-consensual sexual recordings, non-consensual touching/rubbing, and non-consensual penetration. ^{c} Consumption of images of child abuse was assessed with a semi-structured interview (voluntary disclosure of confidential information) in which participants were asked to disclose consumption regardless of whether this was known to the legal system. Any lifetime history of consumption of images of child abuse was coded 1; other responses were coded 0. * p-values < 0.05 were considered significant. † significant after Bonferroni α-correction. In this section p-values < 0.002 (0.05/22) were considered as significant.

3.3. Psychological Characteristics and Comorbidities

Most importantly, men with HD revealed more often psychiatric symptoms such as depression, impulsivity or symptoms of ADHD (see Table 4). Separate analysis of current diagnoses of SCID-I subcategories revealed a higher rate of affective disorders in the HD group (Fisher's exact test ($N = 85$), $p = 0.015$). This increased rate of diagnoses was supported by the psychometric assessment of depressive symptoms with higher symptoms in men with HD (BDI-II; $t(79) = 5.47$, $p < 0.001$, $d = 1.13$). Rates of current SCID-I diagnosis of substance abuse and/or dependency were similar in the two groups (Fisher's exact test ($N = 85$), $p = 1.000$), just as psychometric assessment of alcohol consumption (AUDIT; $t(82) = -0.93$, $p = 0.354$) and nicotine abuse (FTND; $t(83) = 0.73$, $p = 0.471$, $d = 0.16$). However, rates of current anxiety disorders (Fisher's exact test ($N = 85$), $p = 0.690$), obsessive-compulsive disorders (Fisher's exact test ($N = 85$), $p = 1.000$), and somatic symptoms and eating disorders (Fisher's exact test ($N = 85$), $p = 1.000$) did not differ between the groups. Taken together, men with HD and healthy controls showed similar proportions of current SCID-I (Fisher's exact test (N = 80), p = 0.104) and lifetime SCID-I diagnosis (Fisher's exact test (N = 85), p = 0.190). However, men with HD were more likely to display symptoms of ADHD at the time of assessment (ADHS/SB; t(73) = 6.31, p < 0.001, d = 1.37) and to report childhood symptoms of ADHD (WURS-K; t(82) = 3.76, p < 0.001, d = 0.82), Moreover, men with HD revealed greater impulsivity than healthy controls (BIS-11; t(81) = 3.76, p < 0.001, d = 0.83). The results relating to emotion regulation were mixed: men with HD were more likely to use maladaptive emotion regulation strategies (FEEL-E-maladaptive strategies; t(81)= 3.54, p < 0.001, d = 0.78) and "reappraisal" strategies (ERQ: Reappraisal; t(83) = −2.477, p =.015, d = 0.545) but use of adaptive strategies (FEEL-E-adaptive strategies; t(81) = −1.26, p = 0.212) was similar as was use of the "suppression" strategies (ERQ: Suppression; t(83) = 1.852, p = 0.068). Men with HD reported more symptoms of alexithymia (TAS-26; t(79) = 4.11, p < 0.001, d = 0.92) elevated scores in both, attachment-related anxiety (ECR-R anxiety: t(78) = 5.413, p < 0.000, d = 1.245) and attachment-related avoidance (ECR-R avoidance: t(82) = 4.908, p < 0.000, d = 1.064).

Table 4. Psychological characteristics and comorbidities.

	Hypersexual Disorder Group (n = 47)		Healthy Volunteers (n = 38)		p-Value	d
	%	M (SD)	%	M (SD)		
Lifetime Scid-i Diagnosis (yes) [a]	55		39		0.191	
Current Scid-i Diagnosis (yes) [a]	43		25		0.104	
Depression						
Lifetime affective disorders (SCID-I) [a]	50		13		<0.000 †,*	
Current affective disorders (SCID-I) [a]	15		0		0.015 *	
Symptoms of depression (BDI-II) [b,y]		17.25 (11.60)		5.92 (7.72)	<0.001 †,*	1.129
ADHD and impulsivity						
ADHD (ADHS-SB) [c,y]		21.74 (11.26)		8.43 (7.45)	0.001 †,*	1.374
Childhood symptoms of ADHD (WURS-K) [d,y]		26.59 (15.34)		15.00 (12.34)	0.001 †,*	0.824
Impulsivity levels (BIS-11) [e,y]		68.24 (11.22)		59.62 (9.25)	<0.001 †,*	0.83
Substance abuse						
Lifetime substance abuse and/or dependency (SCID-I) [a]	24		24		1	
Current substance abuse and/or dependency (SCID-I) [a]	23		21		1	
Alcohol abuse (AUDIT) [f,y]		6.57 (5.68)		7.68 (4.98)	0.354	
Nicotine dependence (FTND) [g,y]		3.87 (6.23)		2.95 (5.3)	0.471	
Lifetime anxiety disorders (SCID-I) [a]	11		8		0.724	
Current anxiety disorders (SCID-I) [a]	8		5		0.687	
Lifetime obsessive compulsive disorder (SCID-I) [a]	4		3		1	
Current obsessive compulsive disorder (SCID-I) [a]	4		3		1	
Lifetime somatic problems, eating disorder or other (SCID-I) [a]	4		0		0.499	
Current somatic problems, eating disorder or other (SCID-I) [a]	2		0		1	
Emotional Difficulties						
Symptoms of alexithymia (TAS-26) [h,y]		47.56 (10.31)		38.92 (8.35)	0.001 †,*	0.915
Maladaptive emotion regulation strategies (FEEL-E) [i]		107.51 (21.3)		91.68 (18.97)	<0.001 †,*	0.781
Adaptive emotion regulation strategies (FEEL-E) i		115.42 (18.4)		120.77 (20.28)	0.212	
Emotion Regulation: Reappraisal (ERQ) [j]		22.3 (8.62)		26.68 (7.45)	0.015 *	0.545
Emotion Regulation: Suppression (ERQ) [j]		16.19 (5.16)		14.18 (4.72)	0.068	
Attachment style: Anxiety (ECR-R) [k,y]		75.85 (22.84)		50.15 (18.17)	<0.000 †,*	1.245
Attachment style: Avoidance (ECR-R) [k,y]		57.87 (13.7)		41.35(17.16)	<0.000 †,*	1.064

Note. Statistical analysis for SCID-I diagnosis: Fisher's exact test, for all other analysis: t-test. [a] The Structured Clinical Interview for DSM-IV (SCID-I) [56] was used to determine the presence of psychiatric disorders. Presence of a disorder was coded 1, absence was coded 0. [b] Symptoms of depression were assessed using the Beck Depression Inventory-Second Edition [47]. [c] Childhood and adult problems with attention and hyperactivity were assessed using an 18-item self-report scale for the assessment of attention deficit hyperactivity disorder (ADHD) for adults [53]. [d] We screened for attention-deficit disorder using the short version of the Wender Utah Rating Scale [52]. [e] Impulsivity was assessed using the German translation of the Barratt Impulsiveness Scale (Barratt & Patton, 1995). [f] We screened for harmful alcohol consumption using the Alcohol Use Disorders Identification Test [46]. [g] Nicotine dependence was assessed using the Fagerström Test for Nicotine Dependence [45]. [h] Alexithymia was assessed using a German version of the Toronto Alexithymia Scale-26 [49]. [i] Use of adaptive and maladaptive emotion regulation strategies was assessed using the FEEL-E questionnaire [51]. [j] Emotion regulation strategies reappraisal and suppression were assessed using Emotion Regulation Questionnaire [50]. [k] Attachment style was assessed using the attachment-related anxiety and attachment-related avoidance subscales of the Experience in Close Relationships-Revised Scale [48]. [y] Higher values indicate greater problems.

3.4. Logistic Regression Analysis

The variables that differentiated best between men with HD and healthy controls were age at onset of masturbation (OR = 0.55, 95% CI (0.35, 0.86)) and avoidant attachment style (OR = 1.06, 95% CI (1.01,1.11)). Non-significant were child traumata and anxious attachment style. The specified regression model had a good fit (with Nagelkerke R^2 = 0.55 and Hosmer–Lemeshow Test: $\chi^2(7)$ = 11.76, df = 7, p = 0.11) and explained about 55% of the variance between the two groups. The mean classification accuracy was 80.0% (78.1% specificity, 81.4% sensitivity).

4. Discussion

This study is one of the first to analyze phenomenological data from a large sample of individuals who met the proposed criteria for hypersexual disorder [3] and compare them with a group of healthy controls. A considerable number of sociodemographic, neurodevelopmental, and family factors, as well as sexual characteristics, psychological characteristics, and comorbidities were investigated.

Through analysis of an extensive set of variables this study has revealed important differences between people diagnosed with hypersexual disorder and healthy controls.

In summary, men with HD seem to have experienced more difficulties during childhood than healthy controls, being more likely to have had a mother with psychiatric problems, to have experienced various forms of adverse experiences during childhood and to have displayed symptoms of childhood ADHD. Moreover, attachment difficulties with pronounced avoidance in close relationships were higher in men with HD. Onset of masturbation was at an earlier age in men with HD and they experienced higher sexual excitation and less sexual inhibition due to concern about negative consequences, but higher sexual inhibition due to threat of performance failure. Furthermore, men with HD were characterized by problems arising through subjective complaints through their high use of online sexual activities and reported more deviant sexual behaviors, namely higher rates of paraphilia, sexually coercive behavior, and consumption of images of child abuse. Diagnoses of affective disorders and symptoms of a large set of psychiatric comorbidities such as impulsivity, symptoms of adult ADHD, alexithymia, and maladaptive emotion regulation strategies were increased in men with HD.

There were indicators of differences in the childhood of men with HD compared to healthy controls. In our sample, dysfunctional emotion regulation strategies such as a lowered reappraisal and increased maladaptive strategies can be seen in men with HD, as well as increased alexithymia. Men with HD reported a higher rate of adverse childhood experiences; especially the rates of emotional abuse and neglect, as well as sexual abuse were increased, which have been shown to be associated to emotion regulation difficulties [57]. Moreover, maladaptive emotion regulation strategies in men with HD may be fostered by the psychiatric difficulties experienced by the child's mother [58] which were increased in men with HD. We argue that a possible path to HD is via a series of aversive states and experiences in childhood and adolescence which facilitates the development of maladaptive emotion regulation strategies [34]. Moreover, dysfunctional emotion regulation strategies may be associated to the attachment difficulties we observed in men with HD, as children show dysfunctional emotion regulation strategies when they are in a non-secure attachment to their mothers [59]. In a representative survey of the German population, use of online sexual activities was significantly associated to anxiously attached individuals [60]. Our regression analysis showed that avoidance in close relationships differentiated between men with HD and healthy controls, which is in line with Katehakis's [34] suggestion that some HD patients may have disengaged emotionally during childhood. This may lead to impaired development of the limbic system and parts of the prefrontal cortex, due to an adverse interaction involving the central nervous system, autonomic central nervous system, and hypothalamic–pituitary–adrenal axis [34].

Our findings are in line with findings suggesting that men with HD experience deficits in affect regulation and negative affect and may use hypersexual behavior as a maladaptive coping strategy [61]. These neurobiological deficits may develop in early childhood and may impair emotional and intellectual abilities [34]. However, we found only emotional disabilities and no differences in intelligence as measured by WAIS-IV subtests [39] were observed in this study and in a study with a smaller sample [62].

A disposition to hypersexual behavior may manifest early in sexual development, our HD group was characterized by an early onset of masturbation which differentiated significantly between men with HD and healthy controls in logistic regression analysis. Moreover, hypersexual behavior has been associated to early onset of sexual interest [35], and early onset of sexual behavior has been linked to sensation-seeking behavior, depression, and anxiety [63]. Frequency and duration of pornography consumption were higher in men with HD. However, it is important to note that not only the quantity of pornography consumption results in problems but that the relationship between frequency and duration of pornography use and treatment-seeking is not linear, but mediated by the severity of perceived negative symptoms associated with use of pornography [64]. The incentive salience theory of addiction [65,66], which has been applied to HD [26,62], posits that in addiction "wanting" stimuli becomes dissociated from "liking" stimuli. This could explain why men with HD continue with problematic behavior despite the perceived negative consequences. In fact, the men with HD in our sample report more problems due to their increased pornography consumption.

The important role of sexual excitation and inhibition in hypersexual behavior has been shown in large surveys [35,67]. The HD group in our sample reported higher sexual excitation and less sexual inhibition due to perceived threat of performance consequences, and thus higher sexual arousal. We argue that this specific pattern of sexual arousal is a vulnerability factor which, in combination with using sexual behavior as a dysfunctional emotion regulation strategy, increases the likelihood of developing hypersexual disorder. A study of a large online sample that used total number of sexual outlets as an indicator of sex drive found that high sexual interest was associated with self-reported consumption of images of child abuse [68]. In fact, in our sample no healthy control reported to have ever consumed child pornography as opposed to 80% of men with HD. Rates of sexual coercive behavior were increased in men with HD, showing highly increased rates of consumption of child abusive images in men with HD. Based on these results combined with meta-analyses that found hypersexuality to be an empirically supported risk factor in sexual recidivism [69], we encourage clinicians to assess criminal history and potential sexual coercive behavior in patients with HD.

Furthermore, we found increased rates of paraphilic interest in men with HD. To date, there are inconsistent findings on the association of paraphilic interests and HD. Some studies suggest increased rates of paraphilic interests [14], whereas in a field trial for the proposed criteria of HD [9] no connection was found. A possible explanation for divergent rates would be openness to report paraphilic interests, because in Germany information and data gathered in the course of research and treatment situations are protected by confidentiality, even when they include reports on paraphilic interest, child pornography consumption, and sexual coercive behavior. Paraphilic interest by itself (if no others are harmed) does not require or justify clinical intervention [4]; however, paraphilic interests are often associated with relationship difficulties [70]. Generally, the psychological burden represented by HD is one of the main findings to emerge from this study. Our data underline increased symptoms of some psychiatric comorbidities in HD. Especially, the diagnoses of both current and lifetime symptoms of affective disorders are increased in HD group. In our study, the score for symptoms of depression as measured by BDI-II was almost three times as high in men with HD as in healthy controls. In line with our findings, Weiss [71] found that the prevalence of depression was almost 2.5 times higher in men with HD than in the general population. Together the results of a range of studies investigating comorbid affective disorders in hypersexual disorder suggest the prevalence is between 28% and 42% [20,70,71]. Moreover, we suspect that impulsivity, particularly context-specific sexual impulsivity [25] is a characteristic of hypersexual disorder, based on our observation of increased impulsivity in men with HD and future studies should attempt to investigate this. Substance abuse is often connected to increased impulsivity. In our sample we found only increased impulsivity with a large effect size, but the rates of substance abuse did not differ between groups. There are theoretical and empirical studies suggesting that substance abuse plays a role in hypersexual behavior [22,72,73], but the picture remains unclear, since different studies have used different measures and sample sizes. Furthermore, future studies should investigate potential risky sexual behaviors in men with HD, which have been shown to be associated to a large variety of mental disorders [74].

Based on theoretical assumptions and our results, we created a working model for the etiology of hypersexual behavior (Figure 3). While there is no evidence of a monocausal etiology of hypersexual disorder, the model points out multiple components that may increase the possibility of developing hypersexual disorder. This working model may be useful for generating new research questions and adaptions of treatment programs.

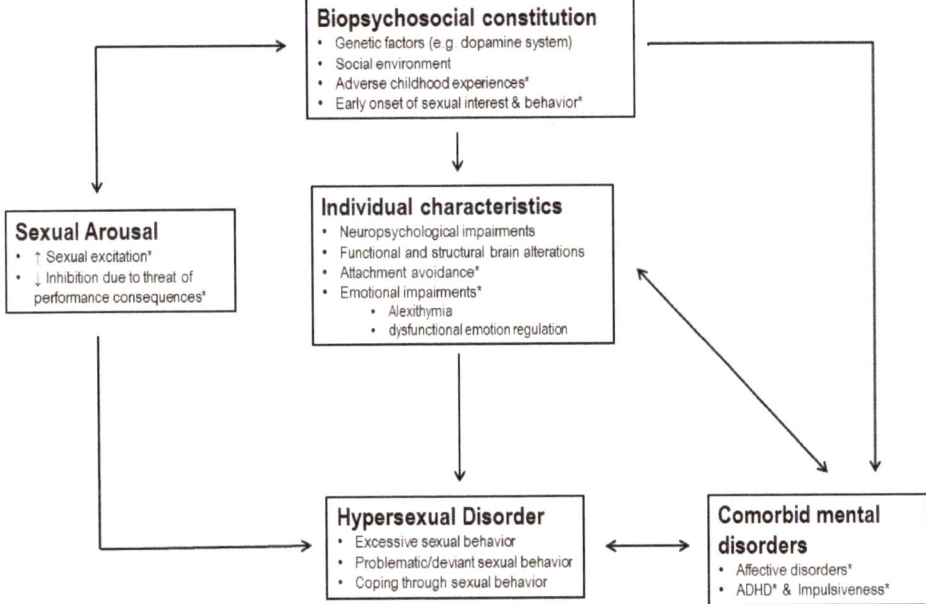

Figure 3. Working model of hypersexual disorder. We assume an underlying combination of genetic and environmental factors that may increase the likelihood of developing hypersexual disorder. A combination of biopsychosocial factors, e.g., genetic and epigenetic factors and adverse childhood events shape individual characteristics and increase the likelihood of developing comorbid psychiatric disorders. A high sexual arousal may be connected to genetic factors and may be both influenced by and influence early onset of sexual experiences. Dysfunctional characteristics of the individual, comorbid disorders, and high sexual arousal may lead to the development of hypersexual disorder. The factors marked with an asterisk were derived a posteriori from our results.

Our data have several implications for treatment. We suggest that clinicians assess possible emotional abuse and neglect, as well as sexual abuse in men with HD. Moreover, our data show that symptoms of comorbid adult ADHD were increased in men with HD and it has been suggested that these patients are likely to benefit from pharmacotherapy and behavioral therapy combined [75]. As a reduction of the use of dysfunctional emotion regulation strategies was seen in our sample, a cognitive-behavioral therapy should also focus on dysphoric mood states and impulsivity in men with HD [76]. A non-judgmental therapeutic approach is needed to tackle paraphilia, which is more frequent in men with HD. We found increased rates of sexual coercive behavior and consumption of child abusive images in men with HD, and if not restricted by limits of confidentiality, we suggest that an assessment by clinicians is strongly advised to prevent possible harmful behavior.

5. Limitation

It is important to note that that this sample consisted of individuals who volunteered to take part in a clinical study and agreed to report intimate details of life events, inner experiences, and sexual behavior. Thus, the characteristics of this sample may not be comparable to those of people with hypersexual disorder who are reluctant to share private information.

Causal explanations about the etiology of HD are difficult to draw, because—with the exception of 2D:4D ratio—we relied on self-report data and clinical interviews in a cross-sectional study and responses may have been affected by social desirability bias.

It is difficult to transfer the conclusions of this study to other cultures. Furthermore, this Western European sample was not representative of the Western European population in terms of, for example, age and educational level.

6. Conclusions

Men with HD appear to have the same neurodevelopment, intelligence levels, sociodemographic background, and family factors compared to healthy controls. However, men with HD report differences in important areas of life, such as adverse experiences in childhood, problematic sexual behavior, and increased psychological difficulties.

Supplementary Materials: The following are available online at http://www.mdpi.com/2077-0383/8/2/157/s1, Additional Analyses.

Author Contributions: Conceptualization, J.E., T.H., U.H., T.H.C.K., J.K.; methodology, J.E., M.V., C.S., I.H., T.H.C.K., formal analysis, J.E., M.V., writing—original draft preparation, J.E., writing—review and editing, J.E., I.H., C.S., M.V., T.H.C.K., U.H., supervision, T.H.C.K., U.H., C.S., T.H., funding acquisition, T.H.C.K., U.H., T.H., J.K.

Funding: The study was supported by a research grant from the European Society for Sexual Medicine.

Acknowledgments: The authors thank Marie-Jean Carstensen, Anna Spielvogel and Julia Liebnau for their assistance in creating the manuscript.

Conflicts of Interest: The material is original research and has not been previously published elsewhere. The authors declare no competing financial interests.

References

1. Derbyshire, K.L.; Grant, J.E. Compulsive sexual behavior: A review of the literature. *J. Behav. Addict.* **2015**, *4*, 37–43. [CrossRef] [PubMed]
2. Fong, T.W.; Reid, R.C.; Parhami, I. Behavioral addictions. Where to draw the lines? *Psychiatr. Clin. N. Am.* **2012**, *35*, 279–296. [CrossRef] [PubMed]
3. Kafka, M.P. Hypersexual Disorder: A Proposed Diagnosis for DSM-V. *Arch. Sex. Behav.* **2010**, *39*, 377–400. [CrossRef] [PubMed]
4. American Psychiatric Association. *Diagnostic and Statistical Manual of Mental Disorders*, 5th ed.; American Psychiatric Association: Washington, DC, USA, 2013; ISBN 089042554X.
5. Kafka, M.P. What happened to hypersexual disorder? *Arch. Sex. Behav.* **2014**, *43*, 1259–1261. [CrossRef] [PubMed]
6. Piquet-Pessôa, M.; Ferreira, G.M.; Melca, I.A.; Fontenelle, L.F. DSM-5 and the decision not to include sex, shopping or stealing as addictions. *Curr. Addict. Reports* **2014**, *1*, 172–176. [CrossRef]
7. Grant, J.E.; Atmaca, M.; Fineberg, N.A.; Fontenelle, L.F.; Matsunaga, H.; Janardhan Reddy, Y.C.; Simpson, H.B.; Thomsen, P.H.; Van Den Heuvel, O.A.; Veale, D.; et al. Impulse control disorders and "behavioural addictions" in the ICD-11. *World Psychiatry* **2014**, *13*, 125–127. [CrossRef]
8. Dickenson, J.A.; Gleason, N.; Coleman, E.; Miner, M.H. Prevalence of Distress Associated With Difficulty Controlling Sexual Urges, Feelings, and Behaviors in the United States. *JAMA Netw. Open* **2018**, *1*, e184468. [CrossRef]

9. Reid, R.C.; Carpenter, B.N.; Hook, J.N.; Garos, S.; Manning, J.C.; Gilliland, R.; Cooper, E.B.; Mckittrick, H.; Davtian, M.; Fong, T. Report of findings in a dsm-5 field trial for hypersexual disorder. *J. Sex. Med.* **2012**, *9*, 2868–2877. [CrossRef]
10. Cooper, A. Sexuality and the Internet: Surfing into the New Millennium. *CyberPsychology Behav.* **1998**, *1*, 187–193. [CrossRef]
11. Cooper, A.; Delmonico, D.L.; Burg, R. Cybersex users, abusers, and compulsives: New findings and implications. *Sex. Addict. Compulsivity J. Treat. Prev.* **2000**, *7*, 5–29. [CrossRef]
12. Döring, N.M. The Internet's impact on sexuality: A critical review of 15 years of research. *Comput. Hum. Behav.* **2009**, *25*, 1089–1101. [CrossRef]
13. Young, K.S. Internet Sex Addiction Risk Factors, Stages of Development, and Treatment. *Am. Behav. Sci.* **2008**, *52*, 21–37. [CrossRef]
14. Wéry, A.; Vogelaere, K.; Challet-Bouju, G.; Poudat, F.-X.; Caillon, J.; Lever, D.; Billieux, J.; Grall-Bronnec, M. Characteristics of self-identified sexual addicts in a behavioral addiction outpatient clinic. *J. Behav. Addict.* **2016**, *5*, 623–630. [CrossRef]
15. Carnes, P.J. Sexual addiction and compulsion: Recognition, treatment & recovery. *CNS Spectr.* **2000**, *5*, 63–72.
16. Carroll, J.S.; Padilla-Walker, L.M.; Nelson, L.J.; Olson, C.D.; Barry, C.M.; Madsen, S.D. Generation XXX: Pornography Acceptance and Use Among Emerging Adults. *J. Adolesc. Res.* **2008**, *23*, 6–30. [CrossRef]
17. Häggström-Nordin, E.; Hanson, U.; Tydén, T. Associations between pornography consumption and sexual practices among adolescents in Sweden. *Int. J. STD AIDS* **2005**, *16*, 102–107. [CrossRef]
18. Kalichman, S.C.; Cain, D. The relationship between indicators of sexual compulsivity and high risk sexual practices among men and women receiving services from a sexually transmitted infection clinic. *J. Sex Res.* **2004**, *41*, 235–241. [CrossRef]
19. Mick, T.M.; Hollander, E. Impulsive-Compulsive Sexual Behavior. *CNS Spectr.* **2006**, *11*, 944–955. [CrossRef]
20. Raymond, N.C.; Coleman, E.; Miner, M.H. Psychiatric comorbidity and compulsive/impulsive traits in compulsive sexual behavior. *Compr. Psychiatry* **2003**, *44*, 370–380. [CrossRef]
21. de Tubino Scanavino, M.; Ventuneac, A.; Abdo, C.H.N.; Tavares, H.; do Amaral, M.L.S.A.; Messina, B.; dos Reis, S.C.; Martins, J.P.L.B.; Parsons, J.T. Compulsive sexual behavior and psychopathology among treatment-seeking men in São Paulo, Brazil. *Psychiatry Res.* **2013**, *209*, 518–524. [CrossRef]
22. *Carnes Don't Call It Love*; Bantam Books: New York, NY, USA, 1991; ISBN 0-553-35138-9.
23. Reid, R.C.; Cyders, M.A.; Moghaddam, J.F.; Fong, T.W. Psychometric properties of the Barratt Impulsiveness Scale in patients with gambling disorders, hypersexuality, and methamphetamine dependence. *Addict. Behav.* **2014**, *39*, 1640–1645. [CrossRef] [PubMed]
24. Reid, R.C.; Dhuffar, M.K.; Parhami, I.; Fong, T.W. Exploring facets of personality in a patient sample of hypersexual women compared with hypersexual men. *J. Psychiatry Pract.* **2012**, *18*, 262–268. [CrossRef] [PubMed]
25. Reid, R.C.; Berlin, H.A.; Kingston, D.A. Sexual impulsivity in hypersexual men. *Curr. Behav. Neurosci. Rep.* **2015**, *2*, 1–8. [CrossRef]
26. Mechelmans, D.J.; Irvine, M.; Banca, P.; Porter, L.; Mitchell, S.; Mole, T.B.; Lapa, T.R.; Harrison, N.A.; Potenza, M.N.; Voon, V. Enhanced attentional bias towards sexually explicit cues in individuals with and without compulsive sexual behaviours. *PLoS ONE* **2014**, *9*, e105476. [CrossRef] [PubMed]
27. Reid, R.C.; Karim, R.; McCrory, E.; Carpenter, B.N. Self-reported differences on measures of executive function and hypersexual behavior in a patient and community sample of men. *Int. J. Neurosci.* **2010**, *120*, 120–127. [CrossRef]
28. Schiebener, J.; Laier, C.; Brand, M. Getting stuck with pornography? Overuse or neglect of cybersex cues in a multitasking situation is related to symptoms of cybersex addiction. *J. Behav. Addict.* **2015**, *4*, 14–21. [CrossRef]
29. Baumeister, R.F.; Catanese, K.R.; Vohs, K.D. Is there a gender difference in strength of sex drive? Theoretical views, conceptual distinctions, and a review of relevant evidence. *Personal. Soc. Psychol. Rev.* **2001**, *5*, 242–273. [CrossRef]
30. Hönekopp, J.; Bartholdt, L.; Beier, L.; Liebert, A. Second to fourth digit length ratio (2D:4D) and adult sex hormone levels: New data and a meta-analytic review. *Psychoneuroendocrinology* **2007**, *32*, 313–321. [CrossRef]
31. Hönekopp, J.; Voracek, M.; Manning, J.T. 2nd to 4th digit ratio (2D:4D) and number of sex partners: Evidence for effects of prenatal testosterone in men. *Psychoneuroendocrinology* **2006**, *31*, 30–37. [CrossRef]

32. Klimek, M.; Andrzej, G.; Nenko, I.; Alvarado, L.C.; Jasienska, G. Digit ratio (2D:4D) as an indicator of body size, testosterone concentration and number of children in human males. *Ann. Hum. Biol.* **2014**, *41*, 518–523. [CrossRef]
33. Varella, M.A.C.; Valentova, J.V.; Pereira, K.J.; Bussab, V.S.R. Promiscuity is related to masculine and feminine body traits in both men and women: Evidence from Brazilian and Czech samples. *Behav. Processes* **2014**, *109*, 34–39. [CrossRef] [PubMed]
34. Katehakis, A. Affective Neuroscience and the Treatment of Sexual Addiction. *Sex. Addict. Compulsivity* **2009**, *16*, 1–31. [CrossRef]
35. Walton, M.T.; Bhullar, N. Compulsive Sexual Behavior as an Impulse Control Disorder: Awaiting Field Studies Data. *Arch. Sex. Behav.* **2018**, *47*, 1327–1831. [CrossRef]
36. Reid, R.C.; Garos, S.; Carpenter, B.N. Reliability, validity, and psychometric development of the hypersexual behavior inventory in an outpatient sample of men. *Sex. Addict. Compulsivity* **2011**, *18*, 30–51. [CrossRef]
37. Bernstein, D.; Fink, L. *Manual for the Childhood Trauma Questionnaire (CTQ)*; The Psychological Corporation: New York, NY, USA, 1998.
38. Oldfield, R.C. The assessment and analysis of handedness: The Edinburgh inventory. *Neuropsychologia* **1971**, *9*, 97–113. [CrossRef]
39. Wechsler, D. *WAIS-IV Wechsler Adult Intelligence Scale Deutschsprachige Adaption*, 4th ed.; Petermann, F., Petermann, U., Eds.; Hogrefe: Göttingen, Germany, 2013.
40. Janssen, E.; Vorst, H.; Finn, P.; Bancroft, J. The sexual inhibition (SIS) and sexual excitation (SES) scales: I. Measuring sexual inhibition and excitation proneness in men. *J. Sex Res.* **2002**, *39*, 114–126. [CrossRef]
41. Pawlikowski, M.; Altstötter-Gleich, C.; Brand, M. Validation and psychometric properties of a short version of Young's Internet Addiction Test. *Comput. Hum. Behav.* **2013**, *29*, 1212–1223. [CrossRef]
42. Carnes, P.; Green, B.; Carnes, S. The same yet different: Refocusing the Sexual Addiction Screening Test (SAST) to reflect orientation and gender. *Sex. Addict. Compulsivity* **2010**, *17*, 7–30. [CrossRef]
43. Wittchen, H.U.; Wunderlich, U.; Gruschwitz, S.; Zaudig, M. *SKID I. Strukturiertes Klinisches Interview für DSM-IV. Achse I: Psychische Störungen. Interviewheft und Beurteilungsheft. Eine deutschsprachige, erweiterte Bearb. d. amerikanischen Originalversion des SKID I*; Hogrefe: Göttingen, Germany, 1997.
44. Patton, J.H.; Stanford, M.S.; Barratt, E.S. Barratt Impulsiveness Scale (BIS-11). *J. Clin. Psychol.* **1995**, *51*, 768–774. [CrossRef]
45. Fagerström, O.K.; Schneider, N.G. Fagerström Test for Nicotine Dependence. *J Behav Med.* **1989**, *12*, 159–181.
46. Saunders, J.B.; Aasland, O.G.; Babor, T.F.; De la Fuente, J.R.; Grant, M. Development of the alcohol use disorders identification test (AUDIT): WHO collaborative project on early detection of persons with harmful alcohol consumption-II. *Addiction* **1993**, *88*, 791–804. [CrossRef] [PubMed]
47. Hautzinger, M.; Keller, F.; Kühner, C. *Beck Depressions-Inventar II. Deutsche Bearbeitung und Handbuch zum BDI II.*; Harcourt Test Services: Frankfurt am Main, Germany, 2006.
48. Fraley, R.C.; Waller, N.G.; Brennan, K.A. An item response theory analysis of self-report measures of adult attachment. *J. Pers. Soc. Psychol.* **2000**, *78*, 350–365. [CrossRef] [PubMed]
49. Kupfer, J.; Brosig, B.; Brähler, E. *TAS-26: Toronto-Alexithymie-Skala-26 (deutsche Version)*; Hogrefe: Göttingen, Germany, 2001.
50. Gross, J.J.; John, O.P. Individual Differences in Two Emotion Regulation Processes: Implications for Affect, Relationships, and Well-Being. *J. Pers. Soc. Psychol.* **2003**, *85*, 348–362. [CrossRef] [PubMed]
51. Petermann, F. Fragebogen zur Erhebung der Emotionsregulation bei Erwachsenen (FEEL-E). *Zeitschrift fur Psychiatry Psychol. Psychother.* **2015**, *63*, 67–68. [CrossRef]
52. Retz-Junginger, P.; Retz, W.; Blocher, D.; Weijers, H.-G.; Trott, G.-E.; Wender, P.H.; Rössler, M. Wender Utah Rating Scale (WURS-k) Die deutsche Kurzform zur retrospektiven erfassung des hyperkinetischen syndroms bei erwachsenen. *Nervenarzt* **2002**, *73*, 830–838. [CrossRef] [PubMed]
53. Rösler, M.; Retz, W.; Retz-Junginger, P.; Thome, J.; Supprian, T.; Nissen, T.; Stieglitz, R.D.; Blocher, D.; Hengesch, G.; Trott, G.E. Instrumente zur Diagnostik der Aufmerksamkeitsdefizit-/Hyperaktivitätsstörung (ADHS) im Erwachsenenalter. *Nervenarzt* **2004**, *75*, 888–895. [CrossRef] [PubMed]
54. Agresti, A. *An Introduction to Categorical Data Analysis*, 2nd ed.; Wiley: Hoboken, NJ, USA, 2018; ISBN 1119405262.
55. Cohen, J. *Statistical Power Analysis for the Behavioral Sciences*, 2nd ed.; Erlbaum Associates: Hillsdale, NJ, USA, 1988; ISBN 9780805802832.

56. First, M.B.; Spitzer, R.L.; Gibbon, M.; Williams, J.B. *Structured Clinical Interview for DSM-IV Axis I Disorder*; New York State Psychiatric Institute: New York, NY, USA, 1995.
57. Carvalho Fernando, S.; Beblo, T.; Schlosser, N.; Terfehr, K.; Otte, C.; Löwe, B.; Wolf, O.T.; Spitzer, C.; Driessen, M.; Wingenfeld, K. The Impact of Self-Reported Childhood Trauma on Emotion Regulation in Borderline Personality Disorder and Major Depression. *J. Trauma Dissociation* **2014**, *15*, 384–401. [CrossRef]
58. Goodman, S.H.; Gotlib, I.H. Risk for Psychopathology in the Children of Depressed Mothers: A Developmental Model for Understanding Mechanisms of Transmission. *Psychol. Rev.* **1999**, *106*, 458–490. [CrossRef]
59. Waters, S.F.; Virmani, E.A.; Thompson, R.A.; Meyer, S.; Raikes, H.A.; Jochem, R. Emotion regulation and attachment: Unpacking two constructs and their association. *J. Psychopathol. Behav. Assess.* **2010**, *32*, 37–47. [CrossRef]
60. Beutel, M.E.; Giralt, S.; Wölfling, K.; Stöbel-Richter, Y.; Subic-Wrana, C.; Reiner, I.; Tibubos, A.N.; Brähler, E. Prevalence and determinants of online-sex use in the German population. *PLoS ONE* **2017**, *12*, 1–12. [CrossRef]
61. Reid, R.C.; Carpenter, B.N.; Spackman, M.; Willes, D.L. Alexithymia, emotional instability, and vulnerability to stress proneness in patients seeking help for hypersexual behavior. *J. Sex Marital Ther.* **2008**, *34*, 133–149. [CrossRef] [PubMed]
62. Voon, V.; Mole, T.B.; Banca, P.; Porter, L.; Morris, L.; Mitchell, S.; Lapa, T.R.; Karr, J.; Harrison, N.A.; Potenza, M.N.; et al. Neural correlates of sexual cue reactivity in individuals with and without compulsive sexual behaviours. *PLoS ONE* **2014**, *9*, e102419. [CrossRef] [PubMed]
63. Harries, M.D.; Paglia, H.A.; Redden, S.A.; Grant, J.E. Age at first sexual activity: Clinical and cognitive associations. *Ann. Clin. Psychiatry Off. J. Am. Acad. Clin. Psychiatry* **2018**, *30*, 102–112.
64. Gola, M.; Lewczuk, K.; Skorko, M. What matters: Quantity or quality of pornography use? Psychological and behavioral factors of seeking treatment for problematic pornography use. *J. Sex. Med.* **2016**, *13*, 815–824. [CrossRef] [PubMed]
65. Robinson, T.E.; Berridge, K.C. The neural basis of drug craving: An incentive-sensitization theory of addiction. *Brain Res. Rev.* **1993**, *18*, 247–291. [CrossRef]
66. Berridge, K.C.; Kringelbach, M.L. Affective neuroscience of pleasure: Reward in humans and animals. *Psychopharmacology* **2008**, *199*, 457–480. [CrossRef] [PubMed]
67. Rettenberger, M.; Klein, V.; Briken, P. The Relationship Between Hypersexual Behavior, Sexual Excitation, Sexual Inhibition, and Personality Traits. *Arch. Sex. Behav.* **2016**, *45*, 219–233. [CrossRef] [PubMed]
68. Klein, V.; Schmidt, A.F.; Turner, D.; Briken, P. Are sex drive and hypersexuality associated with pedophilic interest and child sexual abuse in a male community sample? *PLoS ONE* **2015**, *10*, 1–11. [CrossRef]
69. Mann, R.E.; Hanson, R.K.; Thornton, D. Assessing risk for sexual recidivism: Some proposals on the nature of psychologically meaningful risk factors. *Sex. Abuse J. Res. Treat.* **2010**, *22*, 191–217. [CrossRef]
70. Kafka, M.P.; Hennen, J. A DSM-IV Axis I Comorbidity Study of Males (*n* = 120) With Paraphilias and Paraphilia-Related Disorders. *Sex. Abuse* **2002**, *14*, 349–366. [CrossRef]
71. Weiss, D. The prevalence of depression in male sex addicts residing in the United States. *Sex. Addict. Compulsivity* **2004**, *11*, 57–69. [CrossRef]
72. Hagedorn, W.B. The call for a new Diagnostic and Statistical Manual of Mental Disorders diagnosis: Addictive disorders. *J. Addict. Offender Couns.* **2009**, *29*, 110–127. [CrossRef]
73. Kaplan, M.S.; Krueger, R.B. Diagnosis, assessment, and treatment of hypersexuality. *J. Sex Res.* **2010**, *47*, 181–198. [CrossRef] [PubMed]
74. Maclean, J.C.; Xu, H.; French, M.T.; Ettner, S.L. Mental health and risky sexual behaviors: Evidence from DSM-IV Axis II disorders. *J. Ment. Health Policy Econ.* **2013**, *16*, 187–208. [PubMed]
75. Reid, R.C.; Davtian, M.; Lenartowicz, A.; Torrevillas, R.M.; Fong, T.W. Perspectives on the assessment and treatment of adult ADHD in hypersexual men. *Neuropsychiatry* **2013**, *3*, 295–308. [CrossRef]
76. Hallberg, J.; Kaldo, V.; Arver, S.; Dhejne, C.; Öberg, K.G. A cognitive-behavioral therapy group intervention for hypersexual disorder: A feasibility study. *J. Sex. Med.* **2017**, *14*, 950–958. [CrossRef] [PubMed]

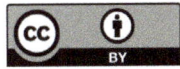

© 2019 by the authors. Licensee MDPI, Basel, Switzerland. This article is an open access article distributed under the terms and conditions of the Creative Commons Attribution (CC BY) license (http://creativecommons.org/licenses/by/4.0/).

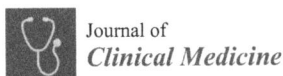

Article

Understanding the Mechanism of Antidepressant-Related Sexual Dysfunction: Inhibition of Tyrosine Hydroxylase in Dopaminergic Neurons after Treatment with Paroxetine but Not with Agomelatine in Male Rats

Yanira Santana [1], Angel L. Montejo [2,*], Javier Martín [3], Ginés LLorca [4], Gloria Bueno [4] and Juan Luis Blázquez [5]

1. Department of Psychiatry, Hospital Universitario de Salamanca, 37007 Salamanca, Spain; doctorayani@hotmail.com
2. University of Salamanca, IBSAL, Nursing School E.U.E.F., 37007 Salamanca, Spain
3. Department of Statistics, School of Medicine, University of Salamanca, 37007 Salamanca, Spain; jmv@usal.es
4. Department of Psychiatry, School of Medicine, University of Salamanca, 37007 Salamanca, Spain; gllorca@usal.es (G.L.); gloriabueno@usal.es (G.B.)
5. Department of Human Anatomy and Histology, IBSAL NEUR-2, School of Medicine, University of Salamanca, 37007 Salamanca, Spain; jlba@usal.es
* Correspondence: amontejo@usal.es; Tel.: +34-639-754-620

Received: 16 November 2018; Accepted: 21 January 2019; Published: 23 January 2019

Abstract: Antidepressant-related sexual dysfunction is a frequent adverse event caused by serotonergic activation that intensely affects quality of life and adherence in depressed patients. The dopamine system has multiple effects promoting sexual behavior, but no studies have been carried out to confirm dopaminergic changes involved in animal models after antidepressant use. Methods: The sexual behavior-related dopaminergic system in the rat was studied by comparing two different antidepressants and placebo for 28 days. The antidepressants used were paroxetine (a serotonergic antidepressant that causes highly frequent sexual dysfunction in humans) and agomelatine (a non-serotonergic antidepressant without associated sexual dysfunction). The tyrosine hydroxylase immunoreactivity (THI) in the substantia nigra pars compacta, the ventral tegmental area, the zona incerta, and the hypothalamic arcuate nucleus, as well as the dopaminergic projections to the striatum, hippocampus, cortex, and median eminence were analyzed. Results: The THI decreased significantly in the substantia nigra and ventral tegmental area after treatment with paroxetine, and the labeling was reduced drastically in the zona incerta and mediobasal hypothalamus. The immunoreactive axons in the target regions (striatum, cortex, hippocampus, and median eminence) almost disappeared only in the paroxetine-treated rats. Conversely, after treatment with agomelatine, a moderate reduction in immunoreactivity in the substantia nigra was found without appreciable modifications in the ventral tegmental area, zona incerta, and mediobasal hypothalamus. Nevertheless, no sexual or copulatory behavior was observed in any of the experimental or control groups. Conclusion: Paroxetine but not agomelatine was associated with important decreased activity in dopaminergic areas such as the substantia nigra and ventral tegmental areas that could be associated with sexual performance impairment in humans after antidepressant treatment.

Keywords: dopaminergic system; paroxetine; agomelatine; immunohistochemical study; sexual dysfunction; male rats

1. Introduction

The dopaminergic (DA) and serotonergic (5-HT) modulatory systems are involved in regulating multiple functions through their abundant projections throughout the Central Nervous System (CNS). These systems are closely related and interact to control motor, cognitive, and affective functions. Dysfunction of these systems results in pathologies as marked as Parkinson's disease, schizophrenia, depressive disorders, and Attention Deficit Hyperactivity Disorder (ADHD) AHDH syndrome.

The dopaminergic neurons are an anatomically and functionally heterogeneous group of cells, located in particular in the diencephalon and mesencephalon. In the murine brain, DA neurons are identified mainly in three structures. The first structure comprises the meso-diencephalic tegmental cell groups (A8–A10). Because these neurons originate from the substantia nigra (SN) and the ventral tegmental area (VTA) of the mesencephalon and diencephalon, we will refer to these neurons as meso-diencephalic dopaminergic (mdDA) neurons. They constitute the largest group of neurons and project to the striatum (nigrostriatal pathway), the limbic system (meso-limbic pathway), and the cerebral cortex (mesocortical pathway). The second structure is the zona incerta cell group (A13) in the ventral thalamus. The third structure comprises the hypothalamic (A12, A14, and A15) cell groups. The A12 group is the largest and provides the tuberoinfundibular and the tuberohypophysial projections involved in neuroendocrine regulation [1,2].

The interaction between DA and 5-HT systems is complex because it involves many types of membrane receptors that have mixed effects. The 5-HT neurons from the raphe nuclei send projections to dopaminergic cells in both the VTA and the SN, and to their terminals in the nucleus accumbens, prefrontal cortex, and striatum [3]. Some experimental data demonstrates that several 5-HT receptors subtypes (1a, 1b, 2a, 3, and 4) act to facilitate neuronal DA function and release, while the 5-HT2c receptor mediates an inhibitory effect on DA neuron activity and on DA release [4–6].

In recent years, antidepressant use has increased rapidly in Western countries because it is widely prescribed by psychiatrists and general practitioners. The introduction of selective serotonin reuptake inhibitors (SSRIs) in the late 1980s facilitated this process because of the alleged safety of these drugs compared with more dangerous drugs that were used previously [7,8]. However, some adverse effects of SSRIs are frequent and underestimated. One example is sexual dysfunction, which affects patients' quality of life and continuity of treatment [9–13]. The incidence of sexual dysfunction is high (50–70%) when the mechanism of action is blocking serotonin reuptake, whereas drugs that act preferably on noradrenaline or dopamine reuptake have a less negative impact on the sexual function [14–16].

A high frequency of treatment discontinuation, close to 40%, has been notified in patients with major depression due to poor tolerance to antidepressant-related sexual dysfunction [15]. Several methods have been described for the therapeutic approach of this adverse event, including dose reduction, change to another antidepressant, or the use of corrective medication; unfortunately, none of these methods is completely effective deteriorating the quality of life of the patient in the long term [16,17].

Although mechanisms that cause sexual dysfunction still are not well understood, a recent study in rats suggests that the inhibitory effects of serotonergic antidepressants are related to the inhibitory effect of serotonin on dopamine release in hypothalamic and mesolimbic areas [18,19].

The inhibitory effect of serotonin on dopaminergic transmission was first shown by a reduction in nigral neuronal activity in response to electrical stimulation of the medial and dorsal raphe nucleus [20,21]. The increase in synaptic serotonin in response to SSRIs could then conceivably result in an amplification of the tonic inhibitory effects of serotonin, thereby leading to a reduction in DA transmission in the striatum [22]. This is supported by recent studies that have demonstrated a reduction in the substantia nigra tyrosine hydroxylase (TH) immunoreactive cell counts in response to SSRI administration [23].

SSRIs can also inhibit the basal activity of DA neurons in the VTA, which is strongly implicated in sexual desire and motivation. Thus, fluoxetine causes a dose-dependent inhibition of the VTA dopaminergic neuron firing rate, but it does not affect the activity of DA cells in other regions [24].

Acute injection of fluvoxamine, paroxetine, and sertraline produces a dose-dependent inhibition of some VTA DA neurons, but it does not affect the basal firing rate of other DA cells.

Agomelatine is a novel antidepressant drug that works on melatonergic (MT1 and MT2), and serotonergic (5-HT 2B and 5-HT2C) receptors [25]. Agomelatine has been used in two randomized studies in healthy male volunteers. These studies showed that agomelatine 25–50 mg/day is similar to placebo in sexual response, showing a lack of sexual dysfunction, whereas paroxetine 20 mg/day is related to a high sexual dysfunction frequency (>80% of patients showed decreased libido and orgasm delay) [26,27].

Our aim in this research is to study the dopaminergic system in male Wistar rats, especially the nuclei where neurons are located in the brainstem (substantia nigra pars compacta (SNc) and VTA), diencephalon (zona incerta (ZI) and hypothalamic arcuate nucleus (Arc)), and their most relevant axonal projections (striatum, hippocampus, hypothalamus, and cortex) in animals treated with paroxetine or agomelatine, which represents two different mechanisms of antidepressant action related to sexual adverse events. We will compare their effects on immunoreactivity to tyrosine hydroxylase, the rate-limiting enzyme of dopamine synthesis. The presence of this enzyme is considered a good marker of dopaminergic neurons in the central nervous system. We hypothesize that if the dopaminergic system is involved in sexual dysfunction caused by SSRIs, different antidepressant treatments will differentially modify TH immunoreactivity.

2. Material and Methods

Male Wistar rats, aged approximately 3 months old, were used. Rats were maintained under a 12 h light/dark cycle and at a constant temperature (20 °C) with free access to food and water. All animals were handled and cared for in accordance with the recommendations of European Commission and Spanish laws (2007/526/EC and RD 1201/2005). Authorization was requested to the Bioethics Committee of the University of Salamanca.

Twenty animals were distributed into the following groups: (1) four normal rats; (2) four rats treated orally with 10% hydroxyl-methyl-cellulose (the vehicle in which agomelatine was dissolved); (3) six rats treated orally with 10 mg/kg/day of paroxetine diluted in aqueous solution; and (4) six rats treated orally with 10 mg/kg/day of agomelatine diluted in 10% hydroxyl-methyl-cellulose. Because agomelatine needs to be dissolved in 10% hydroxyl-methyl-cellulose for absorption, an agomelatine control group was created with four rats that received only 10% hydroxyl-methyl-cellulose to observe its effects on the dopaminergic system. Since no differences were observed with the normal group, both finally were grouped as an only control group with eight rats.

Agomelatine solution was kindly provided by the manufacturer (Servier Lab) and paroxetine was obtained from the pharmacy. All treatments were performed for 28 days at 18:00 h each day. The size of the sample was empirically chosen due to the lack of previous evidence in the scientific literature on this topic.

Twenty-four hours after the end of treatment, rats were euthanized between 10:00 and 13:00 h. The brain was quickly extracted, the front and rear ends of the brain, the brainstem (pons and medulla oblongata), and the cerebellum were removed, and the remaining block was divided into two halves and fixed by immersion in Bouin's fluid. Tissue was embedded in paraffin. The brain block was oriented to obtain coronal sections (8 μm thick). The whole block of tissue from each animal was serially cut and mounted (two sections per slide). Every tenth slide was stained with hematoxylin–eosin for orientation.

In order to observe the copulatory behavior and the possible differences between the experimental and control groups, two Wistar female rats were used. After 28 days, when the period of administration of paroxetine, agomelatine or placebo ended, one of the females was coupled in a new cage with one male from each group successively. Any sexual or approaching behavior was observed for a maximum of 5 min at 18:00 h, once for each male.

2.1. Immunohistochemistry

Selected sections were processed for tyrosine hydroxylase immunohistochemistry using the streptavidin–biotin method (EnVision, Dako, Denmark) with diaminobenzidine (DAB) as the electron donor. The antiserum (anti-tyrosine hydroxylase, GeneTex) was diluted in Tris buffer, pH 7.6, containing 0.7% non-gelling seaweed lambda carrageenan (Sigma) and 0.5% Triton X-100 (Sigma). The antiserum was used at a dilution of 1:300. The conditions and duration of incubation with the various reagents, especially with DAB and H_2O_2, was the same in all cases. Use of preimmune serum and omission of incubation in the primary antiserum during the immunostaining procedure were used as test controls and resulted in no immunostaining.

2.2. Quantification of Immunohistochemical Staining Intensity

Quantification of immunohistochemical staining intensity was performed using the open source software ImageJ (National Institutes of Health). We determined the pixel intensity of 60 immunoreactive neurons in the normal/control and experimental groups (we selected 15 neurons from the VTA nucleus and 15 from the SNc nucleus in four rats from each groups). To avoid possible differences in the pixel intensity resulting from the presence or absence of a cell nucleus, all measured cells had a visible cell nucleus. To determine the intensity of pixels, ImageJ assigns a value of 0 to the color black and a value of 255 to the color white. Thus, a greater staining intensity corresponds to a lower pixel intensity value.

2.3. Statistical Analysis

A two-factor ANOVA was used to analyze the differences in pixel intensity between groups and nuclei (SNc and VTA) and interaction between both factors. If the interaction between factors was statistically significant, one-way ANOVA was used to detect the differences between experimental groups for each level of area followed by Tukey's multiple comparison tests where appropriate. Statistical significance was defined as $p < 0.05$. The mean and 95% confidence intervals (CIs) for each outcome are presented. Statistical analysis was conducted using the IBM SPSS 23 package (IBM, Armonk, NY, USA).

3. Results

In this study, images of the caudate-putamen, nucleus accumbens, and cortex were obtained from sections that correspond approximately with the coronal sections marked as Bregma 1.68–0.72 mm in the Paxinos and Watson atlas of the rat brain. Images of the zona incerta, arcuate nucleus and hippocampus correspond approximately with the coronal planes marked as Bregma −2.04 to −3.24 mm in the same atlas, and images of the VTA and SNc were obtained from sections that correspond approximately with the coronal sections marked as Bregma −4.80 to −5.28 mm in the rat brain atlas. The cortex images refer to the areas S1 (primary somatosensory cortex) and M1 (primary motor cortex) in the same atlas [27,28].

We found no differences in the staining intensity between normal and control rats treated with hydroxy-methyl-cellulose. Therefore, the findings in animals treated with paroxetine and agomelatine were analyzed in relation to the normal/control group of rats.

3.1. Substantia Nigra Compacta and the Ventral Tegmental Area

To identify the nuclei in DA neurons, we used the usual anatomical terms, and also referred to its name in the aminergic classification system by Dahlström and Fuxe (1964), in which the DA system is distributed into the groups A8–A14.

In the substantia nigra (A9) and ventral tegmental area (A10) of control rats, TH neurons and neuronal processes are strongly reactive. Neuron labeling is intense throughout the cytoplasm, so that when the section affects the neuronal nucleus, it appears as a negative zone. TH axons surrounding the A9 and A10 nuclei also show a strong reaction, both penetrating the reticular substantia nigra

(SNR) as located dorsally (Figure 1A). Conversely, in animals treated with paroxetine, the labeling is weak in both neurons and neuronal processes of the SNc and VTA nuclei. In the areas surrounding the nuclei, cited axons are barely visible (Figure 1B). In the SNc and VTA of agomelatine-treated rats, TH reactivity is similar to that described in the control rats, although labeling seems somewhat less intense (Figure 1C).

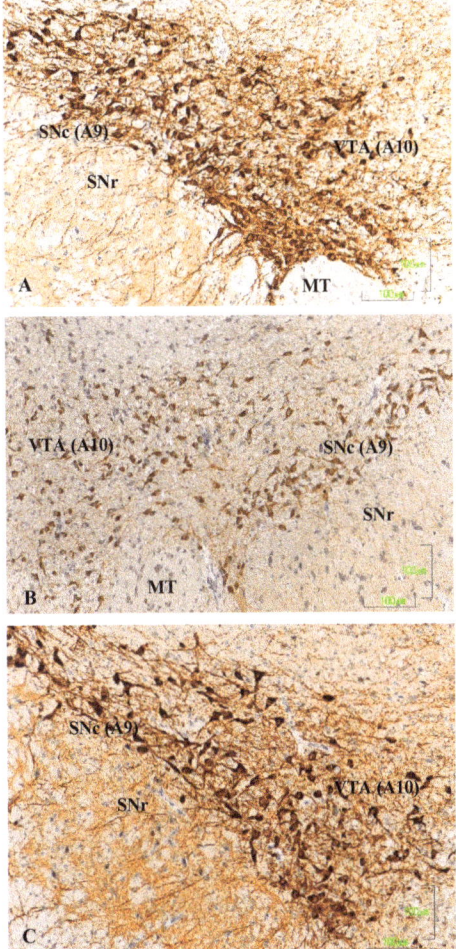

Figure 1. (A–C). Tyrosine hydroxylase immunoreactivity in the meso-diencephalic dopaminergic system of rats from the control (**A**), paroxetine (**B**), and agomelatine (**C**) groups. Bars, 100 m. SNc, substantia nigra pars compacta; SNr, substantia nigra pars reticulate; VTA, ventral tegmental area; MT, mammilothalamic tract.

3.2. Striatum and Nucleus Accumbens

In the striatum (CPu) of the control animals, the labeling is intense and uniform throughout the matrix, but striosomes are negative (Figure 2A). In the nucleus accumbens, dopaminergic fibers are preferentially located in the lateral region. At higher magnifications, labeling is shown as dense dots, corresponding to the axons of the nigrostriatal pathway. We have not seen cell bodies of dopaminergic neurons in this region (Figure 2D).

The dopaminergic projections to the striatum are significantly affected after treatment with paroxetine, with the absence of immunoreactivity throughout the dorsal and medial CPu and significantly reduced immunoreactivity in the remaining area (Figure 2B). At higher magnifications, dopaminergic fibers have mostly disappeared (Figure 2E). In the striatum of animals treated with agomelatine, TH reactivity is reduced compared to the control group, but is more intense than in rats treated with paroxetine (Figure 2C,F). In the nucleus accumbens, the pattern of labeling is uniform throughout the CPu matrix (Figure 2C).

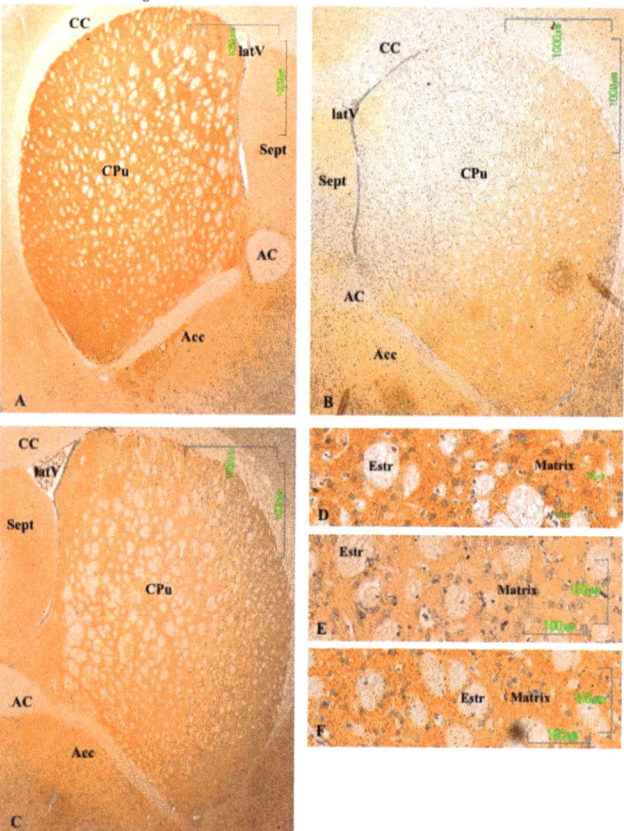

Figure 2. (**A–F**). Tyrosine hydroxylase immunoreactivity in the striatum of control rats (**A,D**), and rats treated with paroxetine (**B,E**) and agomelatine (**C,F**). Bars 1000 m (**A–C**) and 100 m (**D–F**). The reactivity is visible as dotted labeling that is evenly distributed by the matrix of the caudate-putamen (CPu), except in paroxetine-treated rats. CC, corpus callosum; latV, lateral ventriculum; AC, anterior commissure; Acc, nucleus accumbens; Estr, striatum; Sept, septum.

3.3. Hippocampus

In the hippocampus of control animals, there was a strong reaction in the A3 region of the cornu ammonis (CA3; Figure 3A), which was shown by discrete labeling throughout the hippocampal region (Figure 3A lacks a bar, but the magnification is the same as in Figure 3B,C). After treatment with paroxetine, labeling of TH axons was strongly reduced, especially in CA3 (Figure 3B). Immunoreactivity slightly decreased in the agomelatine-treated group, even though reactive axons are observed (Figure 3C). We also detected TH-positive axons in the septum of rats in the control and agomelatine-treated groups, while labeling had also disappeared in paroxetine-treated animals.

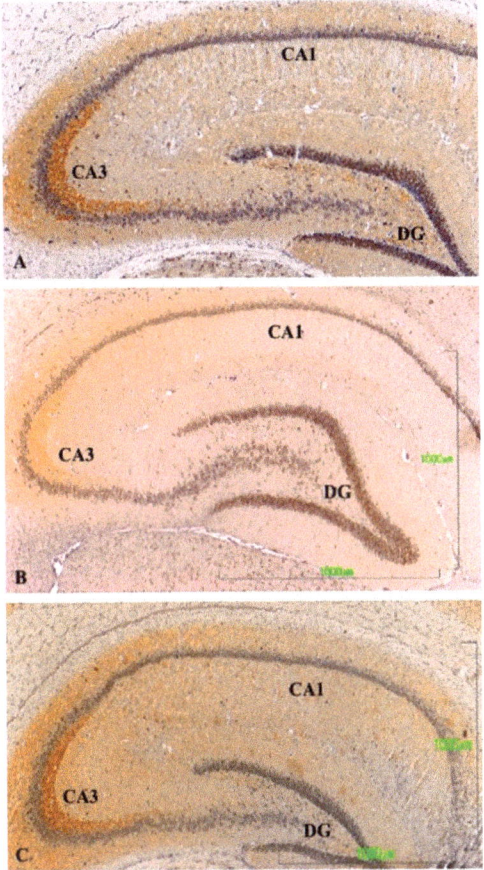

Figure 3. (A–C). Tyrosine hydroxylase immunoreactivity in the hippocampus of rats from the control (**A**), paroxetine (**B**), and agomelatine (**C**) groups. Bars, 1000 m. (Figure 3A is presented at the same magnification as that of Figure 3B,C). The immunoreactivity is limited to the CA3 area and is greatly reduced following treatment with paroxetine. DG, dentate gyrus; CA, cornu ammonis.

3.4. Cerebral Cortex

Figure 4 summarizes our observations on the dopaminergic innervation of the rat primary motor/somatosensory cortex (CM/S). This represents the mesocortical pathway. The reactivity in control rats is limited to axons and is located preferably in layers II/III, and it decreases both beneath and towards the surface (Figure 4A). Similar to other locations in rats treated with paroxetine, the labeling almost completely disappears (Figure 4B), but it is reduced in animals treated with agomelatine (Figure 4C).

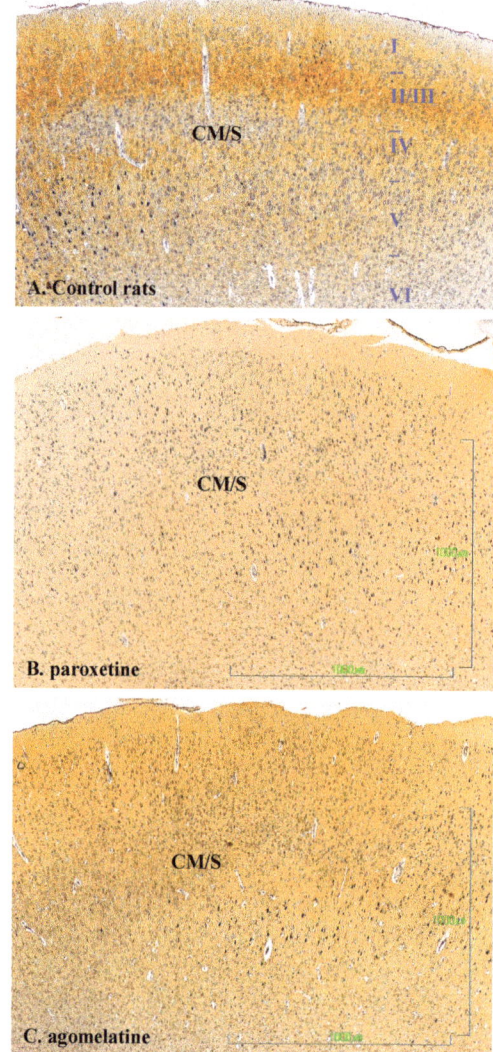

Figure 4. (**A**–**C**). Tyrosine hydroxylase immunoreactivity in the cerebral cortex layers I-VI of rats from the control (**A**), paroxetine (**B**), and agomelatine (**C**) groups. Bars, 1000 m. (Figure 4A is presented at the same magnification as that of Figure 4B,C). CM/S, motor/somatosensory cortex.

3.5. Zona Incerta and Hypothalamus

In the control rats, TH-positive neurons in the zona incerta (A13) and fibers in and around the nucleus show intense labeling (Figure 5A). In rats treated with agomelatine, the appearance and reactivity of dopaminergic neurons is similar to that observed in the control group (Figure 5C). Conversely, in the animals treated with paroxetine, TH immunostaining is low in the neuronal cell bodies and it disappears in the nerve fibers (Figure 5B).

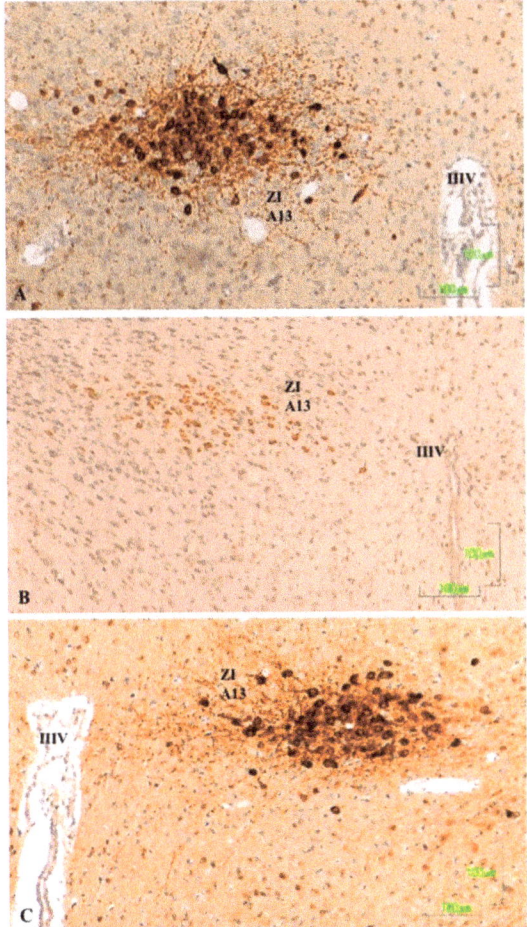

Figure 5. (**A–C**). Tyrosine hydroxylase immunoreactivity in the zona incerta of rats from the control (**A**), paroxetine (**B**), and agomelatine (**C**) groups. Bars, 100 m. In the rats treated with paroxetine, the labeling is weak whereas in animals treated with agomelatine, labeling is similar to that shown the control rats. IIIV, third ventricle; ZI, zona incerta.

In the dopaminergic A12 group in the arcuate nucleus, the hypothalamic neurons behave similarly to those of the zona incerta (Figure 6). In the control group, the neurons show a more intense staining in the cell bodies of the arcuate nucleus (NARC) and in axons in the tuberoinfundibular tract that reach the outer zone of the median eminence (EM) (Figure 6A). Conversely, in the paroxetine-treated group, the arcuate neurons exhibit weak immunoreactivity, and the fibers of the median eminence are nonreactive (Figure 6B). In animals treated with agomelatine, the immunostaining is intense both in the neuronal bodies and in the median eminence, but it is somewhat reduced compared to control rats (Figure 6C).

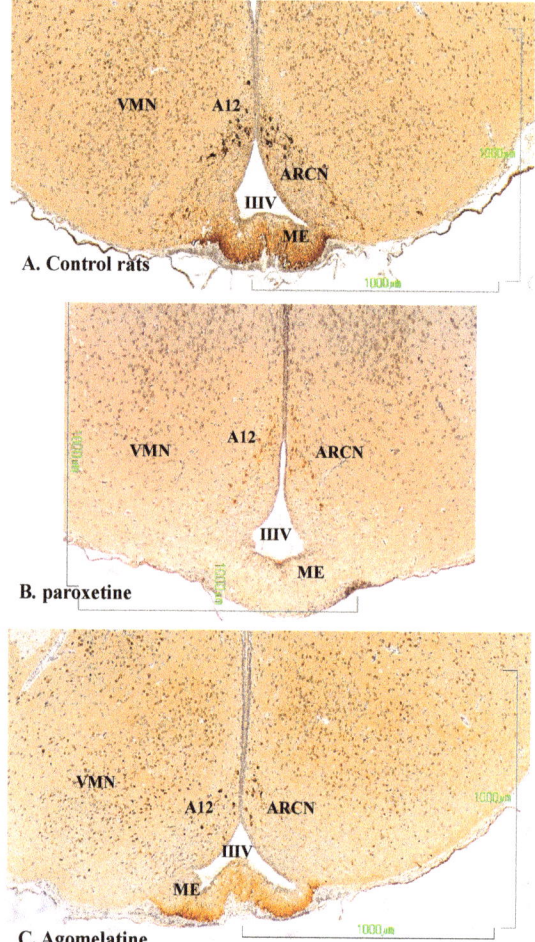

Figure 6. (**A–C**). Tyrosine hydroxylase immunoreactivity in the mediobasal hypothalamus of rats from the control (**A**), paroxetine (**B**), and agomelatine (**C**) groups. Bars, 1000 m. After treatment with paroxetine, TH immunoreactivity is absent from the median eminence. ARCN, arcuate nucleus; ME, median eminence; IIIV, third ventricle; VMN, ventromedial nucleus.

3.6. Quantification of TH Immunoreactivity in the SNc and VTA

As noted in the Materials and methods section, we used the open source software ImageJ to determine the pixel intensity in SNc and VTA neurons. This software assigns a value of 0 to the color black and a value of 255 to the color white. Thus, a greater staining intensity corresponds to a lower pixel value intensity. However, interaction between the experimental group and the area was detected (p-value < 0.0001, Figure 7). To analyze the interacction, we compared the differences between experimental groups by each area. There were statistical differences between the three experimental groups ($p < 0.0001$) in SNc, and between control and paroxetine groups in the VTA ($p = 0.001$).

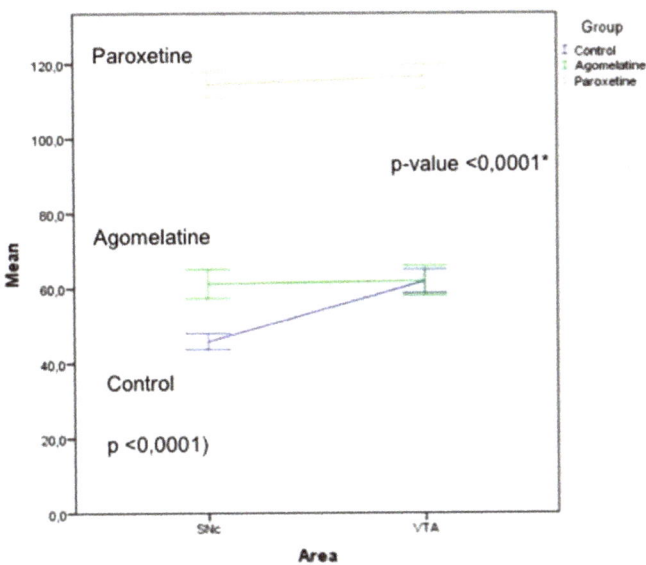

p-value <0,0001*) in VTA between control versus paroxetine

Figure 7. Pixel intensity was determined using open source software ImageJ. There are significant differences between all groups in the SNc, but no statistical difference between the control group and rats treated with agomelatine in the VTA.

3.7. Observation of Sexual and Mating Behaviour

The possible sexual or approaching behavior was observed for a maximum of 5 min, at 18:00 h. just once for each male and female couple. It was observed that the female rats were receptive for riding when meeting the male. However, the males in both experimental and control groups behaved sexually indifferent, showing stereotyped behaviors such as running around the cage and raising on their hind legs. No animals performed coitus with the female; therefore, we cannot draw any conclusions from this observation.

4. Discussion

To explain sexual dysfunction caused by treatment with SSRIs, various mechanisms have been proposed, among which is the inhibition of the dopaminergic system [18].

Given that the antidepressant-induced effects on sexual parameters in Wistar rats correspond well with their known effects in humans [14,15,29], we conducted a comparative experimental study on the dopaminergic system in male rats treated with paroxetine and agomelatine. This research improves our understanding of the mechanisms that explain sexual dysfunction, focusing on the meso-diencephalic dopaminergic system.

Recently, MacGillivray et al. (2011) examined the effects of two different SSRIs, citalopram and fluoxetine, on cells containing tyrosine hydroxylase (TH) in nigrostriatal dopamine neurons and showed that both antidepressants induced a significant reduction in the number of TH cells in the Substantia Nigra. Our experimental model includes DA neurons from the substantia nigra and the VTA, and DA neurons of the zona incerta (ZI) and the tuberoinfundibular system. In this research, we did not count the immunoreactive TH cells, but we determined the intensity of staining in SNc and VTA TH cells.

TH is the rate-limiting enzyme of dopamine synthesis, and it is considered one of the major agents in determining dopamine levels. When need for neurotransmitter increases at a DA synapse, TH is activated to make more DOPA. TH activity must be sustained until the need reduces and its activity must be turned off when the need for neurotransmitters has passed [30].

We believe it is relevant to clarify the meaning of changes in TH immunoreactivity regarding the available dopamine and dopaminergic system activity. What we show by immunohistochemical staining is the approximate number of immunoreactive TH molecules (the rate-limiting enzymes of catecholamine synthesis) in the areas studied, which is a good marker of dopamine neurons and fibers. Thus, under controlled staining conditions such as those in this study, more intense labeling means more TH molecules, which leads to an increased dopamine synthesis rate. Conversely, a reduction in the intensity of the labeling means generally fewer TH molecules and a decrease in DA synthesis.

If we consider the large number of known 5-HT and DA receptors and the many factors that can influence regulation of sexual behavior, it is almost impossible to draw accurate conclusions. However, our data can complement those obtained using other methodologies and from human clinical studies. To our knowledge, paroxetine and agomelatine have not been explored in this field until now.

DA has multiple effects that promote sexual behavior by stimulating the copulatory capacity and genital reflexes. In the nigrostriatal pathway, DA influences motor activity; in the mesolimbic pathway, DA activates motivated behavior, including copulation; and in the medial preoptic area, DA controls genital reflexes, copulation patterns, and sexual motivation [31].

4.1. Paroxetine Reduces TH Immunoreactivity in All Meso-Diencephalic Dopaminergic Systems

Treatment with paroxetine frequently causes sexual dysfunction in humans for short, medium, and long durations [32], and this adverse effect is related to the hypofunction of the dopaminergic system in nigrostriatal and mesolimbic/mesocortical pathways, as reported in various publications [18,31,33,34]. Similar results have been observed after the administration of fluoxetine or escitalopram, which induce a decrease in DA neuron firing rate in the VTA [35]. It is suggested that this class of antidepressant acts through 5-HT2C receptors [17]. Recently, Demireva et al. (2018) [36] have demonstrated that SSRI-induced motor deficits in mice can be reversed by systemic or SNr-localized 5-HT2C receptor antagonism. SSRIs induce SNr hyperactivity and SNc (dopaminergic) hypoactivity that can also be reversed by systemic 5-HT2C receptor antagonism. Considering the critical role of DA in hedonic processes, the decrease in firing activity by SSRIs might contribute to the resistance to antidepressants in some patients.

Our results additionally show a general decrease in TH immunoreactivity in these dopaminergic systems after treatment with paroxetine, which is consistent with the results of the authors cited above, and which could result in a reduction in motivated behavior, including copulation (mesolimbic pathway) and overall sexual dysfunction.

We also showed a previously unreported reduction of TH reactivity in DA neurons of the ZI. These neurons originate the incerto-hypothalamic tract, which innervates the anterior hypothalamus and the dorsomedial and paraventricular nuclei, and which is thought to have a stimulatory role in the release of LH [37]. More recently, other authors have proposed that ZI dopamine stimulates the release of LH and prolactin acting through glutamatergic NMDA receptors [38]. The incerto-hypothalamic pathway is involved in coordination of genital reflexes necessary for erection [39]. Therefore, the important decrease in the intensity of TH staining in ZI neurons of paroxetine-treated rats, must correspond to a decrease in the available DA and its stimulatory effect on the release of LH and sexual behavior.

Our study also shows that TH immunoreactivity is weak in the tuberoinfundibular dopaminergic neurons, and that labeling disappears from the median eminence dopaminergic axons after treatment with paroxetine. These observations are consistent with data from Lyons et al. (2016) [40], which showed that fluoxetine and sertraline, directly suppress tuberoinfundibular dopamine (TIDA) neuron activity. The hypo-function of this dopaminergic inhibitory system will be accompanied by hyperprolactinemia, as in treatment with other antidepressants or antipsychotics. Among the consequences of hyperprolactinemia in men are erectile dysfunction, with reduced sexual desire, and sometimes ejaculatory and orgasmic disorder [41–43].

Our findings of decreased immunoreactivity to TH after treatment with paroxetine are consistent with other published data reporting a reduction of TH gene expression in VTA and SN areas after fluoxetine administration for 16 and 31 days [44], or a decrease in TH mRNA in the locus ceruleus after chronic paroxetine administration [45].

The sexual dysfunction linked to antidepressant treatment has also been studied in humans via neuroimaging, showing that paroxetine and other SSRIs reduce the activity of brain networks involved in processing the motivational and emotional aspects of sexual function [46,47].

To summarize, many clinical and experimental studies show that SSRI antidepressants (including paroxetine) can alter all phases of sexual activity, from desire to arousal, orgasm, and ejaculation. Sexual dysfunction in males results in the inability to achieve erection or reach orgasm, while in women the problem is usually a decrease in sexual desire and delay or difficulty in reaching orgasm. In addition, there is growing experimental evidence that inhibition of meso-diencephalic dopaminergic systems is a determining factor in the aforementioned effects [18].

Our research shows that treatment with paroxetine reduces TH labeling in the incerto-hypothalamic and tuberoinfundibular dopaminergic systems. Hypo-function in these systems probably leads to a decrease in hypothalamic-pituitary-gonadal axis activity, which has been shown in clinical studies after treatment with antidepressants [48,49].

4.2. Agomelatine Treatment Also Slightly Reduces Dopaminergic Activity but Less Than Paroxetine

This study also shows that treatment with agomelatine for 28 days reduces immunoreactivity to TH in the SNc, although the effect is less intense than after treatment with paroxetine. Moreover, our data show no difference in immunoreactivity for TH in the VTA between control rats and those treated with agomelatine, which suggests that agomelatine does not affect the activity of the SNc and VTA dopaminergic neurons in the same way.

Agomelatine has an antidopaminergic action similar to melatonin [50], although the decrease in immunoreactivity to TH produced by agomelatine is not as intense as that produced by paroxetine. However, agomelatine increases levels of DA and NA in the frontal cortex (via mesocortical) by 5HT2C receptor blockade, but it does not affect the DA in the striatum and accumbens (nigrostriatal and mesolimbic pathways) [4,51]. Our data shows moderate reactivity of dopaminergic axons in the striatum as well as an intense TH labeling in the mesocortical fibers (not shown), which is consistent with previously published results.

It has also been reported that agomelatine stimulates tuberoinfundibular dopaminergic neurons, thereby inhibiting the lactotrope cell activity [52]. We found no difference in TH staining intensity in the ZI and in the tuberoinfundibular dopaminergic system between the control rats and those treated with agomelatine. Thus, we cannot confirm or reject this assertion.

In summary, treatment with agomelatine has a moderate inhibitory effect on the dopaminergic nigrostriatal system, but its action on the meso-limbic and meso-cortical pathways is barely noticeable and is much lower than that produced by paroxetine administration. Additionally, agomelatine does not seem to inhibit the incerto-hypothalamic and tuberoinfundibular dopaminergic systems.

These data are consistent with previous observations that show notable differences in the impact of various antidepressants on the dopaminergic system. The differential effects of paroxetine and agomelatine on the TH immunoreactivity and dopaminergic systems may partly explain the impact that the tested treatments have on sexual function, including the high frequency of sexual dysfunction in paroxetine-treated patients.

The observations on sexual behavior were negative and no mating behavior was observed. These negative results could be due to some limitations in the experimental design, even though the rat was ovulating and sexually receptive during the contact with the male. The lack of mating behavior could be due to the sexual encounter that took place in a new cage and not in the female's usual cage.

On the other hand, the observation took place at 18:00 h, which was the same time of usual contact with the observer who had previously administered the drugs. Additionally, the observation period of 5 min was perhaps scarce, and the observation method could have been different, for example using a recording without the presence of the observer.

5. Limitations.

The ImageJ data could only be used for statistical analysis on the substantia nigra and the VTA since these areas are nuclei in which many neurons are observed in each microscopic cut. However, this method could not be applied to the other brain territories analyzed because the neuronal population is much smaller and the representativeness of the statistical analysis in the cuttings could not be guaranteed.

The presence of negative results in the observation of sexual behavior could be due to some methodological limitations of the design that should be taken into account for future studies in order to reproduce suitable results in this field.

Author Contributions: Conceptualization Y.S., A.L.M., G.L., G.B. and J.B.; methodology, Y.S., A.L.M., G.L. and J.B.; formal analysis, J.M.; investigation, Y.S. and J.B.; resources, A.L.M.; data curation, Y.S., G.B. and J.B.; writing—original draft preparation, J.B., Y.S. writing—review and editing, J.L.B. and A.L.M.; funding acquisition, A.L.M.

Funding: This research received partial external funding from the Asociación Española de Sexualidad y Salud Mental.

Acknowledgments: We acknowledge the donation of solution of agomelatine for this experimental research given by Servier Laboratories (France).

Conflicts of Interest: Dr. Montejo has received consultancy fees or honoraria/research grants in the last 5 years from Eli Lilly, Forum Pharmaceuticals, Rovi, Servier, Lundbeck, Otsuka, Janssen Cilag, Pfizer, Roche, Instituto de Salud Carlos III, and the Junta de Castilla y León. The rests of the authors declare no conflict of interest.

References

1. Chinta, S.J.; Andersen, J.K. Dopaminergic neurons. *Int. J. Biochem. Cell Biol.* **2005**, *37*, 942–946. [CrossRef] [PubMed]
2. Smits, S.M.; Burbach, J.P.H.; Smidt, M.P. Developmental origin and fate of meso-diencephalic dopamine neurons. *Prog. Neurobiol.* **2006**, *78*, 1–16. [CrossRef] [PubMed]
3. Steinbusch, H.W.M. Serotonin immunoreactive neurons and their projections in the CNS. In *Handbook of Chemical Anatomy: Classical Transmitters and Transmitter Receptors in the CNS Part II*, 1st ed.; Björklung, A., Hökfelt, T., Kuhar, M.J., Eds.; Elsevier: New York, NY, USA, 1984; Volume 3, pp. 68–125.
4. Alex, K.D.; Pehek, E.A. Pharmacologic mechanisms of serotonergic regulation of dopamine neurotransmission. *Pharmacol. Ther.* **2007**, *113*, 296–320. [CrossRef]
5. Di Matteo, V.; Di Giovanni, G.; Pierucci, M.; Esposito, E. Serotonin control of central dopaminergic function: Focus on in vivo microdialysis studies. *Prog. Brain Res.* **2008**, *172*, 7–44. [CrossRef]
6. Esposito, E.; Di Matteo, V.; Di Giovanni, G. Serotonin-dopamine interaction: An overview. *Prog. Brain Res.* **2008**, *172*, 3–6. [CrossRef]
7. Barth, M.; Kriston, L.; Klostermann, S.; Barbui, C.; Cipriani, A.; Linde, K. Efficacy of selective serotonin reuptake inhibitors and adverse events: Meta-regression and mediation analysis of placebo-controlled trials. *Br. J. Psychiatry* **2016**, *208*, 114–119. [CrossRef] [PubMed]
8. Linde, K.; Kriston, L.; Rücker, G.; Jamil, S.; Schumann, I.; Meissner, K.; Sigterman, K.; Schneider, A. Efficacy and acceptability of pharmacological treatments for depressive disorders in primary care: Systematic review and network meta-analysis. *Ann. Fam. Med.* **2015**, *13*, 69–79. [CrossRef]
9. Montejo, A.; Majadas, S.; Rizvi, S.J.; Kennedy, S.H. The effects of agomelatine on sexual function in depressed patients and healthy volunteers. *Hum. Psychopharmacol.* **2011**, *26*, 537–542. [CrossRef]
10. Baldwin, D.S.; Foong, T. Antidepressant drugs and sexual dysfunction. *Br. J. Psychiatry* **2013**, *202*, 396–397. [CrossRef]

11. Montejo-González, A.L.; Llorca, G.; Izquierdo, J.A.; Ledesma, A.; Bousoño, M.; Calcedo, A.; Carrasco, J.L.; Ciudad, J.; Daniel, E.; De la Gandara, J.; et al. SSRI-induced sexual dysfunction: Fluoxetine, paroxetine, sertraline, and fluvoxamine in a prospective, multicenter, and descriptive clinical study of 344 patients. *J. Sex Marital Ther.* **1997**, *23*, 176–194. [CrossRef]
12. Montejo, A.L.; Montejo, L.; Navarro-Cremades, F. Sexual side-effects of antidepressant and antipsychotic drugs. *Curr. Opin. Psychiatry* **2015**, *28*, 418–423. [CrossRef]
13. Montejo, A.L.; Llorca, G.; Izquierdo, J.A.; Rico-Villademoros, F. Incidence of sexual dysfunction associated with antidepressant agents: A prospective multicenter study of 1022 outpatients. Spanish Working Group for the Study of Psychotropic-Related Sexual Dysfunction. *J. Clin. Psychiatry* **2001**, *62* (Suppl. 3), 10–21.
14. Clayton, A.H.; Alkis, A.R.; Parikh, N.B.; Votta, J.G. Sexual Dysfunction Due to Psychotropic Medications. *Psychiatr. Clin. N. Am.* **2016**, *39*, 427–463. [CrossRef] [PubMed]
15. Montejo, A.L.; Montejo, L.; Baldwin, D.S. The impact of severe mental disorders and psychotropic medications on sexual health and its implications for clinical management. *World Psychiatry* **2018**, *17*, 3–11. [CrossRef] [PubMed]
16. Montejo, A.L.; Perahia, D.G.; Spann, M.E.; Wang, F.; Walker, D.J.; Yang, C.R.; Detke, M.J. Sexual function during long-term duloxetine treatment in patients with recurrent major depressive disorder. *J. Sex. Med.* **2011**, *8*, 773–782. [CrossRef] [PubMed]
17. Farnia, V.; Shirzadifar, M.; Shakeri, J.; Rezaei, M.; Bajoghli, H.; Holsboer-Trachsler, E.; Brand, S. Rosa damascena oil improves SSRI-induced sexual dysfunction in male patients suffering from major depressive disorders: Results from a double-blind, randomized, and placebo-controlled clinical trial. *Neuropsychiatr. Dis. Treat.* **2015**, *11*, 625–635. [CrossRef]
18. Bijlsma, E.Y.; Chan, J.S.; Olivier, B.; Veening, J.G.; Millan, M.J.; Waldinger, M.D.; Oosting, R.S. Sexual side effects of serotonergic antidepressants: Mediated by inhibition of serotonin on central dopamine release? *Pharmacol. Biochem. Behav.* **2014**, *121*, 88–101. [CrossRef]
19. Boureau, Y.L.; Dayan, P. Opponency revisited: Competition and cooperation between dopamine and serotonin. *Neuropsychopharmacology* **2011**, *36*, 74–97. [CrossRef]
20. Dray, A.; Gonye, T.J.; Oakley, N.R.; Tanner, T. Evidence for the existence of a raphe projection to the substantia nigra in rat. *Brain Res.* **1976**, *113*, 45–57. [CrossRef]
21. Dray, A.; Davies, J.; Oakley, N.R.; Tongroach, P.; Vellucci, S. The dorsal and medial raphe projections to the substantia nigra in the rat: Electrophysiological, biochemical and behavioural observations. *Brain Res.* **1978**, *151*, 431–442. [CrossRef]
22. MacGillivray, L.; Reynolds, K.B.; Sickand, M.; Rosebush, P.I.; Mazurek, M.F. Inhibition of the serotonin transporter induces microglial activation and downregulation of dopaminergic neurons in the substantia nigra. *Synapse* **2011**, *65*, 1166–1172. [CrossRef] [PubMed]
23. Seshadri, K.G. The neuroendocrinology of love. *Indian J. Endocrinol. Metab.* **2016**, *20*, 558–563. [CrossRef] [PubMed]
24. Prisco, S.; Esposito, E. Differential effects of acute and chronic fluoxetine administration on the spontaneous activity of dopaminergic neurones in the ventral tegmental area. *Br. J. Pharmacol.* **1995**, *116*, 1923–1931. [CrossRef] [PubMed]
25. De Bodinat, C.; Guardiola-Lemaitre, B.; Mocaër, E.; Renard, P.; Muñoz, C.; Millan, M.J. Agomelatine, the first melatonergic antidepressant: Discovery, characterization and development. *Nat. Rev. Drug Discov.* **2010**, *9*, 628–642. [CrossRef] [PubMed]
26. Montejo, A.L.; Prieto, N.; Terleira, A.; Matias, J.; Alonso, S.; Paniagua, G.; Naval, S.; Parra, D.G.; Gabriel, C.; Mocaër, E.; Portolés, A. Better sexual acceptability of agomelatine (25 and 50 mg) compared with paroxetine (20 mg) in healthy male volunteers. An 8-week, placebo-controlled study using the PRSEXDQ-SALSEX scale. *J. Psychopharmacol.* **2010**, *24*, 111–120. [CrossRef] [PubMed]
27. Montejo, A.L.; Deakin, J.F.; Gaillard, R.; Harmer, C.; Meyniel, F.; Jabourian, A.; Gabriel, C.; Gruget, C.; Klinge, C.; MacFayden, C.; et al. Better sexual acceptability of agomelatine (25 and 50 mg) compared to escitalopram (20 mg) in healthy volunteers. A 9-week, placebo-controlled study using the PRSexDQ scale. *J. Psychopharmacol.* **2015**, *29*, 1119–1128. [CrossRef]
28. Paxinos, G.; Watson, C. *The Rat Brain in Stereotaxic Coordinates*, 5th ed.; Elsevier: San Diego, CA, USA, 2005.

29. Kennedy, S.H.; Eisfeld, B.S.; Dickens, S.E.; Bacchiochi, J.R.; Bagby, R.M. Antidepressant-induced sexual dysfunction during treatment with moclobemide, paroxetine, sertraline, and venlafaxine. *J. Clin. Psychiatry* **2000**, *61*, 276–281. [CrossRef]
30. Daubner, S.C.; Le, T.; Wang, S. Tyrosine hydroxylase and regulation of dopamine synthesis. *Arch. Biochem. Biophys.* **2011**, *508*, 1–12. [CrossRef]
31. Hull, E.M.; Muschamp, J.W.; Sato, S. Dopamine and serotonin: Influences on male sexual behavior. *Physiol. Behav.* **2004**, *83*, 291–307. [CrossRef]
32. Serretti, A.; Chiesa, A. Treatment-emergent sexual dysfunction related to antidepressants: A meta-analysis. *J. Clin. Psychopharmacol.* **2009**, *29*, 259–266. [CrossRef]
33. Baldessarini, R.J.; Marsh, E. Fluoxetine and side effects. *Arch. Gen. Psychiatry* **1990**, *47*, 191–192. [CrossRef]
34. Bala, A.; Nguyen, H.M.T.; Hellstrom, W.J.G. Post-SSRI Sexual Dysfunction: A Literature Review. *Sex. Med. Rev.* **2018**, *6*, 29–34. [CrossRef] [PubMed]
35. Belujon, P.; Grace, A.A. Dopamine System Dysregulation in Major Depressive Disorders. *Int. J. Neuropsychopharmacol.* **2017**, *20*, 1036–1046. [CrossRef] [PubMed]
36. Demireva, E.Y.; Suri, D.; Morelli, E.; Mahadevia, D.; Chuhma, N.; Teixeira, C.M.; Ziolkowski, A.; Hersh, M.; Fifer, J.; Bagchi, S.; et al. 5-HT2C receptor blockade reverses SSRI-associated basal ganglia dysfunction and potentiates therapeutic efficacy. *Mol. Psychiatry* **2018**. [CrossRef]
37. MacKenzie, F.J.; Hunter, A.J.; Daly, C.; Wilson, C.A. Evidence that the dopaminergic incerto-hypothalamic tract has a stimulatory effect on ovulation and gonadotrophin release. *Neuroendocrinology* **1984**, *39*, 289–295. [CrossRef] [PubMed]
38. Bregonzio, C.; Moreno, G.N.; Cabrera, R.J.; Donoso, A.O. NMDA receptors in the medial zona incerta stimulate luteinizing hormone and prolactin release. *Cell. Mol. Neurobiol.* **2004**, *24*, 331–342. [CrossRef] [PubMed]
39. Ferretti, A.; Caulo, M.; Del Gratta, C.; Di Matteo, R.; Merla, A.; Montorsi, F. Dynamics of male sexual arousal: Distinct components of brain activation revealed by fMRI. *Neuroimage* **2005**, *26*, 1086–1096. [CrossRef]
40. Lyons, D.J.; Ammari, R.; Hellysaz, A.; Broberger, C. Serotonin and Antidepressant SSRIs Inhibit Rat Neuroendocrine Dopamine Neurons: Parallel Actions in the Lactotrophic Axis. *J. Neurosci.* **2016**, *36*, 7392–7406. [CrossRef]
41. Buvat, J. Hyperprolactinemia and sexual function in men: A short review. *Int. J. Impot. Res.* **2003**, *15*, 373–377. [CrossRef]
42. Montejo, A.L.; Arango, C.; Bernardo, M.; Carrasco, J.L.; Crespo-Facorro, B.; Cruz, J.J.; del Pino, J.; García-Escudero, M.A.; García-Rizo, C.; González-Pinto, A.; et al. Spanish consensus on the risks and detection of antipsychotic drug-related hyperprolactinaemia. *Rev. Psiquiatr. Salud Ment. (Engl. Ed.)* **2016**, *9*, 158–173. [CrossRef]
43. Montejo, A.L.; Arango, C.; Bernardo, M.; Carrasco, J.L.; Crespo-Facorro, B.; Cruz, J.J.; Del Pino-Montes, J.; García-Escudero, M.A.; García-Rizo, C.; González-Pinto, A.; et al. Multidisciplinary consensus on the therapeutic recommendations for iatrogenic hyperprolactinemia secondary to antipsychotics. *Front. Neuroendocrinol.* **2017**, *45*, 25–34. [CrossRef] [PubMed]
44. Oliva, J.M.; Uriguën, L.; Pérez-Rial, S.; Manzanares, J. Time course of opioid and cannabinoid gene transcription alterations induced by repeated administration with fluoxetine in the rat brain. *Neuropharmacology* **2005**, *49*, 618–626. [CrossRef] [PubMed]
45. Rovin, M.L.; Boss-Williams, K.A.; Alisch, R.S.; Ritchie, J.C.; Weinshenker, D.; West, C.H.; Weiss, J.M. Influence of chronic administration of antidepressant drugs on mRNA for galanin, galanin receptors, and tyrosine hydroxylase in catecholaminergic and serotonergic cell-body regions in rat brain. *Neuropeptides* **2012**, *46*, 81–91. [CrossRef] [PubMed]
46. Abler, B.; Seeringer, A.; Hartmann, A.; Grön, G.; Metzger, C.; Walter, M.; Stingl, J. Neural correlates of antidepressant-related sexual dysfunction: A placebo-controlled fMRI study on healthy males under subchronic paroxetine and bupropion. *Neuropsychopharmacology* **2011**, *36*, 1837–1847. [CrossRef] [PubMed]
47. Graf, H.; Walter, M.; Metzger, C.D.; Abler, B. Antidepressant-related sexual dysfunction—Perspectives from neuroimaging. *Pharmacol. Biochem. Behav.* **2014**, *121*, 138–145. [CrossRef] [PubMed]
48. Hendrick, V.; Gitlin, M.; Altshuler, L.; Korenman, S. Antidepressant medications, mood and male fertility. *Psychoneuroendocrinology* **2000**, *25*, 37–51. [CrossRef]

49. Safarinejad, M.R. Evaluation of endocrine profile and hypothalamic-pituitary-testis axis in selective serotonin reuptake inhibitor-induced male sexual dysfunction. *J. Clin. Psychopharmacol.* **2008**, *28*, 418–423. [CrossRef] [PubMed]
50. Fornaro, M.; Prestia, D.; Colicchio, S.; Perugi, G. A systematic, updated review on the antidepressant agomelatine focusing on its melatonergic modulation. *Curr. Neuropharmacol.* **2010**, *8*, 287–304. [CrossRef]
51. Millan, M.J.; Gobert, A.; Lejeune, F.; Dekeyne, A.; Newman-Tancredi, A.; Pasteau, V.; Rivet, J.M.; Cussac, D. The novel melatonin agonist agomelatine (S20098) is an antagonist at 5-hydroxytryptamine2C receptors, blockade of which enhances the activity of frontocortical dopaminergic and adrenergic pathways. *J. Pharmacol. Exp. Ther.* **2003**, *306*, 954–964. [CrossRef]
52. Chu, Y.S.; Shieh, K.R.; Yuan, Z.F.; Pan, J.T. Stimulatory and entraining effect of melatonin on tuberoinfundibular dopaminergic neuron activity and inhibition on prolactin secretion. *J. Pineal Res.* **2000**, *28*, 219–226. [CrossRef]

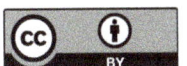

© 2019 by the authors. Licensee MDPI, Basel, Switzerland. This article is an open access article distributed under the terms and conditions of the Creative Commons Attribution (CC BY) license (http://creativecommons.org/licenses/by/4.0/).

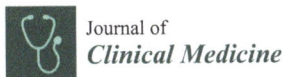

Review

The Potential Associations of Pornography Use with Sexual Dysfunctions: An Integrative Literature Review of Observational Studies

Aleksandra Diana Dwulit and Piotr Rzymski *

Department of Environmental Medicine, Poznan University of Medical Sciences, 60-806 Poznan, Poland
* Correspondence: rzymskipiotr@ump.edu.pl; Tel.: +48-61854-7604

Received: 30 May 2019; Accepted: 24 June 2019; Published: 26 June 2019

Abstract: This paper reviews the associations between pornography use and sexual dysfunction based on evidence from observational studies. The existing data in this regard mostly derive from cross-sectional investigations and case reports. There is little if no evidence that pornography use may induce delayed ejaculation and erectile dysfunction, although longitudinal studies that control for confounding variables are required for a full assessment. The associations between pornography use and sexual desire may differ between women and men although the existing data is contradictory and causal relationships cannot be established. The strongest evidence is available for the relation of pornography use with decreased sexual satisfaction, although the results of prospective studies are inconsistent. The paper outlines future research prospects beneficial in understanding the nature of associations between pornography use and sexual dysfunctions in men and women.

Keywords: pornography; sexual dysfunction; erectile dysfunction; delayed ejaculation; sexual desire; sexual satisfaction

1. Introduction

The existing literature provides a number of varying descriptions of the term pornography. According to the Final Report of the Attorney General's Commission on Pornography, it can be defined as any material that is predominantly sexually explicit and intended primarily for the purpose of sexual arousal [1]. Currently, pornography represents an important economic venture [2,3]. Its greatest development has occurred along with the emergence of computer technologies and the expansion of the Internet [4,5]. Due to a high sense of anonymity and almost unrestricted access, the Internet has become the most important medium of dissemination of pornographic content (known as online pornography), particularly in the form of images and videos [6,7]. The ease, arousal strength, and diversity with which pornography can be reached online indicates that it may operate as a supernormal stimulus [8].

According to various epidemiological studies, a relatively large number of adults have been exposed to pornography [9–12]. Recent representative surveys demonstrate that in developed countries with unrestricted Internet access, such as the United States and Australia, the majority of men (64–70%) and approx. one quarter/third (23–33%) of women are using pornography [13,14]. However, the number of pornography users is also relatively high in developing countries—recent surveys have shown that over half of students in Ethiopia and Bangladesh have been exposed to it [11,15]. The extensive use of pornography is also supported by data provided by Pornhub, one of the largest online pornographic websites, which clearly indicate that it is primarily men that are associated with content of this type (74%), and that the number of visitors to pornographic sites is growing from year to year (Figure 1). Some men deal with pornography on a regular, daily basis [16]. At the same time, the percentage of women interested in using this type of content is growing [17]. The Pornhub service is usually visited by young people under the age 34 from the United States, the United Kingdom and India. An emerging and as yet not fully assessed issue is the unintentional contact from advertising or spam e-mail messages both of which may sometimes be difficult to avoid [18].

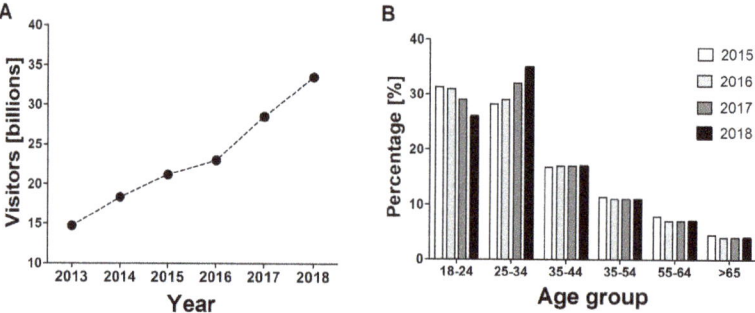

Figure 1. Statistics of pornography use in the period of 2013–2018 according to data shared by Pornhub: (**a**) annual number of visitors to Pornhub, (**b**) visitors to Pornhub by age.

Although interest in pornographic content can be partially considered as a natural element in the development of sexual experience in young people, the multiplicity and diversity of available online pornographic materials as well as the difficulty of restricting access to them lead to a question on the potential effects of pornography consumption. There is a steady increase in number of studies addressing the prevalence, patterns, outcomes, and various other aspects related to pornography use as clearly indicated by a systematic search of English language papers indexed in the PubMed/Medline database—a key term "pornography" yields 142 papers published in the period 1980–1989, 238 papers in 1990–1999, 524 papers in 2000–2009, and as many as 949 papers in 2010–2018. However, despite a continuous interest in the study of various aspects of pornography use, there are number of unresolved issues regarding the nature and magnitude of these effects. For example, some investigations demonstrate that pornography may fit into the addiction framework via mechanisms similar to chemical compounds [19,20] although controversies in this regard exist [21–24]. An addiction to pornography is not recognized in the DSM-5 and ICD-11 classifications (although the latter specifies a diagnostic category of Compulsive Sexual Behavior Disorder under impulse control disorders that may be used to diagnose problematic pornography use), various studies refer to it rather as "self-perceived pornography addiction" [12,16,25–27], and some alternative models based on moral incongruence, compulsivity, or impulsivity were also proposed to describe problematic pornography use [21,28,29]. Whether pornography may be associated with changes in sexual function is also a subject open to wide discussion. However, there are number of recognized risk factors for sexual dysfunction encompassing medical conditions, substance abuse, medication use, as well as cultural and social factors [30] which are difficult to address in studies focusing solely on pornography use. In the general population, the most frequently identified sexual dysfunctions include premature ejaculation and erectile dysfunction in men and desire and arousal dysfunction in women [31], and a number of studies have aimed to evaluate the potential associations between the occurrence of these effects and pornography use. At the same time, the potential effects of pornography use are the subject of a number of nonacademic discussions, and some publicly expressed opinions in this regard appear to be politically and ideologically driven. All in all, this creates a need to critically assess the existing evidence, outline study limitations and shortcomings, and highlight the future research prospects in the field of pornography use and its associations with sexual function.

The aim of this paper was to review the cross-sectional and longitudinal studies as well as case reports on potential associations between the use of pornography and sexual dysfunctions, namely erectile dysfunction, delayed ejaculation, and decrease in sexual desire and sexual satisfaction. These conditions are among the most often identified sexual dysfunctions in men and women [30–32]. Both quantitative (addressing the frequency of use) and qualitative (addressing the patterns of use) research was taken into account as these two approaches complement each other in understanding the complex nature of factors associated with pornography [33,34]. For this purpose, a systematic search for original research published since 2000 in peer-reviewed journals was performed using the PubMed/Medline and Scopus database, and by hand-searching reference lists from identified papers. The limitations of the conducted studies and future research prospects are also outlined.

2. Delayed Ejaculation

Delayed ejaculation describes a sexual dysfunction occurring in men, manifested by prolonged time required to ejaculate or complete inability to achieve it. Due to the complexity of psychosexual and psychosocial factors that contribute to its pathogenesis, there are no universal methods of treatment [35]. Its potential causes include, among many, frequent masturbation and the occurrence of significant discrepancies between real sexual intercourse with a partner and sexual fantasy preferred during masturbation [35,36]. Both masturbation and sexual fantasy are often associated with pornography use thus its potential relationship with the onset of delayed ejaculation is hypothetically plausible. A systematic search with key terms "pornography and ejaculation" and "pornography and delayed ejaculation" identified five original papers, including three cross-sectional studies and two case studies.

The first study to address the potential impact of pornography use on ejaculatory dysfunction was conducted on a group of 115 hypersexual, predominantly heterosexual men (mean age 41 years, range 19–76 years) [37]. As reported, a relatively significant percentage of subjects (23.5%; $n = 27$) masturbated chronically (at least 1 h/day or >7 h/week), usually while viewing pornography. In comparison with other subjects, this particular group was characterized by a higher anxiety level and was less likely to establish partner relationships or to persevere in them, even if they were established. These subjects frequently (19/27; 71%) reported some sexual dysfunctions with delayed ejaculation being reported the most often (in over 30% of cases). There are, however, a number of limitations to this study in the context of understanding the potential role of pornography in the occurrence of delayed ejaculation: (1) it only included hypersexual male subjects who represent a group that generally often masturbates and views pornography [38], and it remains unknown how these findings may be representative of the general population; (2) the onset of delayed ejaculation may result exclusively from the frequent masturbation or subjects with delayed ejaculation may tend to masturbate more often—in both cases, pornography use may remain unrelated; (3) it was unestablished whether the pornography use in hypersexual subjects facing delayed ejaculation preceded problems with this sexual dysfunction, therefore its role as a causative factor in delayed ejaculation cannot be established.

Two other cross-sectional studies involving young subjects do not support the potential existence of a relationship between pornography use and delayed ejaculation. The first of them surveyed Italian students attending their final year of high school ($n = 1492$; aged 18–19 years) who frequently admitted to using pornography (78%, including 8% using it on daily basis) and observed that ejaculatory issues were reported in 1% of surveyed, regardless of the frequency of pornography consumption [39]. In the second study, two large-scale samples of heterosexual men (aged 18–40 years) from three European countries, Croatia, Norway, and Portugal ($n = 3948$), were analyzed and, as demonstrated using multivariate logistic regression, no significant association between delayed ejaculation and pornography was detected [40].

In addition to cross-sectional studies, Park et al. [41] and Blair [36] reported cases in which delayed ejaculation appeared in some way to be related to pornography use. The former report described a case of a 20-year-old man with no chronic or mental disorder who used pornography for a long duration at a high frequency (1–2 times/day), gradually reaching for content that deviated progressively further from the standard. He also admitted to using an artificial vagina that supposedly allowed him to reach orgasm much faster. He self-reported the difficulty in maintaining an erection and ejaculating during masturbation and sexual intercourse, which contributed to disturbances in partner relations with his fiancée. As the authors emphasize, despite the fact that the man felt a physical and mental attraction to his partner, he preferred to use a more stimulating erotic toy (artificial vagina). The authors suggest that excessive pornography use could trigger changes in the nervous pathways responsible for sexual desire and erection, as well as changes in the functioning of the reward system, and subsequently caused delayed ejaculation [41]. These suggestions, however, remain purely speculative as no evidence to justify them was provided. As found, the delayed ejaculation was fully resolved after cessation of online pornography use and the quality of partner relationship was improved. However, the use of the artificial vagina was simultaneously discontinued. It therefore remains unestablished whether the delayed ejaculation was in any way related to the use of pornography, the artificial vagina, or both.

The case reported by Blair [36] included a 19-year-old male who could not achieve ejaculation during sexual penetration. The man started using pornographic content at the age of 12; a year later, he used it regularly, and at the age of 15 he began to reach for more and more thematic content (depicting the so-called bondage and acts of domination). Cessation of pornography and advice to avoid masturbation using a firm grip and switch to a more gentle style of penile stimulation were reported to be an effective therapy enabling the subject to achieve orgasm during an intercourse [36]. Therefore, this case also cannot be used as sole evidence for pornography-induced ejaculation impairment as it could just as well result from penile desensitization, a consequence of frequent masturbation. Some studies have reported that masturbation frequency and style, particularly the so-called "idiosyncratic" pattern that due to speed, pressure, and duration is difficult to be replicated by a partner, may be a predisposition for retarded ejaculation [42–44]. Therefore, the extent to which pornography use may contribute to such phenomenon remains unclear.

In summary, there is currently little evidence that an association between pornography use and delayed ejaculation exists and no indication that pornography use can be a cause of this sexual dysfunction. However, the assessment in this regard is only based on cross-sectional studies and case reports. Future research, particularly more extensive cohort studies and case-control observations, is therefore required.

3. Erectile Dysfunction

Erectile dysfunction is defined as a chronic inability to maintain an erection which prevents the introduction of the penis into the vagina. Its most common causes include age, diabetes, depression, cardiovascular and neurological diseases, selected psychogenic factors (including stress and abuse of psychoactive substances), and using selected pharmaceuticals [45]. Considering that some studies indicated a significant correlation between hypersexuality and problems with erectile function [46], it is plausible that some association in this respect may also exist for pornography use. A systematic search with key terms "pornography and erectile dysfunction", "pornography and erectile function", and "pornography and erection" identified a total of seven papers overall encompassing two case reports [41], six cross-sectional studies [28,39,40,47–49] and one longitudinal study [28].

Two interesting cases were presented by Park et al. [41]. In the first, a 40-year-old man with difficulty in maintaining an erection and achieving orgasm was described. During the period preceding the study he had intensively undertaken masturbation associated with the frequent use of online pornography, which was reported to be associated with an increasing amount of time required to achieve orgasm. He had also begun to view his wife as becoming gradually less sexually attractive. His physical parameters (including state of genitals) were in good condition. The patient was advised that his dysfunctions could have arisen from increased sexual stimulation, frequent masturbation, and change in the stimulation threshold due to exposure to strong pornographic content. The man, however, was unable to refrain from masturbation and watching pornography and did not initiate the treatment [41]. Another case described by the same authors concerns a 24-year-old man who was abusing alcohol and antidepressants, and had attempted suicide. He also reported to using online pornography at a frequency estimated at 5 h daily during the 6 months preceding the treatment. He experienced a weakened sexual interest in his wife, which was manifested by his inability to maintain an erection and preference to watching pornography, during which he experienced no erection problems. After discontinuing the use of pornography, according to the therapist's recommendation, his erectile dysfunction disappeared [41]. Both of these cases are complicated with confounding variables and no casual relation between pornography use and erectile dysfunction can be seen. In the first, it is not possible to separate the potential effects of frequent pornography use and excessive masturbation, although one should note that these two phenomena can often be highly correlated in men [50]. The second case is complicated by psychiatric history (use of antidepressants and suicide attempt) as well as by the reported alcohol abuse which itself is a common cause of sexual dysfunctions such as erectile retardation [51].

As found in a pilot observational study conducted in 2006 on a small group of young adult men ($n = 25$; mean age 29 years), nearly half of them ($n = 12$) showed no signs of sexual arousal, including erections while watching an erotic film (penile rigidity < 5%; and 0% in eight subjects) [47]. These observations were initially associated with a potentially high level of exposure to pornographic content, lowering the responsiveness to sexual stimuli associated with the presentation of sex in a more standard edition (vanilla sex). In the second stage of the study, a larger number of men were recruited ($n = 80$) and exposed to longer and more diverse erotic films. Nineteen percent of them ($n = 15$) failed to respond sexually. It appeared that the risk of sexual dysfunction increased along with the number of pornographic films that had been viewed by the respondents during the previous year [47]. Another study of a larger range was conducted in 2016 on a group of 434 men (mean age 29.5 years, range 18–72). Using the International Index of Erectile Function questionnaire, the ability to achieve an erection and orgasm, the degree of sexual desire, satisfaction with sexual intercourse, and general sexual satisfaction were evaluated in 276 subjects who had had sexual intercourse during the last month. The study concluded that problematic online sexual behavior (defined as compulsive, persistent, uncontrolled use of pornographic content) was a significant predictor of a low level of erection [49].

In turn, the study surveying Italian high school students ($n = 1429$; age 18–19 years) did not show that erection problems were more frequently admitted by teenagers watching pornography, regardless of the self-reported frequency of its use [39]. A cross-sectional study conducted in two-large scale samples on heterosexual men (aged 18–40 years): the first in 2011 on Croatian, Norwegian, and Portuguese heterosexual men ($n = 2727$) and the second in 2014 on another sample of Croatian men ($n = 1211$) identified a positive relationship between pornography use and erectile dysfunction in the first subset of individuals from Croatia although the effect was small and not confirmed in other groups [40]. Another study reported that instead of erectile dysfunction, pornography use in 280 heterosexual men (mean age 23 years) was positively correlated with sexual arousal which was self-reported when watching visual stimuli in the laboratory [48]. Furthermore, subjects indicating higher pornography consumption also reported a greater desire for solo and partnered sexual behaviors. However, this study had a number of limitations: a high number of monogamous individuals (which may be more sexually exploratory, particularly if young), a rather limited frequency of pornography use in the studied group (individuals were divided into three groups using pornography 0, 1–2, and >2 h per week but the maximum frequency remained unreported), and an unknown period of pornography use in the investigated individuals prior to the study.

The most recent study performed by Grubbs and Gola [28] reported a positive association between self-reported erectile dysfunction and self-reported problematic pornography use but not mere pornography use in a cross-sectional sample of 147 undergraduate men (mean age 20 years) in the United States as well as in a sample of 433 men (mean age 33 years) matched to the demographic norms of this country. The one-year, four-wave longitudinal study that was based on these two samples, completed across all four time points by 117 participants, and with two point-data collected for 278 subjects, also found that baseline pornography use and problematic pornography use was positively associated with prospective erectile dysfunction. However, latent growth modelling indicated that no baseline variables served as predictors of the trajectory of erectile functioning over time. Although these results support the existence of an association between erectile dysfunction and problematic pornography use, they fail to show a causal relationship. It is thus plausible that men with erectile dysfunction may tend to use more pornography, including patterns they self-perceive as problematic [28].

As yet, there is little or no evidence on a causal relationship between erectile dysfunction and frequency of pornography use. It cannot be ruled out that subjects with erectile dysfunction may be more prone to using pornography more frequently. One should note that cross-sectional and longitudinal studies performed so far are solely based on self-reported data introducing a significant limitation. Some research clearly indicates that the prevalence of self-reporting of erectile dysfunction may vary considerably from the prevalence identified by objective methods such as the International Index of Erectile Function to the extent that the former might be unreliable in assessing the real presence of this sexual dysfunction [52]. There is a need for further longitudinal exploration of associations between erectile dysfunction and pornography use that would include individuals of different age and with various baseline pornography use and employ a diverse methodology encompassing physiological measures and partner reports.

4. Changes in Sexual Desire

From the perspective of biological sciences, the term libido is used to describe sexual desire, a trait controlled by central nervous system associated with the sexual drive and wish to engage in sexual activities [53]. As highlighted, it should not be mistaken for sexual arousal which manifests itself physiologically and may not always be positively correlated with sexual desire [54]. This said, it can be hypothesized whether pornography use increases or decreases libido, and if frequency and duration of pornography consumption may modify such responses. One can also consider different responses in males and females due to varying sex roles and sexually differentiated neural activity in response to sexual stimuli [55]. To explore it, a systematic search for original studies was performed with the key terms "pornography and libido" and "pornography and sexual desire". A total of five papers associated with this subject were identified and included cross-sectional studies [39,40,50,56,57].

Carvalheira, Træen, & Stulhofer [50] analyzed the relationship between masturbation and the use of pornography and sexual desire in a group of European heterosexual men (mean age 40 years, range 21–73) who had reported a problem of reduced sexual desire (n = 596). As found, more than half of the studied subjects who had experienced a significant decrease in libido within six months before the examination were involved with pornographic materials at least once a week. The study further found that frequency of masturbation and pornography use are strongly correlated in men with decreased sexual desire. One should note that the cross-sectional nature of this study does not allow any causation between pornography consumption and decreased libido to be established, and that interpretation of the obtained data is also limited by the lack of a control group constituted by men with no sexual dysfunctions. Although it is generally an interesting or even counterintuitive observation that men with an impaired libido may watch more pornography and masturbate often, it is important to highlight that men with lower sexual desire (contrary to women with lower libido) tend to increase the frequency of masturbation in a manner unrelated to pornography consumption [58,59]. Considering the high accessibility of online pornography, it is no surprise that men who tend to masturbate often will also constitute a group using it as sexual stimuli.

Cross-sectional observations in Italian students attending the last year of high school (n = 1492, aged 18–19 years) indicated that as many as 78% of them admitted to using pornographic content, with 8% indicating doing so on a daily basis. A decrease in sexual desire was reported by 10% of pornography users, and appeared to increase with the frequency of consumption: among students exposed at least once a week, it accounted for 16%, while in the case of those exposed less often it was 6%; the nonusers did not report it at all [39].

The findings of Carvalheira, Træen, & Stulhofer [50] and Pizzol, Beroldo, & Foresta [39] were not confirmed in a large study encompassing large-scale samples of heterosexual men (aged 18–40 years) from Croatia, Norway, and Portugal (n = 3948) and applying multivariate logistic regression [40]. In turn, a study on women ($n = 754$; aged 18 = 76 years) reported that those involved in a long-term relationship that use pornography more frequently may reveal increased sexual desire towards their partners and report a higher desire for sexual variety [56]. This is a relatively important finding indicating the potential difference in patterns of pornography use between men and women, although one should note that the cross-sectional nature of the study does not imply causation. It remains to be explored whether a pornography-induced increase in libido exists in women or women with higher sexual desire are also more open to watching pornography more frequently. Moreover, the potential role of sexual partner (in terms of sexual desire and satisfaction) and satisfaction from a relationship may represent important factors for inclusion in multivariate analyses conducted in the future. Interestingly, a recent cross-sectional survey of 240 committed heterosexual couples (mean age of males and females 35 and 33 years, respectively) confirmed the positive correlation of pornography use by women with their sexual desire but also found a similar but weaker relation in men [57].

Neurobiological research indicates that the potentially negative effect of long-term pornography use on sexual desire may result from changes in the responsiveness of the reward system to sexual stimuli, preferentially more active as a result of stimuli associated with pornography than with real sexual intercourse [60,61]. However, observational studies do not provide consistent data to support the hypothesis that use of pornography is a causative factor for a decrease in sexual desire and rather provide a contradictory observation as regards the existence and direction of correlations between pornography use and libido. These contradictions may potentially arise from the complex nature of sexual desire in both men and women, which is influenced by a number of biological, psychological, relational, sexual and cultural factors [62,63]. Considering that some studies have reported that subjects with higher sexual boredom and lower libido may tend to masturbate more frequently [50], it is important to elucidate the role the pornography use and pornography-associated masturbation may play in fulfilling the need for sexual gratification. Further cross-sectional studies as well as prospective investigations that control for these factors are greatly required to draw some final conclusions on the relation of pornography use and level of sexual desire.

5. Changes in Sexual Satisfaction

It could be hypothesized that the frequent exposure to pornography can potentially impact sexual satisfaction. The potential reasons for its decrease may include: (1) a comparison of real partners to idealized acting roles in pornographic films [64,65], (2) disappointment when the actual partner is not interested in recreating the scenes observed in pornographic material, (3) disappointment due to the inability to obtain such a broad spectrum of sexual novelties, with a real partner as presented in pornographic material [66,67] and (4) contact with pornography chosen instead of sexual intercourse with a real partner [68,69].

On the other hand, one could also hypothesize that in some cases, use of pornography may increase sexual satisfaction by providing inspiration for real sex. However, the magnitude of these effects may differ between men and women, and may also be potentially modified by frequency and time of pornography use, as well as type of pornography consumed. Moreover, it may also be hypothesized that shared pornography use in couples may have a positive impact on sexual satisfaction as it could stimulate partners for more sexual exploration during real intercourse [70].

A systematic search with the key term "pornography and sexual satisfaction" identified a total of 23 papers reporting observational studies among which 20 cross-sectional surveys (Table 1) and four prospective investigations were reported [65,71–73].

As found, the associations of pornography use on sexual satisfaction may differ across gender (Table 1). In general, its decrease was more often observed in men than women. Moreover, the frequency of pornography use may also be differentially associated with sexual satisfaction in both genders—in men, its decrease was already reported at a rate of use estimated at a few times per year while in women at a frequency of once a month [74]. As demonstrated in both women and men, age of first exposure may also be associated with decrease in sexual satisfaction, with a two-fold increase in the odds if such exposure occurred ≤ 12 years in reference to individuals exposed for the first time >16 years. Nonreligious individuals and those in a relationship were also found to reveal weaker associations between pornography use and sexual satisfaction [74,75]. Interestingly, one study reported that, in men, the negative association between pornography use and sexual satisfaction appeared to diminish once masturbation frequency was controlled [76]. However, one should note that pornography consumption and masturbation are usually highly associated in men [50]. Altogether, it highlights that the context of pornography use may highly moderate the nature of associated effects and should be taken into account in further assessments. As recently indicated, length of relationship was negatively associated with pornography use in women, thus mitigating its effects on sexual satisfaction [77]. In turn, in newly married couples, pornography use was demonstrated to be negatively correlated with sexual satisfaction [73]. One study demonstrated that the association between pornography use and sexual satisfaction may be differentiated according to the attachment styles of the studied subjects: with no association found in secure individuals (neither anxious nor avoidant), a negative association among preoccupied (high anxiety but low avoidance) and dismissing (low avoidance and high anxiety) subjects and a positive one among fearful persons (simultaneously highly anxious and avoiding) [78]. This puts an association between pornography use and sexual satisfaction in a wider psychological context in which it may arise from early interactions with caregivers that, via internalization of operative cognitive models, guide behavior and cognition, in relation with sexuality in adulthood. This is particularly interesting in the light of the research of Szymanski and Stewart-Richardson [79] who demonstrated that frequency of pornography use as well as problematic pornography use in heterosexual men is related to more avoidant and more anxious attachment styles. The authors hypothesize that these men use pornography as it allows them to experience emotional and/or sexual gratification without having to risk interpersonal rejection or intimacy [79]. Altogether, these findings suggest that the nature of associations between pornography use and sexual satisfaction may depend on various variables encompassing gender, relationship status, cultural/religious factors, and psychological background, and this, in addition to quantitative data, should be taken into account in future studies.

Overall, it appears that individuals, particularly men, who use pornography more often also tend to report lower satisfaction with their sex life. The limitations of cross-sectional studies do not allow us to distinguish whether pornography induces a decrease in sexual satisfaction or whether low sexual satisfaction predicts more frequent pornography consumption, or both. The first longitudinal, three-wave (six months between waves) panel study in this regard conducted on a population of Dutch adolescents ($n = 1052$; aged 13–20 years) revealed that pornography use consistently reduced sexual satisfaction but also that low sexual satisfaction led to increase in pornography use [65]. This highlights that these bidirectional relationships must be taken into account, and that other factors contributing to lower sexual satisfaction (that may potentially include sexual or psychosocial dysfunctions) should be addressed to fully elucidate the reasons for pornography use. Gender was not demonstrated to be a moderator of observed effects in this study. However, another four-wave panel study (six months between waves) which was also conducted on a sample of Dutch adolescents ($n = 1132$; aged 11–18 years) indicated that more frequent pornography use at baseline predicted less sexual satisfaction at the last study point in males, while in females, sexual satisfaction was negatively associated with an increase in pornography use [71]. The findings by Peter & Valkenburg [65] and Doornwaard et al. [71] were not replicated in the other, three-wave longitudinal study (one year between waves) that surveyed 190 newly married heterosexual couples [73]. As demonstrated, the frequency of pornography use in women and men failed to predict changes in sexual satisfaction and pre-existing sexual satisfaction did not predict changes in pornography consumption. More recently, a longitudinal six-wave study (six months between waves) of females ($n = 775$) and males ($n = 514$) aged 15–18 years, also found no significant association between frequency of pornography use and sexual satisfaction, regardless of gender [72]. Further prospective studies will be necessary before any definite conclusions can be drawn.

Table 1. Cross-sectional studies on association between pornography use and sexual satisfaction in women and men.

Study Type	Group	Age of Subjects Mean ± SD (range) years	Method	Observation	Reference
Online survey	373 heterosexual men	19 ± 2 (18–29)	Multidimensional Sexuality Questionnaire	Frequency of PU and PPU correlated with ↓ sexual satisfaction	[79]
Online survey	217 heterosexual couples	37 ± 11 ♂; 35 ± 10 ♀	Index of Sexual Satisfaction	Frequency of PU correlated with ↓ sexual satisfaction only in male	[80]
Online survey	650 men	(18–25)	Snell's Index of Sexual Satisfaction	Earlier exposure to P correlated with ↓ sexual satisfaction	[81]
Online survey	326 heterosexual men; 456 heterosexual women	20 (18–30)	One-item question	Frequency of PU correlated with ↓ sexual satisfaction only in male	[82]
Online survey	221 women; 75 men; (97% heterosexual)	29 ± 9 (18–87)	Index of Sexual Satisfaction	No correlation between frequency of PU and sexual satisfaction	[83]
Online survey	1513 heterosexual adults	23 ± 8	Two-item question	Frequency of PU correlated with ↓ sexual satisfaction	[74]
Online survey	240 heterosexual couples	35 ± 9 (18–72) ♂; 33 ± 9 (18–60) ♀	Golombok Rust Inventory of Sexual Satisfaction	Couple PU correlated with ↑ sexual satisfaction Unknown individual use correlated with ↓ sexual satisfaction	[57]
Pen-and-paper survey	1501 randomly selected adults	50 ± 18 (17–98)	One-item question	Frequency of PU correlated with ↓ sexual satisfaction only in male	[75]
Online survey	565 women; 471 men	(18–55)	One-item question	Frequency of PU correlated with ↓ sexual satisfaction only in male	[77]
Online survey	894 heterosexual adults	30 ± 9	Two-item question	Frequency of PU correlated with ↓ sexual satisfaction with no gender differences	[84]
Online survey	596 women; 234 men	25 ± 8 (18–78)	Global Measure of Sexual Satisfaction	Frequency of PU correlated with ↓ sexual satisfaction, particularly lower scores were seen in compulsive users.	[85]
Online survey	587 women; 232 men	25 ± 8 (18–78)	Global Measure of Sexual Satisfaction	Frequency of PU correlated with ↓ sexual satisfaction in both gender	[86]
Online survey	1471 women; 1109 men	(18–60)	New Scale of Sexual Satisfaction	Frequency of PU correlated with ↓ sexual satisfaction in both gender	[87]
Pen-and-paper survey	190 newly married heterosexual couples	34 ♂; 31 ♀	Perceived Relationship Quality Components (PRQC) Inventory	Frequency of PU correlated with ↓ sexual satisfaction in both gender	[73]
Face-to-face interviews	2610 married adults	53 ± 14 (25–80)	One-item question	Frequency of PU correlated with ↓ sexual satisfaction in studied group	[88]
Online survey	433 heterosexual married couples	38 (22–59) ♂; 35 (20–44) ♀	One-item question	No correlation between frequency of PU and sexual satisfaction in husbands and wives	[79]
Pen-and-paper survey	326 heterosexual couples	38 ± 10 ♂; 36 ± 10 ♀	Golombok Rust Inventory of Sexual Satisfaction	Frequency of PU correlated with ↓ sexual satisfaction in both gender	[89]
Pen-and-paper survey	460 women; 130 men	24 ± 7 (18–64)	One-item question with Likert scale	PU correlated with ↓ sexual satisfaction. The association was differentiated by attachment styles: negative among anxious/avoidant subjects, positive among fearful individuals	[78]
Online survey	3004 women; 2079 men	22 ± 1 (18–26)	One-item question	Earlier age of exposure to P increased odds for ↓sexual satisfaction	[12]
Online survey	470 men	27 ± 11	Global Measure of Sexual Satisfaction	Frequency of PU correlated with ↓ sexual satisfaction	[76]
Online survey	378 men	47 ± 14	Global Measure of Sexual Satisfaction	Frequency of PU correlated with ↓ sexual satisfaction	[76]

P—pornography PU—pornography use; PPU—problematic pornography use; SD—standard deviation.

Importantly, the majority of cross-sectional studies summarized in Table 1 only assessed individual pornography use. As shown by Willoughby & Leonhardt [57], shared viewing of pornography in heterosexual couples is correlated with higher sexual satisfaction. As demonstrated, women using pornography may more often experience guilt, disgust, and embarrassment [90], which are rather not experienced when this use is shared with their partners—such a scenario may promote positive sexual interactions in couples. One should note, however, that the findings of Willoughby & Leonhardt [57] are derived from a cross-sectional study and no causality can be established. It can be hypothesized that shared pornography use increases sexual satisfaction in partners or that partners experiencing higher sexual satisfaction may tend to view pornography together more often.

Additionally, interesting associations between pornography use and a partner's sexual satisfaction have been reported. For example, Yucel and Gassanov [91] who surveyed 433 heterosexual married couples observed that a husband's pornography consumption was negatively correlated with his wife's sexual satisfaction while a wife's pornography use was not associated with her husband's satisfaction. In turn, the longitudinal observations made in 190 newlywed couples found that increased sexual satisfaction in men was a predictor of a decline in pornography viewing by their wives [73]. These bivariate associations suggest that gender patterns in pornography consumption in couple relationships may mutually affect sexual satisfaction and may be important to consider in future works on the effects of pornography use on the quality of sex life.

In conclusion, the accumulating evidence from cross-sectional studies supports the hypothesis that pornography use is associated with lower sexual satisfaction. However, the magnitude of this association appears to depend on a number of factors, including gender, relationship status, frequency, duration, and pattern of pornography use, and the age at which pornography use was initiated. One should also note that although much attention is paid to associations with lower sexual satisfaction, some studies not only report no associations of pornography consumption in this regard in large number of surveyed subjects but also indicate that some individuals experience an increase in sexual satisfaction. For example, in a recent cross-sectional study of Polish students who admit to current pornography use, respectively 68% and 7% associated its consumption with no effect and a beneficial effect on sexual satisfaction [12]. Moreover, studies in couples demonstrate that use of pornography may not necessarily be associated with less sexual satisfaction, and that in some cases, a positive correlation can be observed [57]. As already shown in relation to relationship quality, it is highly plausible that the nature of the association between pornography use and sexual satisfaction in individuals in romantic relationships may not only depend solely on the frequency of use but the context in which it is consumed, such as concordance or discrepancy in partners' use, levels of acceptance of pornography use from both partners, known or hidden use, and individual or shared use [70,92]. Moreover, the longitudinal studies conducted so far have failed to fully confirm that pornography use is a causative factor in impaired sexual satisfaction. It remains to be explored whether the potential effect of pornography in this regard can be influenced by: (i) sexual orientation: the majority of studies have focused on heterosexual individuals while homo- and bisexual individuals may even be more frequent pornography users as preliminarily found in men [93], (ii) physical disabilities as they may also influence a baseline sexual satisfaction [94], and (iii) co-occurrence of other sexual dysfunctions, as some authors have indicated that pornography use may be a continuation of pre-existing compulsive sexual behaviors [64,95].

6. Future Research Prospects and Conclusions

Increasing access to the Internet has opened a completely new chapter for the pornographic industry, simultaneously increasing both the time and strength of exposure to pornographic content, and its potential effects on health. The studies conducted so far indicate a correlational relationship between pornography consumption and selected sexual dysfunctions with the strongest evidence for a decrease in sexual satisfaction. It should be noted that the vast majority of observations are based on cross-sectional studies or case reports and without future research based on extensive case-control and/or prospective cohort studies, causality cannot be comprehensively assessed. One should also note that assessment of pornography use in studies is mostly based on self-reporting and that objective confirmation of exposure is not possible. Moreover, the presence of sexual dysfunctions such as erectile dysfunction is also often self-reported and creates the risk of their being underestimated; thus, when possible, the use of validated tools is advised. There are number of recognized risk factors for sexual dysfunctions which need to be considered when evaluating the potential effects of pornography use in future studies. The frequency of pornography use may in turn be potentially modulated by various parameters such as gender, cultural/religious factors, relationship status, and psychological background. Further research on associations between pornography consumption and sexual dysfunction should also take these into account. Unlike the effect of psychoactive substances or binge eating, the potential effects of pornography use cannot be recreated using experimental animal models, while the scope of experimental research involving human volunteers is rather limited and can often only be used to assess short-term outcomes. This in turn highlights the need for more, well-designed observational, particularly prospective studies. To provide a broad insight into the potential associations of pornography use with sexual dysfunctions, it would be best for future studies to provide a definition of pornography, specify the type of pornographic content consumed by the studied subjects (e.g., violent, nonviolent, mainstream, and paraphilic), control for the frequency of masturbation, consider the sexual orientation of participants, whether they are in a relationship or not, and if they are what is their relationship satisfaction and whether they consume pornography individually or in a shared manner. The context in which pornography is consumed rather than the mere use may moderate the associated effects, and such context must be taken into account in further assessments. The complexity of factors influencing pornography use and modulating its associated effects, as well as the susceptibility of research models to methodological biases and difficulties in overcoming the limitations of studies strongly justify a need for further investigation on the associations between sexual functionality and pornography consumption, which is particularly important given the high rates of the latter.

Conflicts of Interest: The authors declare no conflict of interest.

References

1. McManus, M. *Final Report of the Attorney General's Commission on Pornography*; Rutledge Hill Press: Nashville, TN, USA, 1986.
2. Wilkinson, E. The diverse economies of online pornography: From paranoid readings to post-capitalist futures. *Sexualities* **2017**, *20*, 981–998. [CrossRef]
3. Cannatelli, B.L.; Smith, B.R.; Sydow, A. Entrepreneurship in the controversial economy: Toward a research agenda. *J. Bus. Ethics* **2019**, *155*, 837–851. [CrossRef]
4. Paasonen, S. Online Porn. In *The SAGE Handbook of Web History, Niels Brügger, Ian Milligan and Megan Ankerson*; Sage Publications: Thousand Oaks, CA, USA, 2018; pp. 551–563.
5. D'Orlando, F. The demand for pornography. *J. Happiness Stud.* **2011**, *12*, 51–75. [CrossRef]
6. Cooper, A.; Putnam, D.E.; Planchon, L.S.; Boies, S.C. Online sexual compulsivity: Getting tangled in the net. *Sex. Addict. Compulsivity* **1999**, *6*, 79–104. [CrossRef]
7. Boies, S.C.; Cooper, A.; Osborne, C.S. Variations in internet-related problems and psychosocial functioning in online sexual activities: Implications for social and sexual development of young adults. *Cyberpsychol. Behav.* **2004**, *7*, 207–230. [CrossRef]
8. Goodwin, B.C.; Browne, M.; Rockloff, M. Measuring preference for supernormal over natural rewards: A two-dimensional anticipatory pleasure scale. *Evolut. Psychol.* **2015**. [CrossRef]
9. Habesha, T.; Aderaw, Z.; Lakew, S. Assessment of exposure to sexually explicit materials and factors associated with exposure among preparatory school youths in Hawassa City, Southern Ethiopia: A cross-sectional institution based survey. *Reprod. Health* **2015**, *12*, 86. [CrossRef] [PubMed]
10. Peter, J.; Valkenburg, P.M. Adolescents and pornography: A review of 20 years of research. *J. Sex Res.* **2016**, *53*, 509–531. [CrossRef] [PubMed]

11. Chowdhury, M.R.H.K.; Chowdhury, M.R.K.; Kabir, R.; Perera, N.K.P.; Kader, M. Does the addiction in online pornography affect the behavioral pattern of undergrad private university students in Bangladesh? *Int. J. Health Sci.* **2018**, *12*, 67–74.
12. Dwulit, A.D.; Rzymski, P. Prevalence, Patterns and Self-Perceived Effects of Pornography Consumption in Polish University Students: A Cross-Sectional Study. *Int. J. Environ. Res. Public Health* **2019**, *16*, 1861. [CrossRef] [PubMed]
13. Rissel, C.; Richters, J.; De Visser, R.O.; Mckee, A.; Yeung, A.; Rissel, C.; Caruana, T. A profile of pornography users in Australia: Findings from the second Australian study of health and relationships. *J. Sex Res.* **2016**, *54*, 227–240. [CrossRef] [PubMed]
14. Grubbs, J.B.; Kraus, S.W.; Perry, S.L. Self-reported addiction to pornography in a nationally representative sample: The roles of use habits, religiousness, and moral incongruence. *J. Behav. Addict.* **2018**, *8*, 88–93. [CrossRef] [PubMed]
15. Abrha, K.; Worku, A.; Lerebo, W.; Berhane, Y. Sexting and high sexual risk-taking behaviours among school youth in northern Ethiopia: Estimating using prevalence ratio. *BMJ Sex. Reprod. Health* **2019**. [CrossRef] [PubMed]
16. Duffy, A.; Dawson, D.L.; das Nair, R. Pornography addiction in adults: A systematic review of definitions and reported impact. *J. Sex. Med.* **2016**, *13*, 760–777. [CrossRef] [PubMed]
17. Wright, P.J.; Bae, S.; Funk, M. United States women and pornography through four decades: Exposure, attitudes, behaviors, individual differences. *Arch. Sex. Behav.* **2013**, *42*, 1131–1144. [CrossRef] [PubMed]
18. Flood, M. Exposure to pornography among youth in Australia. *J. Sociol.* **2007**, *43*, 45–60. [CrossRef]
19. Brand, M.; Young, K.S.; Laier, C.; Wölfling, K.; Potenza, M.N. Integrating psychological and neurobiological considerations regarding the development and maintenance of specific Internet-use disorders: An Interaction of Person-Affect-Cognition-Execution (I-PACE) model. *Neurosci. Biobehav. Rev.* **2016**, *71*, 252–266. [CrossRef]
20. Gola, M.; Wordecha, M.; Marchewka, A.; Sescousse, G. Visual sexual stimuli—Cue or reward? A perspective for interpreting brain imaging findings on human sexual behaviors. *Front. Hum. Neurosci.* **2016**, *10*, 1–7.
21. Ley, D.; Prause, N.; Finn, P. The Emperor has no clothes: A review of the "pornography addiction" model. *Curr. Sex. Health Rep.* **2014**, *6*, 94–105. [CrossRef]
22. Love, T.; Laier, C.; Brand, M.; Hatch, L.; Hajela, R. Neuroscience of Internet pornography addiction: A review and update. *Behav. Sci.* **2015**, *5*, 388–433. [CrossRef]
23. de Alarcón, R.; de la Iglesia, J.I.; Casado, N.M.; Montejo, A.L. Online Porn Addiction: What We Know and What We Don't—A Systematic Review. *J. Clin. Med.* **2019**, *8*, 91. [CrossRef] [PubMed]
24. Kraus, S.W.; Voon, V.; Potenza, M.N. Should compulsive sexual behavior be considered an addiction? *Addiction* **2016**, *111*, 2097–2106. [CrossRef] [PubMed]
25. Bradley, D.F.; Grubbs, J.B.; Uzdavines, A.; Exline, J.J.; Pargament, K.I. Perceived addiction to internet pornography among religious believers and nonbelievers. *Sex. Addict. Compulsivity* **2016**, *23*, 225–243. [CrossRef]
26. Grubbs, J.B.; Perry, S.L. Moral incongruence and pornography use: A critical review and integration. *J. Sex Res.* **2018**, *7*, 1–9. [CrossRef] [PubMed]
27. Sniewski, L.; Farvid, P.; Carter, P. The assessment and treatment of adult heterosexual men with self-perceived problematic pornography use: A review. *Addict. Behav.* **2018**, *77*, 217–224. [CrossRef] [PubMed]
28. Grubbs, J.B.; Gola, M. Is pornography use related to erectile functioning? Results from cross-sectional and latent growth curve analyses. *J. Sex. Med.* **2019**, *16*, 111–125. [CrossRef] [PubMed]
29. Bőthe, B.; Tóth-Király, I.; Potenza, M.N.; Griffiths, M.D.; Orosz, G.; Demetrovics, Z. Revisiting the role of impulsivity and compulsivity in problematic sexual behaviors. *J. Sex Res.* **2019**, *56*, 166–179. [CrossRef] [PubMed]
30. McCabe, M.P.; Sharlip, I.D.; Lewis, R.; Atalla, E.; Balon, R.; Fisher, A.D.; Segraves, R.T. Risk factors for sexual dysfunction among women and men: A consensus statement from the fourth international consultation on sexual medicine 2015. *J. Sex. Med.* **2015**, *13*, 153–167. [CrossRef]
31. McCabe, M.P.; Sharlip, I.D.; Atalla, E.; Balon, R.; Fisher, A.D.; Laumann, E.; Lee, S.W.; Lewis, R.; Segraves, R.T. Definitions of sexual dysfunctions in women and men: A consensus statement from the fourth international consultation on sexual medicine. *J. Sex. Med.* **2016**, *13*, 135–143. [CrossRef]
32. Di Sante, S.; Mollaioli, D.; Gravina, G.L.; Ciocca, G.; Limoncin, E.; Carosa, E.; Lenzi, A.; Jannini, E.A. Epidemiology of delayed ejaculation. *Transl. Androl. Urol.* **2016**, *5*, 541–548. [CrossRef]

33. Gola, M.; Lewczuk, K.; Skorko, M. What matters: Quantity or quality of pornography use? Psychological and behavioral factors of seeking treatment for problematic pornography use. *J. Sex. Med.* **2016**, *13*, 815–824. [CrossRef] [PubMed]
34. Lewczuk, K.; Szmyd, J.; Skorko, M.; Gola, M. Treatment seeking for problematic pornography use among women. *J. Behav. Addict.* **2017**, *6*, 445–456. [CrossRef] [PubMed]
35. Abdel-Hamid, I.A.; Ali, O.I. Delayed ejaculation: Pathophysiology, diagnosis, and treatment. *World J. Men's Health* **2018**, *36*, 22–40. [CrossRef] [PubMed]
36. Blair, L. How difficult is it to treat delayed ejaculation within a short-term psychosexual model? A case study comparison. *Sex. Relatsh. Ther.* **2018**, *33*, 298–308. [CrossRef]
37. Sutton, K.S.; Stratton, N.; Pytyck, J.; Kolla, N.J.; Cantor, J.M. Patient characteristics by type of hypersexuality referral: A quantitative chart review of 115 consecutive male cases. *J. Sex Marital Ther.* **2015**, *41*, 563–580. [CrossRef] [PubMed]
38. Öberg, K.G.; Hallberg, J.; Kaldo, V.; Dhejne, C.; Arver, S. Hypersexual disorder according to the hypersexual disorder screening inventory in help-seeking Swedish men and women with self-identified hypersexual behavior. *Sex. Med.* **2017**, *5*, e229–e236. [CrossRef] [PubMed]
39. Pizzol, D.; Bertoldo, A.; Foresta, C. Adolescents and web porn: A new era of sexuality. *Int. J. Adolesc. Med. Health* **2016**, *28*, 169–173. [CrossRef] [PubMed]
40. Landripet, I.; Stulhofer, A. Is pornography use associated with sexual difficulties and dysfunctions among younger heterosexual men? *J. Sex. Med.* **2015**, *12*, 1136–1139. [CrossRef]
41. Park, B.Y.; Wilson, G.; Berger, J.; Christman, M.; Reina, B.; Bishop, F.; Klam, W.P.; Doan, A.P. Is internet pornography causing sexual dysfunctions? A review with clinical reports. *Behav. Sci.* **2016**, *6*, 3. [CrossRef]
42. Perelman, M.A.; Rowland, D.L. Retarded ejaculation. *World J. Urol.* **2006**, *24*, 645–652. [CrossRef]
43. Perelman, M.A. Psychosexual therapy for delayed ejaculation based on the sexual tipping point model. *Transl. Androl. Urol.* **2016**, *5*, 563–575. [CrossRef] [PubMed]
44. Bronner, G.; Ben-Zion, I.Z. Unusual masturbatory practice as an etiological factor in the diagnosis and treatment of sexual dysfunction in young men. *J. Sex. Med.* **2014**, *11*, 1798–1806. [CrossRef] [PubMed]
45. Mobley, D.F.; Khera, M.; Baum, N. Recent advances in the treatment of erectile dysfunction. *Postgrad. Med. J.* **2017**, *93*, 679–685. [CrossRef] [PubMed]
46. Klein, V.; Jurin, T.; Briken, P.; Štulhofer, A. Erectile dysfunction, boredom, and hypersexuality among coupled men from two European countries. *J. Sex. Med.* **2015**, *12*, 2160–2167. [CrossRef] [PubMed]
47. Janssen, E.; Bancroft, J. The Dual-control model: The role of sexual inhibition excitation in sexual arousal and behavior. In *The Psychophysiology of Sex*; Janssen, E., Ed.; Indiana University Press: Bloomington, IN, USA, 2006; pp. 197–222.
48. Prause, N.; Pfaus, J. Viewing sexual stimuli associated with greater sexual responsiveness, not erectile dysfunction. *Sex. Med.* **2015**, *3*, 90–98. [CrossRef] [PubMed]
49. Wéry, A.; Billieux, J. Online sexual activities: An exploratory study of problematic and non-problematic usage patterns in a sample of men. *Comput. Hum. Behav.* **2016**, *56*, 257–266. [CrossRef]
50. Carvalheira, A.; Træen, B.; Stulhofer, A. Masturbation and pornography use among coupled heterosexual men with decreased sexual desire: How many roles of masturbation? *J. Sex Marital Ther.* **2015**, *41*, 626–635. [CrossRef] [PubMed]
51. Arackal, B.S.; Benegal, V. Prevalence of sexual dysfunction in male subjects with alcohol dependence. *Indian J. Psychiatry* **2007**, *49*, 109–112.
52. Wu, C.J.; Hsieh, J.T.; Lin, J.S.; Hwang, T.I.; Jiann, B.P.; Huang, S.T.; Wang, C.J.; Lee, S.S.; Chiang, H.S.; Chen, K.K.; et al. Comparison of prevalence between self-reported erectile dysfunction and erectile dysfunction as defined by five-item International Index of Erectile Function in Taiwanese men older than 40 years. *Urology* **2017**, *69*, 743–747. [CrossRef]
53. Mark, K.P.; Lasslo, J.A. Maintaining sexual desire in long-term relationships: A systematic review and conceptual model. *J. Sex Res.* **2018**, *55*, 563–581. [CrossRef]
54. Santtila, P.; Wager, I.; Witting, K.; Harlaar, N.; Jern, P.; Johansson, A.; Varjonen, M.; Sandnabba, N.K. Discrepancies between sexual desire and sexual activity: Gender differences and associations with relationship satisfaction. *J. Sex Marital Ther.* **2008**, *34*, 31–44. [CrossRef] [PubMed]
55. Rupp, H.A.; Wallen, K. Sex differences in response to visual sexual stimuli: A review. *Arch. Sex. Behav.* **2008**, *37*, 206–218. [CrossRef] [PubMed]

56. Krejcova, L.; Chovanec, M.; Weiss, P.; Klapilova, K. Pornography consumption in women and its association with sexual desire and sexual satisfaction. *J. Sex. Med.* **2017**, *5* (Suppl. 4), e243.
57. Willoughby, B.J.; Leonhardt, N.D. Behind closed doors: Individual and joint pornography use among romantic couples. *J. Sex Res.* **2018**. [CrossRef] [PubMed]
58. Nutter, D.E.; Condron, M.K. Sexual fantasy and activity patterns of females with inhibited sexual desire versus normal controls. *J. Sex Marital Ther.* **1983**, *9*, 276–282. [CrossRef]
59. Nutter, D.E.; Condron, M.K. Sexual fantasy and activity patterns of males with inhibited sexual desire and males with erectile dysfunction versus normal controls. *J. Sex Marital Ther.* **1985**, *11*, 91–98. [CrossRef]
60. Steele, V.R.; Staley, C.; Fong, T.; Prause, N. Sexual desire, not hypersexuality, is related to neurophysiological responses elicited by sexual images. *Socioaffect. Neurosci. Psychol.* **2013**, *3*, 20770. [CrossRef]
61. Voon, V.; Mole, T.B.; Banca, P.; Porter, L.; Morris, L.; Mitchell, S.; Lapa, T.R.; Karr, J.; Harrison, N.A.; Potenza, M.N.; et al. Neural correlates of sexual cue reactivity in individuals with and without compulsive sexual behaviours. *PLoS ONE* **2014**, *9*, e102419. [CrossRef]
62. Nimbi, F.M.; Tripodi, F.; Rossi, R.; Navarro-Cremades, F.; Simonelli, C. Male sexual desire: An overview of biological, psychological, sexual, relational, and cultural factors influencing desire. *Sex. Med. Rev.* **2019**. [CrossRef]
63. McCabe, M.P.; Goldhammer, D.L. Demographic and psychological factors related to sexual desire among heterosexual women in a relationship. *J. Sex Res.* **2012**, *49*, 78–87. [CrossRef]
64. Schneider, J.P. Effects of cybersex addiction on the family: Results of a survey. *Sex. Addict. Compulsivity* **2000**, *7*, 31–58. [CrossRef]
65. Peter, J.; Valkenburg, P.M. Adolescents' exposure to sexually explicit internet material and sexual satisfaction: A longitudinal study. *Hum. Commun. Res.* **2009**, *35*, 171–194. [CrossRef]
66. Braun-Courville, D.K.; Rojas, M. Exposure to sexually explicit web sites and adolescent sexual attitude and behaviors. *J. Adolesc. Health* **2009**, *45*, 156–162. [CrossRef] [PubMed]
67. DeKeseredy, W.S.; Hall-Sanchez, A. Adult pornography and violence against women in the heartland. *Violence Against Women* **2017**, *23*, 830–849. [CrossRef] [PubMed]
68. Brooks, G.R. *The Centerfold Syndrome*; Jossey-Bass: San Francisco, CA, USA, 1995.
69. Schneider, J.; Weiss, R. *Cybersex Exposed*; Hazelden: Center City, MN, USA, 2001.
70. Vaillancourt-Morel, M.P.; Daspe, M.È.; Charbonneau-Lefebvre, V.; Bosisio, M.; Bergeron, S. Pornography Use in Adult Mixed-Sex Romantic Relationships: Context and Correlates. *Curr. Sex. Health Rep.* **2019**, *11*, 35–43. [CrossRef]
71. Doornwaard, S.M.; Bickham, D.S.; Rich, M.; Vanwesenbeeck, I.; van den Eijnden, R.J.; Ter Bogt, T.F. Sex-related online behaviors and adolescents' body and sexual self-perceptions. *Pediatrics* **2014**, *134*, 1103–1110. [CrossRef] [PubMed]
72. Milas, G.; Wright, P.; Štulhofer, A. Longitudinal Assessment of the Association Between Pornography Use and Sexual Satisfaction in Adolescence. *J. Sex Res.* **2019**, 1–13. [CrossRef]
73. Muusses, L.D.; Kerkhof, P.; Finkenauer, C. Internet pornography and relationship quality: A longitudinal study of within and between partner effects of adjustment, sexual satisfaction and sexually explicit internet material among newly-weds. *Comput. Hum. Behav.* **2015**, *45*, 77–84. [CrossRef]
74. Wright, P.J.; Bridges, A.J.; Sun, C.; Ezzell, M.B.; Johnson, J.A. Personal pornography viewing and sexual satisfaction: A quadratic analysis. *J. Sex Marital Ther.* **2018**, *44*, 308–315. [CrossRef]
75. Perry, S.L.; Whitehead, A.L. Only bad for believers? Religion, pornography use, and sexual satisfaction among American men. *J. Sex Res.* **2019**, *56*, 50–61. [CrossRef]
76. Miller, D.J.; McBain, K.A.; Wendy, W.L.; Raggat, P.T.F. Pornography, preference for porn-like sex, masturbation, and men's sexual and relationship satisfaction. *Pers. Relatsh.* **2019**, *26*, 93–113. [CrossRef]
77. Daspe, M.-E.; Vaillancourt-Morel, M.-P.; Lussier, Y.; Sabourin, S.; Ferron, A. When pornography use feels out of control: The moderation effect of relationship and sexual satisfaction. *J. Sex Marital Ther.* **2018**, *44*, 343–353. [CrossRef] [PubMed]
78. Gouvernet, B.; Rebelo, T.; Sebbe, F.; Hentati, Y.; Yougbaré, S.; Combaluzier, S.; Rezrazi, A. Is pornography pathogen by itself? Study of the role of attachment profiles on the relationship between pornography and sexual satisfaction. *Sexologies* **2017**, *26*, 27–33. [CrossRef]
79. Szymanski, D.M.; Stewart-Richardson, D.N.L. Psychological, relational, and sexual correlates of pornography use on young adult heterosexual men in romantic relationships. *J. Men's Stud.* **2014**, *22*, 64–82. [CrossRef]

80. Bridges, A.J.; Morokoff, P.J. Sexual media use and relational satisfaction in heterosexual couples. *Pers. Relatsh.* **2011**, *18*, 562–585. [CrossRef]
81. Štulhofer, A.; Buško, V.; Landripet, I. Pornography, sexual socialization, and satisfaction among young men. *Arch. Sex. Behav.* **2008**, *39*, 168–178. [CrossRef] [PubMed]
82. Morgan, E.M. Associations between young adults' use of sexually explicit materials and their sexual preferences, behaviors, and satisfaction. *J. Sex Res.* **2011**, *48*, 520–530. [CrossRef] [PubMed]
83. Minarcik, J.; Wetterneck, C.T.; Short, M.B. The effects of sexually explicit material use on romantic relationship dynamics. *J. Behav. Addict.* **2016**, *5*, 700–707. [CrossRef] [PubMed]
84. Wright, P.J.; Steffen, N.J.; Sun, C. Is the relationship between pornography consumption frequency and lower sexual satisfaction curvilinear? Results from England and Germany. *J. Sex Res.* **2019**, *56*, 9–15. [CrossRef] [PubMed]
85. Vaillancourt-Morel, M.-P.; Blais-Lecours, S.; Labadie, C.; Bergeron, S.; Sabourin, S.; Godbout, N. Profiles of cyberpornography use and sexual well-being in adults. *J. Sex. Med.* **2017**, *14*, 78–85. [CrossRef] [PubMed]
86. Blais-Lecours, S.; Vaillancourt-Morel, M.-P.; Sabourin, S.; Godbout, N. Cyberpornography: Time use, perceived addiction, sexual functioning, and sexual satisfaction. *Cyberpsychol. Behav. Soc. Netw.* **2016**, *19*, 649–655. [CrossRef] [PubMed]
87. Cranney, S.; Stulhofer, A. Whosoever looketh on a person to lust after them: Religiosity, the use of mainstream and nonmainstream sexually explicit material, and sexual satisfaction in heterosexual men and women. *J. Sex Res.* **2017**, *54*, 694–705. [CrossRef] [PubMed]
88. Perry, S.L. Does viewing pornography reduce marital quality over time? evidence from longitudinal data. *Arch. Sex. Behav.* **2017**, *46*, 549–559. [CrossRef] [PubMed]
89. Brown, C.C.; Carroll, J.S.; Yorgason, J.B.; Busby, D.M.; Willoughby, B.J.; Larson, J.H. A common-fate analysis of pornography acceptance, use, and sexual satisfaction among heterosexual married couples. *Arch. Sex. Behav.* **2017**, *46*, 575–584. [CrossRef] [PubMed]
90. Sabina, C.; Wolak, J.; Finkelhor, D. The nature and dynamics of Internet pornography exposure for youth. *CyberPscyhol. Behav.* **2008**, *11*, 691–693. [CrossRef] [PubMed]
91. Yucel, D.; Gassanov, M.A. Exploring actor and partner correlates of sexual satisfaction among married couples. *Soc. Sci. Res.* **2010**, *3*, 725–738. [CrossRef]
92. Wright, P.J.; Tokunaga, R.S.; Kraus, A.; Klann, E. Pornography consumption and satisfaction: A meta-analysis. *Hum. Commun. Res.* **2017**, *43*, 315–343. [CrossRef]
93. Downing, M.J.; Schrimshaw, E.W.; Scheinmann, R.; Antebi-Gruszka, N.; Hirshfield, S. Sexually explicit media use by sexual identity: A comparative analysis of gay, bisexual, and heterosexual men in the United States. *Arch. Sex. Behav.* **2017**, *46*, 1763–1776. [CrossRef] [PubMed]
94. McCabe, M.; Taleporos, G. Sexual esteem, sexual satisfaction and sexual behavior among people with physical disability. *Arch. Sex. Behav.* **2003**, *32*, 359–369. [CrossRef] [PubMed]
95. Schneider, J.P. A qualitative study of cybersex participants: Gender differences, recovery issues, and implications for therapists. *Sex. Addict. Compulsivity* **2000**, *7*, 249–278. [CrossRef]

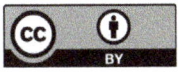

© 2019 by the authors. Licensee MDPI, Basel, Switzerland. This article is an open access article distributed under the terms and conditions of the Creative Commons Attribution (CC BY) license (http://creativecommons.org/licenses/by/4.0/).

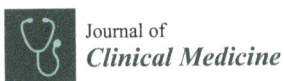

Review

Hormonal Contraceptives, Female Sexual Dysfunction, and Managing Strategies: A Review

Nerea M. Casado-Espada [1], Rubén de Alarcón [1], Javier I. de la Iglesia-Larrad [1], Berta Bote-Bonaechea [1] and Ángel L. Montejo [1,2,*]

[1] Psychiatry Service, Institute of Biomedical Research of Salamanca (IBSAL), University Clinical Hospital of Salamanca, Paseo San Vicente, SN 37007 Salamanca, Spain; nmcasado91@gmail.com (N.M.C.-E.); ruperghost@gmail.com (R.d.A.); javidelaiglesia.jdli@gmail.com (J.I.d.l.I.-L.); bertabot@yahoo.es (B.B.-B.)
[2] Nursing School E.U.E.F., University of Salamanca, Av. Donantes de Sangre SN 37007 Salamanca, Spain
* Correspondence: amontejo@usal.es; Tel.:+34639754620

Received: 12 May 2019; Accepted: 24 June 2019; Published: 25 June 2019

Abstract: In recent decades, hormonal contraceptives (HC) has made a difference in the control of female fertility, taking an unequivocal role in improving contraceptive efficacy. Some side effects of hormonal treatments have been carefully studied. However, the influence of these drugs on female sexual functioning is not so clear, although variations in the plasma levels of sexual hormones could be associated with sexual dysfunction. Permanent hormonal modifications, during menopause or caused by some endocrine pathologies, could be directly related to sexual dysfunction in some cases but not in all of them. HC use seems to be responsible for a decrease of circulating androgen, estradiol, and progesterone levels, as well as for the inhibition of oxytocin functioning. Hormonal contraceptive use could alter women's pair-bonding behavior, reduce neural response to the expectation of erotic stimuli, and increase sexual jealousy. There are contradictory results from different studies regarding the association between sexual dysfunction and hormonal contraceptives, so it could be firmly said that additional research is needed. When contraceptive-related female sexual dysfunction is suspected, the recommended therapy is the discontinuation of contraceptives with consideration of an alternative method, such as levonorgestrel-releasing intrauterine systems, copper intrauterine contraceptives, etonogestrel implants, the permanent sterilization of either partner (when future fertility is not desired), or a contraceptive ring.

Keywords: female sexual dysfunction; hormonal contraceptive; libido; desire; sex life; orgasm; vaginal ring; depot medroxyprogesterone acetate

1. Introduction

In recent decades, hormonal contraception (HC) has made a difference in the control of female fertility, taking an unequivocal role in improving contraceptive efficacy. Moreover, there are numerous studies that state that the use of hormonal contraceptives is very prevalent in the female population of childbearing age [1–8]. In a study carried out by Hall et al. in 2012, it was estimated that 63% of women of reproductive age worldwide who were married or in a relationship were using some type of contraception, with the contraceptive pill as the third most commonly used method (9% of women aged 15–19 years) [3,9]. Combined oral contraception seems to be the most popular form of reversible contraception in Europe and the United States [7,8].

The popularity and widespread use of hormonal contraceptives is partly due to their benefits, such as: (1) Being a highly effective and reversible form of contraception; (2) the woman has control over this method of contraception; (3) the failure rate is less than 1%; and (4) they have a well-established safety profile [1].

However, the use of hormonal contraceptives is relatively recent: In 1956, an oral contraceptive pill (mestranol in combination with norethynodrel) was used for the first time in a clinical trial; a year later, in 1957, the formulation of 150 µg mestranol and 10 mg norethynodrel received approval for the treatment of "female disorders" (menstrual irregularities, etc.) [1]. It was three years later, in 1960, when the Food and Drug Administration (FDA) approved the use of the pill as a contraceptive, containing 75 mestranol and 5 mg norethynodrel [1,10]. At the beginning, oral contraceptives were available only to married women, and, in 1972, the pill also began to be available for single women in all states [1]. Since the approval of the use of the pill in 1960, it has undergone many evolutions in dosage, hormone type, and regimen. It has been used by more than 100 million women worldwide and has the widest geographic distribution of any method of contraception [10].

The use of hormonal contraceptives is widespread, with a significant percentage of healthy population among its users. Some of its side effects are well known, such as the increased prothrombotic and cardiovascular risk (estrogen dependent) [10]. On the other hand, non-contraceptive benefits of hormonal contraceptives, such as as cycle regulation with predictable withdrawal bleeds, decreased menstrual flow, and decreased anemia, have been widely documented [10]. However, the influence of these drugs on female sexual function is not as clear, although it is mentioned in the technical prospects of the contraceptive pills. Additionally, there are very few controlled studies in this field.

Conversely, despite the widespread use of contraceptives in the general population, there are many other drugs that have been widely studied and associated with frequent iatrogenic sexual dysfunction. Antihypertensive drugs, diuretics, and beta-blockers seem to exert a detrimental impact on sexual function [11], as do antipsychotics [12–14], antidepressants [12,13,15], and others. In addition, there are endocrine disorders that are also associated with alterations in sexual function, such as diabetes [16], obesity, and metabolic syndrome [17]. On top of this, sexual dysfunction is a possible symptom associated with other hormonal alterations such as those that take place during menopause [18] or postpartum [19]. There are differences regarding which aspects of sexual function were most affected by menopause. The Massachusetts Women's Health Study, the Melbourne Women's Midlife Health project, the Penn Ovarian Aging Study and the Study of Women's Health Across the Nation (SWAN) are some of the pieces of research that were carried out in this regard. Notably, three out of four of these studies noted declines in sexual desire during the menopause transition [18].

In this review, first of all, detailed information has been included about the hormonal contraceptive methods, focusing on the type of administration, hormonal composition, mechanism of action, and expected effects on hormonal function in women. Second, an approximation is given to the concept and significance of sexual dysfunction, in addition to its prevalence in the female population. These first sections have the objective of contextualizing and favoring the understanding of the next ones; the main aim of this study is to clarify whether there is evidence of the effect of hormonal contraceptives on female sexual function. In this review, we attempt to provide a summary of the existing data about the impact of hormonal contraceptives on sexuality. We differentiate between studies that claim that there are no effects of hormonal contraceptives on sexual function and others that defend that there are. Within the latter, we differentiate between those that show positive and negative effects on female sexual function. Likewise, in this review, some treatment options are proposed according to the studies reviewed.

This review provides a compilation of the existing evidence about the relationship between female sexual function and hormonal contraceptives, in addition to the existing therapeutic management strategies. This is the first review that includes a summary table, which allows the clinician to access to the most relevant information at a glance. Likewise, it is the only study that proposes a therapeutic algorithm for the management of hormonal contraceptives-related sexual dysfunction.

2. Materials and Methods

The aim of this review is developing, assimilating, and synthesizing the existing evidence about the influence of hormonal contraception on female sexual function. In addition, we intended to identify gaps in knowledge in this field in order to design new studies that may fill those gaps in the future. Our review focuses on the use of hormonal contraceptives in women of childbearing age and on the influence of these drugs on female sexual function [1,2]. In addition, the study reviews the differences in the influence of the HCs on female sexual function (FSF) according to the hormonal composition and the mechanism of action of the different HCs in order to determine which one has the lowest profile of secondary effects in the sexual area. On the other hand, to our knowledge, this is the latest effort to offer an overview of the recommended strategies in cases in which the use of HCs is associated with sexual dysfunction. To achieve this purpose, we performed a scoping review following PRISMA guidelines (Preferred Reporting Items for Systematic Reviews and Meta-Analyses) (Figure 1). In this review, we selected key articles based on hormonal contraception and female sexual function. PubMed and Cochrane were chosen as the main databases used due to the extensive contents of biomedical research they offer, their free access, and their ease of use. Our search term combinations were: "Hormonal contraception" AND "female sexual function" OR "female sexual dysfunction." The filters "publication date: From 2000/01/01 to 2019/01/31" and "review" were applied in the search in order to limit the amount of material available. No language restrictions were applied. Similar and related articles that were considered of special interest for our review were also included, and they were compiled though cross-referencing. Similarly, some relevant clinical practice guidelines were included. The 64 papers that were included were chosen because they fit the topic of the review (presenting information about female sexual dysfunction, hormonal contraception, hormonal variations, and their relationship with female sexual function; directly treating the impact of hormonal contraceptives in female sexual function; or providing relevant information about the management strategies of female sexual dysfunction associated with the use of HCs). We reviewed six prospective observational studies, eight clinical trials, 19 cross-sectional studies, 22 reviews, and nine other works that include consensus and clinical practice guidelines. Most of the studies were carried out in European countries, although there were also studies carried out in the US, Asia, Australia, and South America. The population of the studies reviewed varied between 40 and 18,787, although in the case of clinical trials, the largest population analyzed was 600 subjects.

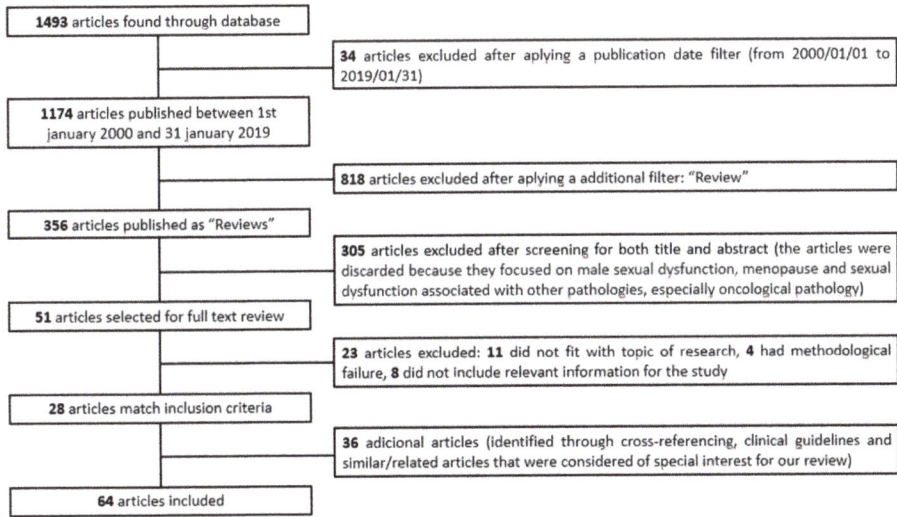

Figure 1. PRISMA flow diagram. (Preferred Reporting Items for Systematic Reviews and Meta-Analyses).

We summarized the findings and best practice recommendations for addressing a woman's contraception and its potential association with sexual function. We excluded those articles that focused on male sexual dysfunction, menopause, and sexual dysfunction related to medical disease, such as oncological pathology. Every attempt was made to combine as much similar data as possible. Institutional review board approval was not needed for this review.

3. Results

3.1. Hormonal Contraceptives

The combined oral contraceptive (COC) was first approved in 1960. Since then, it has undergone many evolutions in dosage, hormone type, and regimen. It has been used by more than 100 million women worldwide and has the widest geographic distribution of any method of contraception [10]. In this section, we will provide detailed information about hormonal contraceptives in terms of the existing types, their hormonal composition, their mechanism of action, and the alterations in hormonal function that derive from them.

3.1.1. Types

At present, there are twenty different contraceptive methods approved by the FDA [20], ten of which are female hormonal contraceptive methods: Eight are reversible contraceptive methods, and two are emergency contraceptive methods. In Table 1, we can see the different categories of hormonal contraceptives mentioned.

Table 1. Hormonal contraceptives. Route of administration, dosing frequency, mechanism of action, and association with sexual effects.

Hormonal Contraceptives	Route of Administration	Dosing Frequency	Mechanism of Action	Sexual Effects
Levonorgesetrel-realising intrauterine systems (LNG-IUDs)	Intrauterine	Inserted by a healthcare provider. Lasts up to 3–5 years, depending on the type. LARC.	• Prevention of fertilization: produces a weak foreign body reaction and endometrial decidualization and glandular atrophy • changes in the amount and the viscosity of cervical mucus → barrier to sperm penetration • Ovulation is likely inhibited in some women but is preserved in most study subjects • Endometrial estrogen and progesterone receptors are suppressed	Positive effects. However, more studies are needed
"The implant". Etonorgestrel implant.	Subdermal	Inserted by a healthcare provider. Lasts up to 3 years. LARC.	• Inhibition of the ovulation and consistently does so until the beginning of the third year of use. • Ovarian activity, including estradiol synthesis, is still present. • The ENG implant causes thickening of the cervical mucus and changes in the endometrial lining	Negative effects. However, more studies are needed.
Depot Medroxyprogesterone Acetate (DMPA)	Intramuscularly	Every three months. SARC/LARC.	• Inhibition of the secretion of pituitary gonadotropins → suppressing ovulation • Increase of the viscosity of cervical mucus and induction of endometrial atrophy	Mixed results. More studies are needed.

Table 1. Cont.

Hormonal Contraceptives	Route of Administration	Dosing Frequency	Mechanism of Action	Sexual Effects
"The Pill". Combined oral contraceptive	Oral	Must swallow a pill every day.	• Suppression of pituitary gonadotropin secretion → inhibiting ovulation • Increase of cervical mucus viscosity → impairing sperm transport • Effects on tubal transport → narrowing or eliminating the potential fertilization window • Possible endometrial effects • Folliculogenesis impairment	Mixed results. More studies are needed.
"The Mini pill". Progestin-Only Pills (POPs)	Oral	Must swallow a pill at the same time every day.	• Alteration of the cervical mucus: more viscid, less copious → inhibits sperm penetration • Possible impairment of sperm motility and decreased tubal cilia activity • Negative luteinizing hormone (LH) feedback leads to suppression of ovulation in up to 50% of users	Mixed results. More studies are needed.
Contraceptive Patch	Dermal. Is placed on 1 of 4 sites: the buttocks, upper outer arm, lower abdomen, or upper torso, excluding the breast.	Put on a new patch each week for 3 weeks (21 total days). Do not put on a patch during the fourth week.	• Similar to the Combined Oral Contraception. • Following the first application of the patch, serum hormone levels increase gradually over the first 48 to 72 hours, reach a plateau, and then remain constant during the remainder of the 21-day period. • Compared with COCs plasma hormone levels remain constant and the peak levels are lower because first-pass hepatic metabolism and gastrointestinal enzyme degradation are avoided.	Positive effects. Slight increases in sexual function scores were noted with contraceptive patch, but not clinically significant.
Vaginal Contraceptive Ring	Vaginal	Put the ring into the vagina yourself. Keep the ring in you r vagina for 3 weeks	• Similar to the Combined Oral Contraception • Serum hormone levels increase immediately after ring insertion and then decrease slowly over the cycle • Gastrointestinal absorption and the hepatic first-pass effect are avoided	Mixed results. More studies are needed.
Emergency contraceptives	Route of administration	Dosing frequency		
Levonorgestrel 1.5 mg	Oral	Swallow the pills as soon as possible within 3 days after having unprotected sex.		
Ulipristal Acetate	Oral	Swallow the pills within 5 days after having unprotected sex.		

Reversible contraceptive methods include: Combined hormonal contraceptives (CHCs), progestin-only contraceptives, and intrauterine contraceptives (IUCs). COCs include the "pill" or combined oral contraceptives (COCs), the contraceptive patch, and the vaginal ring. When talking about progestin-only contraceptives, we can differentiate between progestin-only-pills (POPs), depot medroxyprogesterone acetate (DMPA), and the "implant" or single rod etonogestrel subdermal implant. IUCs include copper intrauterine devices (Cu-IUDs) and levonorgestrel-releasing intrauterine systems (LNG-IUS) [10,21,22]. Emergency hormonal contraceptives (ECs) are: Levonorgestrel of 1.5 mg (1 pill) or 0.75 mg (2 pills) and ulipristal acetate [20]. Permanent contraceptive methods that are approved by the FDA are: Sterilization surgery for women, a sterilization implant for women, and sterilization surgery for men [20].

3.1.2. Hormones

The hormonal composition of hormonal contraceptives is based on progestins alone or on a combination of progestogens and estrogens [10,20–24]. Several different progestins are used in combined oral contraceptives (COCs). These progestins may also have estrogenic, antiestrogenic, androgenic, antiandrogenic, or antimineralocorticoid activity [10]. Most progestins are 19-nortestosterone derivatives. Progestins may be classified according to their chemical structure as an estrane (norethindrone, norethindrone acetate, ethynodiol diacetate) or as a gonane (LNG, desogestrel, norgestimate). In general, gonane progestins appear to be more potent than the estrane derivatives (smaller doses can be used), but other differences between the estrane and gonane compounds are difficult to characterize [10]. Table 2 shows the classification of progestogens used in hormonal contraception according to their androgenic potency. Among the contraceptive progestins available in the United States, norgestrel and levonorgestrel are the most androgenic; norethindrone and norethindrone acetate are less androgenic; and desogestrel, etonogestrel, norgestimate, dienogest, and drospirenone are the least androgenic [2]. Newer progestins (norgestimate and desogestrel) have little or no androgenic activity, whereas other progestins (cyproterone acetate, drospirenone, and dienogest) have antiandrogenic activity [10]. The varying progestational "potencies" attributed to different COC preparations are based on pharmacological experimental models. Many variables affect the potency of COCs (including dosage, bioavailability, protein binding, receptor binding affinity, and interindividual variability), making it difficult to extrapolate the results of isolated experiments to provide clinically relevant information in humans. There is no clear clinical or epidemiological evidence that compares the relative potencies of currently available COCs [10]. Systemic progestins may be associated with a loss of sexual desire due to the suppression of ovarian function and endogenous estrogen production [6]. Along the same line of reasoning, in their study about women's self-reported sexual desire across natural cycles, Roney and Simmons observed that levels of salivary progesterone negatively predicted women's sexual desire [25,26]. Furthermore, based on the findings by Grebe et al., effective dosages of progestin should be associated with a stronger positive linkage between women's loyalty/faithfulness to their relationship partners and the frequency with which they engaged in sexual intercourse with their partners [26,27]. However, contraceptive pills with progestogens with antiandrogenic effect do not affect sexual desire, according to some reports [28,29]. In recent studies, drospirenone and dienogest have reported a positive effect on sexual response as well as attraction, desire, satisfaction, and coital frequency [28,30], perhaps due to the ability to reduce the activity of 5-alpha reductase [31].

Table 2. Classification of progestogens used in contraception according to their androgenic potency.

Most Androgenic	Less Androgenic	The Least Androgenic	Antiandrogenic
Norgestrel levonorgestrel	Norethindrone Norethindrone acetate Ethynodiol diacetate	Desogestrel Etonogestrel Norgestimate	Cyproterona acetato Drospirenona Dienogest

With regard to estrogens as hormonal components of hormonal contraceptive methods, three types of estrogens are used in COCs (as it can be seen in Figure 2): Ethinylestradiol (EE), estradiol valerate (E2V), and 17 beta-estradiol (E2). E2V is rapidly metabolized to E2 [10]. Due to its biochemical structure, estradiol has less impact on the synthesis of hepatic proteins than ethinyl estradiol, which is likely to result in a better metabolic and vascular profile [3]. The new formulations of launched COCs have lower doses of estrogen, and EE has been replaced by more "physiological" forms of estrogen, such as 17β-estradiol (E2) or E2-Valerate (E2 V) [32]. There is some evidence to suggest that estrogens play an essential role in female sexuality, and prior research has found that declining sexual functioning in women is most closely related to declining estrogen levels [6,33] Similarly, levels of salivary estradiol positively predicted women's sexual desire, conversely to progesterone [25,26]. Regarding loyalty and faithfulness, dosages of estradiol should predict a weaker positive linkage between women's loyalty/faithfulness to their relationship partners and frequency of sexual intercourse (not including masturbation and sexual fantasies; independently of androgenicity of sexual hormones) [26,27].

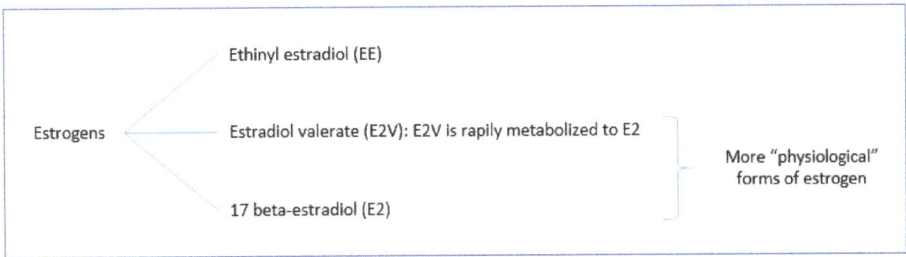

Figure 2. Types of estrogens used in combined oral contraceptives (COCs).

3.1.3. Mechanism of Action of Hormonal Contraceptives

In Table 1, we can see a summary of the different categories of hormonal contraceptives mentioned with their respective mechanism of action of hormonal contraceptives. The mechanism of action of hormonal contraceptives depends on their hormonal composition and the route of administration.

Combined hormonal contraceptives (CHCs) encompass oral contraceptives (pill), patch, and the vaginal ring. Their mechanism of action is similar.

With regard to combined oral contraceptives (COCs), they have multiple mechanisms of action due to both their estrogenic and progestational components: The suppression of pituitary gonadotropin secretion (inhibiting ovulation), the increase of cervical mucus viscosity (impairing sperm transport), the suppression of the luteinizing hormone (LH), and the impairment of ovulation [10].

The patch is a 20 cm^2 square matrix system that delivers 200 mg of norelgestromin (the primary active metabolite of norgestimate) and 35 mg of ethinylestradiol (EE) daily to the systemic circulation. Following the first application of the patch, serum hormone levels increase gradually over the first 48–72 h, reach a plateau, and then remain constant during the remainder of the 21-day period. Compared with COC, plasma hormone levels remain constant, and the peak levels are lower because first-pass hepatic metabolism and gastrointestinal enzyme degradation are avoided. Curiously, although peak levels are lower, the area under the curve, which represents overall EE exposure, is larger. One patch is applied weekly for three consecutive weeks, followed by a one patch-free week. The patch can be placed on one of four sites: The buttocks, upper outer arm, lower abdomen, or upper torso, excluding the breast [10].

The ring releases 15 mg of EE and 120 mg of the progestin etonogestrel (ENG) (the active metabolite of desogestrel) per day, which is absorbed through the vaginal epithelium. Serum hormone levels increase immediately after ring insertion and then decrease slowly over the cycle [10]. The vaginal route is an ideal method of drug administration, and the advantages of this method are well established. By avoiding gastrointestinal absorption and the hepatic first-pass effect, the vaginal administration of contraceptives enables the use of lower hormonal doses and the achievement of steady drug concentrations [34].

There is another group of hormonal contraceptives only composed of progesterone. This group can include the progestin-only pill, depot medroxyprogesterone acetate (DMPA), and the etonogestrel implant. Progestin-only pills (POPs, the "mini-pill") provide reliable, reversible contraception and have very few contraindications. The main mechanism of action is the alteration of the cervical mucus (more viscid, less copious) and the inhibition of sperm penetration. Negative luteinizing hormone (LH) feedback leads to the suppression of ovulation in up to 50% of users. POPs containing desogestrel may inhibit ovulation more consistently [21].

DMPA is administered intramuscularly at three-month intervals (every 12–13 weeks) and is thus considered a long-acting reversible contraceptive (LARC) by some and a short-acting reversible contraceptive (SARC) by others. DMPA works primarily by inhibiting the secretion of pituitary gonadotropins, thereby suppressing ovulation. Women enter a hypoestrogenic state, and their progesterone is low due to anovulation. DMPA also increases the viscosity of cervical mucus (minor mechanism of action) and induces endometrial atrophy [21].

The single-rod etonogestrel subdermal implant (Implanon/Implanon NXT/Nexplanon) is a LARC. The single-rod implant contains 68 mg of the progestin etonogestrel (ENG) and provides contraception for three years. The ENG implant works primarily by inhibiting ovulation and consistently does so until the beginning of the third year of use. Ovarian activity, including estradiol synthesis, is still present. The ENG implant causes a thickening of the cervical mucus and changes in the endometrial lining [21].

The last group is formed by intrauterine contraceptives (IUCs). This group includes copper intrauterine devices (Cu-IUDs) and levonorgestrel-releasing intrauterine systems (LNG-IUS). Only LNG-IUS are explained in this section, because Cu-IUDs do not have a hormonal component. The chief mechanism of action of all IUCs is the prevention of fertilization; they may also have post-fertilization effects, including the potential inhibition of implantation. The LNG-IUS produce a weak foreign body reaction and endometrial changes that include endometrial decidualization and glandular atrophy. The primary mechanism of action is via changes in the amount and the viscosity of cervical mucus, which acts as a barrier to sperm penetration. Ovulation is likely inhibited in some women, but it is preserved in most study subjects. Endometrial estrogen and progesterone receptors are suppressed, which results in changes in bleeding patterns and may contribute to its contraceptive effect [22].

3.1.4. Hormonal Alterations of Hormonal Contraceptives and Their Influence on Female Sexual Function

In contrast to animal species in which linear relationships exist between hormonal status and sexual behavior, sexuality in the human population is remarkably complex and is not determined so simply by the level of sexual steroids [29].

Hormonal contraceptives (HCs) are responsible for a decrease of circulating androgen levels [1,2,29,35], as well as a decrease of the baseline serum levels of estradiol [6,29,35] and progesterone [35] and the inhibition of oxytocin functioning [35]. However, the concentrations of the follicle-stimulating and luteinizing hormones are similar in freely cycling women and in women using HCs [35]. Decreased circulating androgen levels with oral combined hormonal contraceptive (CHC) use, and its negative effects on sexual life, occur by two mechanisms, as follows: (1) An oral CHC increases sex hormone-binding globulin (SHBG) and decreases free testosterone, and (2) androgen production from the ovary is suppressed with an oral CHC. This antiandrogenic effect may be magnified with an oral CHC containing an antiandrogenic progestin [2]. Thus, all CHCs are antiandrogenic, although some formulations, depending on the specific progestin, are more so than others. The patch and the vaginal ring are more antiandrogenic than the pill [1]. As expected, the baseline serum levels of estradiol and progesterone are significantly higher in freely cycling women than in women using an HC. Nevertheless, the concentrations of the follicle-stimulating and luteinizing hormones are similar in both groups [35]. In respect of oxytocin, its functioning is likely to be altered by this variation in the peripheral estradiol and progesterone levels that were found to be altered in women using HCs, and, therefore, a potential mechanism could be related to the direct binding of progesterone to oxytocin receptors (OXTRs), thereby inhibiting OXTR functioning.

The association between hormones and sexuality is multidimensional, as several hormones are important in the regulation of sexual behavior [29].

Though some evidence shows that testosterone has a role in sexual function for women, these conclusions are derived primarily from studies involving postmenopausal women reporting sexual dysfunction [2]. It has been established that sexual desire, autoeroticism, and sexual fantasies in women depend on androgen levels [29]. However, the relevance of changes in androgen levels for an individual woman is unclear, and some women may be more sensitive to androgen level alteration than others [2]. The review by Casey et al. mentioned that most of the studies showed alterations in SHBG and testosterone levels; however, an overall lack of association was found between CHCs and sexual desire [2]. In other studies, decreased levels of estrogen and testosterone in older women have been associated with decreased libido, sensitivity, and erotic stimuli [29]. In addition, it has been found that patients using birth control pills may present with decreased libido. On the other hand, there are reports that suggest that progestogens with antiandrogenic effects in contraceptive pills do not affect sexual desire [29]. While there is conflicting evidence concerning a link between progestins and libido, there is some evidence to suggest that estrogens play an essential role in female sexuality. In this respect, prior research has found that declining sexual functioning in women is most closely related to declining estrogen levels [6].

Finally, with regard to oxytocin, Scheele et al. [35] describe in their work the possible functional implications of oxytocin in female sexuality and the alterations that occur in women who take hormonal contraceptives. Multiple lines of evidence suggest that the hypothalamic peptide oxytocin (OXT) is a key factor modulating pair-bonding behaviors, which means a strong affinity that develops in humans and some species between a mating couple.

In humans, peripheral OXT concentrations are significantly higher in new lovers compared with singles. Likewise, OXT reduces jealousy ratings and neural responses in an imagery task of sexual partner infidelity. OXT also increases the arousal induced by infant photos in nulliparous women and promotes responsiveness to infant crying and laughter by reducing activation in anxiety-related neural circuits. Moreover, OXT has been found to increase the intensity of orgasm and contentment after copulation. Nevertheless, OXT seems to not have an effect on vital signs. The results of the research by Scheele et al. [35] indicate that endogenous OXT concentrations at baseline positively predicted striatal responses to the romantic partners' faces in all female participants. This mechanism was disturbed in those women using an HC, indicating that the partner-specific modulatory effects of OXT are antagonized by gonadal steroids. HC use alters women's pair-bonding behavior (evident in decreased attractiveness ratings of masculine faces), reduced neural response to the expectation of erotic stimuli (a preference shift towards olfactory cues of genetic similarity), and increased sexual jealousy. Furthermore, women who use an HC while choosing partners are more likely to initiate an eventual separation, and wives who discontinue HC use tend to be less satisfied with marriage if they perceive their husband's face to be less attractive. On the other hand, women prefer masculine faces and exhibit higher levels of intersexual competition related to attractiveness at peak fertility in the menstrual cycle; however, these cyclical shifts were found to be diminished in women using an HC. In conclusion, OXT interacts with the brain reward system to reinforce partner value representations in both sexes, a mechanism which may significantly contribute to stable pair-bonding in humans and appears to be altered in women using an HC.

3.2. Sexual Dysfunction

To talk about the effects on sexual function, it is first convenient to define the concept of sexual dysfunction, as well as the types of female sexual dysfunction that are currently described. In this section, the methods used and validated to quantify the degree of sexual dysfunction are also briefly discussed. In addition, an estimate of the prevalence of sexual dysfunction in the female population of childbearing age is shown.

According to the DSM-5 (Diagnostic and Statistical Manual of Mental Disorders, Fifth Edition), sexual dysfunctions are a heterogeneous group of disorders that are typically characterized by a clinically significant disturbance in a person's ability to respond sexually or to experience sexual pleasure [18,36]. On the contrary, we would define "sexual health" as a state of physical, emotional, mental, and social well-being related to sexuality; it is not merely the absence of disease, dysfunction, or infirmary. Sexual health requires a positive and respectful approach to sexuality and sexual relationships, as well as the possibility of having pleasurable and safe sexual experiences, free of coercion, discrimination, and violence [37].

Therefore, optimal sexual function transcends the simple absence of dysfunction [18]. In this regard too, multiple studies have shown a strong positive association between sexual function and the health-related quality of life [18]. Having said that, it can be gathered that the female sexual function is complex and multifactorial, and it is influenced by many biological, psychological, and environmental factors [2,5,18,29]. Therefore, a complete understanding of women's sexual function requires the individual assessment of these factors. The biopsychosocial approach recognizes that biological, psychological, interpersonal, and sociocultural factors can all affect female sexual function, and these factors interact with each other in a dynamic system over time. Biological factors may include hormonal changes that affect the libido or medical/anatomical problems that affect genital sexual response. Psychological factors include mood symptoms, like depression or anxiety, or negative behaviors such as critical self-monitoring during sexual activity. Some examples of interpersonal factors include general satisfaction in the woman's relationship with her partner, which is closely tied to overall sexual satisfaction, as well as quality of communication in the relationship. Finally, some sociocultural factors to consider include the woman's attitudes about menopause and aging, as well as religious, cultural, and other social values regarding sex [18].

When assessing alterations of sexual function possibly related to hormonal contraceptives, other factors that may also affect it should be taken into account. For example, sex hormones (mainly low levels of estradiol), physical and mental well-being, availability of a partner, feeling for her partner, illness and its treatments, changes in social circumstances, and low socioeconomic status could have an impact on women's desire and sexual responsiveness [5,18]. Therefore, there are several factors that can affect female sexual function which should be explored by health providers for an adequate diagnostic and therapeutic approach to sexual dysfunction. However, there are studies that show in their results that sexual health is not a widely explored area for health providers in general. Mercer et al. showed that only 21% of women with persistent sexual problems discuss it with their healthcare provider [18,38]. Furthermore, a recent survey in the USA reported that the majority of gynecologists routinely ask patients about their sexual activities, but most other areas of patients' sexuality, such as sexual problems, including pleasure and satisfaction, are not routinely discussed [34,39].

Theoretical models of women's sexual response can provide a framework for a better understanding female sexual dysfunction. Three of these models are briefly explained here. First, according to the Masters–Johnson model, sexual response progresses predictably and linearly from excitement to plateau, orgasm, and resolution. The main focus of this model is on the physical response of the genitals. Secondly, Helen Singer Kaplan noted that many individuals had problems with sexual desire, denoting the importance of desire to sexual response. In the 1970s, she modified the Masters–Johnson model to a three-phase model of desire, excitement, and orgasm. Thirdly, in 2000, Rosemary Basson and colleagues proposed an alternative circular model of female sexual response. This model has several distinguishing features. On the one hand, spontaneous desire (or "sexual drive") on the part of the woman is not always the starting point for sexual activity. On the other hand, this model emphasizes that sexual stimuli often precede physical arousal and desire, and sexual arousal and desire often co-occur. Finally, the Basson model acknowledges that both physical and emotional satisfaction are important outcomes of engaging in sexual activity. This physical and emotional satisfaction can lead to higher emotional intimacy, which, in turn, can lead to greater receptivity and seeking out of sexual stimuli—hence, the circular model [18].

There has been debate regarding which model best reflects the experiences of women. In a study of 133 women, most of whom were in their 40s and 50s, women who had Female Sexual Function Index (FSFI) scores falling into the "dysfunctional" range and postmenopausal women were more likely to endorse the Basson model [18,40].

With the concept of sexual dysfunction now developed, we may now discuss the types of sexual dysfunction that are described. Four types of female sexual dysfunction are currently recognized: (1) Female orgasmic disorder, (2) female sexual interest/arousal disorder, (3) genito-pelvic pain/penetration disorder, and (4) substance/medication-induced sexual dysfunction. In order to quantify sexual dysfunction in a fairly objective way, there are two commonly used instruments in sexual function studies: The Female Sexual Function Index (FSFI) and the Female Sexual Distress

Scale-Revised (FSDS-R) [18]. The Female Sexual Function Index (FSFI) is a 19 item scale with six domains: Desire, arousal, lubrication, orgasm, pain, and satisfaction. In this scale, questions are graded on a Likert scale, and domains are weighted and summed to give a total score ranging from 2–36, with a cutoff of less than 26.55 suggesting sexual dysfunction. The FSFI has been validated in multiple languages, across age groups, and for multiple sexual disorders [18,41].

Why is it important to read up on sexual dysfunction? Sexual problems are common, estimated to affect 22–43% of women worldwide [18]. Overall, 27% of all reproductive-age US women (aged 18–44 years) report sexual dysfunction, with low sexual desire being the most common, and 10.8% of these women also experience related distress [2]. The prevalence of sexual dysfunction peaks at midlife, with 14% of women aged 45–64 reporting at least one sexual problem associated with significant distress [18]. The proportion with a notable or severe problem in desire, arousal, activity, or satisfaction ranges from 19–25% [5].

3.3. The Effects of Hormonal Contraceptives on Sexuality

This section presents different results found in the literature about the effects of hormonal contraceptives (HCs) on female sexuality (including results that advocate for positive or negative effects or the absence of sexual effects). It also discusses the peculiarities of the different types of HCs on sexuality.

3.3.1. Hormonal Contraceptives Do Not Have Sexual Effects

Some studies have found no change in sexual function with some hormonal contraceptives (HC) [2,3,6,10,42–46]. A recent systematic review of 36 studies involving more than 13,000 women reported no significant changes in sexual desire with the use of oral combined hormonal contraception (CHC) [43]. Another study [47] also reported high satisfaction rates with both LNG-IUS and copper IUC but no difference in sexual function overall or within psychological domains. In another recent study, no association was found between any LARC method and sexual satisfaction scores [48].

On the other hand, Reed et al. explored the relationship between oral contraceptive (OC) use and the risk of developing vulvodynia [49]. Further analysis showed no association between vulvodynia and previous OC use (HR 1.08, 95% CI 0.81–1.43, $p = 0.60$). In a study by Iliadou et al. [50], patients reporting mixed urinary incontinence (MUI) were divided into three groups according to contraceptive use. Of 196 women with MUI, 16 were currently using OC, and 178 reported no current use. Among the 8493 controls, 6321 were not using OC, and 2056 were ($p < 0.0001$). A systematic review of the literature found that sex drive is unaffected in most women taking OC, 3.5% of women taking OC reported a decrease in sexual desire, 12.0% reported an increase, and most of them (84.6%) reported no change [43]. However, the effects of other forms of hormonal contraception on sex drive have not been studied as comprehensively as OC [1].

3.3.2. Hormonal Contraceptives Have Sexual Effects

Positive Effects

According to the studies reviewed, hormonal contraceptives have a series of non-contraceptive effects which can influence and improve different areas of female sexual function. Some of these non-contraceptive effects are: Relief of gynecologic pain [1]; improved appearance, self-confidence, and self-esteem [2]; decrease of anxiety and discomfort [2]; loss of fear of having an unwanted pregnancy [6]; more stable levels of hormones throughout the cycle [51]; and less bleeding with the consequent lower risk of anemia [51]. All these effects contribute to the well-being of women and, consequently, to a possible improvement in the female sexual function. Similarly, hormonal contraceptives have described positive effects on some areas of female sexuality. The most frequently affected areas are: Sexual desire, orgasm number and intensity, satisfaction, and arousal. As mentioned, HCs may help to eliminate the fear of pregnancy, presumably providing a more relaxed and enjoyable sexual experience [1]. Similarly, it is reasonable to consider that an improved appearance would promote self-confidence and increase self-esteem, thereby having a positive effect on sexual function [2]. In a comparison between the vaginal ring, an oral CHC containing a third-generation progestin, subdermal contraception, and no hormonal contraception (control group), the three groups using an HC had increased positive indicators of sexual function (sexual interest and fantasies, orgasm number and intensity, and satisfaction) and decreased negative indicators (anxiety and discomfort). The same results were obtained in a comparison between etonogestrel implant and no contraception [2,52]. LNG-IUS have also been positively associated with sexual desire, arousal, orgasm, and overall sexual function compared with no contraception [2,53].

Furthermore, it may be advantageous for women to have more stable levels of hormones throughout the cycle. Because of the monthly fluctuations in estrogens, progesterone and androgens are associated with a range of symptoms, both genital (i.e., vaginal bleeding, heavy menstrual bleeding (HMB), dysmenorrhea, and pelvic pain) and systemic (i.e., depression, fatigue, headache, irritable bowel symptoms (IBS), asthma, and allergy), triggered by a local and systemic rise in inflammatory molecules released by mast cells when estrogen levels drop [51].

Negative Effects

To begin with, diminished sexual pleasure experienced by some women who use hormonal contraceptive methods may also be a barrier for their use [54], and this could imply an increase in the woman's vulnerability to unintended pregnancy [54]. Consequently, it is important to keep in mind that hormonal contraceptives could have associated side effects that have an influence on female sexual function. Some of these effects could be: Vaginal dryness [2,10,51], a decrease of lubrication [2,51], and pelvic floor symptoms such as dyspareunia [3,51], urinary incontinence, vestibulodynia, and interstitial cystitis [3]. COCs have been also associated with long- and short-term anatomical changes, such as atrophic vulvovaginitis and a decrease of thickness of the labia minora and vaginal introitus area [1]. Negative effects on some areas of female sexuality have been described with HCs, such as: Decreased sexual desire [2,6,10,54], frequency of intercourse [2,54], arousal [2,54], pleasure [2,54], orgasm [2,54], sexual thoughts [54], interest, and enjoyment [6,54].

In contrast to the above section, Elaut et al. [46] and Li et al. [55] defend in their studies that desire and coital frequency naturally increase around ovulation and premenstrually, and COC-associated ovulation inhibition and cycle regulation may blunt this effect, with the corresponding negative impact on libido [10]. Furthermore, longer durations of oral CHC use and younger ages at initiation have been associated with a higher relative risk of vestibulodynia [2], with the resulting negative impact on female sexual function.

3.3.3. Effects on Sexual Function According to the Type of Hormonal Contraceptive

Combined oral contraceptives are widely studied. Nevertheless, other hormonal contraception methods have fewer studies about their influence on sexual function. In this section, the results obtained from the studies reviewed for each type of hormonal contraceptive will be presented. Table 1 shows a summary of this information.

Contraceptive Patch

Concerning patch-related sexual effects, this could be considered the most innocuous CHC. Gracia et al. [56] found that among recent COC users, slight increases in sexual function scores were noted with patch use. However, they concluded that for both products, these changes are not likely to be clinically significant [1,34]. Therefore, it would be advisable to expand the research in this regard.

Contraceptive Ring

With regard to ring-related sexual effects, there are mixed results. On the one hand, two studies showed a decrease in sexual function with vaginal ring compared with COCs [56,57], and one study showed similar results but compared with the patch [58]. However, an improvement in sexual function including sexual desire, fantasies, and satisfaction, accompanied by a reduction of sexual distress, has been described with the vaginal ring [1,2,10,34]. In another study [34], compared with nonusers of hormonal contraception, both vaginal ring and COC users reported significant improvements for anxiousness, sexual pleasure, frequency and intensity of orgasm, satisfaction (all $p < 0.001$), sexual interest, and complicity ($p < 0.01$). However, only women in the vaginal ring group reported a significant increase in sexual fantasies ($p < 0.001$ versus nonusers), while ratings for sexual interest and complicity were significantly higher in ring users versus COC users [34]. As suggested by the researchers, these data indicate that both oral and vaginal contraception seem to improve to some extent the sexual life of women and their partners, whereas the vaginal ring seems to exert a further beneficial effect on the psychological aspects of sexual functioning [59].

Vaginal contraception offers many benefits, including high efficacy, good tolerability, ease of use, once-a-month dosing, and a favorable pharmacokinetic profile, with the added benefits of positive effects on the vaginal microbiome and on sexual parameters [34]. In addition, good cycle control and less fluctuating serum hormonal levels could contribute to the high degree of users' acceptability and satisfaction. Most importantly, a discussion about the vaginal delivery of contraceptive hormones offers the opportunity to stimulate an open dialogue about vaginal functions, thus ultimately contributing to enhancing women's sexual well-being and reproductive health [34]. Consequently, it could be a good hormonal contraceptive option.

Depot Medroxyprogesterone Acetate (DMPA)

DMPA is a highly effective method of contraception. It has been used as a contraceptive agent since 1967 by millions of women worldwide, particularly in less developed regions [21]. In respect of DMPA-related sexual effects, there are mixed results. Despite decreased libido being a common complaint among DMPA users and the fact that progestins have been observed to decrease interest in sex [6], positive sexual effects are also described with this method [6,60]—some reviews even reveal that DMPA is unlikely to be associated with sexual function in women [1,2,6]. However, further research would be needed to support these claims.

Etonogestrel Implant

Etonogestrel implant-related sexual effects are described as negative effects. It has been associated with a lack of interest in sex, a decreased libido, and a reduced sex drive. In addition, a decreased libido has been observed as a significant cause for implant discontinuation [1,6].

Levonorgestrel-Releasing Intrauterine Systems (LNG-IUS)

Intrauterine contraceptives (IUCs) are long-acting reversible contraceptive (LARC) methods that are used by over 150 million women worldwide. IUCs are highly effective methods of contraception that can be used by women of all ages. Rates of IUC use vary throughout the world, from a maximum of 41% in China to a minimum of 0.8% in sub-Saharan Africa [22]. They have generally been associated with positive sexual effects. They have been reported to improve desire, sexual function, and arousal [1,2,60]. Moreover, they seem to improve the health-related quality of life through the improvement of dysmenorrhea and symptoms in patients with endometriosis and adenomyosis, among other things [22].

3.3.4. Other Non-Hormonal Methods of Contraception and Their Effect on Sexual Function

Copper Intrauterine Devices (Cu-IUDs)

There has been no evidence to suggest that the copper IUD is associated with an altered libido [6].

Vasectomy/Tubal Ligation

As a non-hormonal contraceptive method, the effect of sterilization on sexual function extends beyond a simple hormonal effect into the psychological aspects of permanent pregnancy prevention, whether positive (i.e., relief and comfort in the knowledge that sexual activity will not result in pregnancy) or negative (i.e., regret that pregnancy is no longer possible) [2].

Nonuse of Contraception

Female sexual function is complex and multifactorial and is influenced by many biological, psychological, and environmental factors [2,5,18,29]. Therefore, a complete understanding of women's sexual function requires the individual assessment of these factors. Consequently, sexual dysfunction does not have to be associated with hormonal contraception. The use of no contraception was associated with a higher rate of the FSD than the use of either CHCs or nonhormonal methods. Furthermore, lower rates of sexual dysfunction were noted among women using either copper IUC (21%) or a levonorgestrel intrauterine systems (LNG-IUS) (10%) than among women using no contraception (35%). Among other reasons, diminished sexual function perceived to be related to contraception may lead to the nonuse of effective contraception, and, conversely, the nonuse of contraception may in itself be a factor in sexual dysfunction, perhaps owing to concerns about unintended pregnancy [2].

3.3.5. The Sexual Side Effects of Hormonal Contraceptives are not Well Studied

Existing evidence for an association between sexual dysfunction and contraception is inconsistent, and additional research is needed [2]. Findings from studies comparing women using non hormonal contraception with those using hormonal methods have shown mixed results [2]. The sexual side effects of hormonal contraceptives are not well studied, particularly with regard to their impact on libido [1]. Similarly, there is no clear information about the effect of HCs on pelvic symptoms and sexual function, nor on how they affect a woman's quality of life in relation to bowel and bladder symptoms, regardless of period control and menstrual bleeding. Moreover, the association between COC use and the presence of any type of urinary incontinence (UI) is unclear, and results suggest that the effect of current COC use on dyspareunia per se is inconsistent [3].

Healthcare care providers must be aware that hormonal contraceptives can have negative effects on female sexuality so they can counsel and care for their patients appropriately [1]. In order to better evaluate any possible effect on mood or libido, practitioners should assess patients prior to initiation of hormonal contraception to establish their baseline [60]. The lack of consistency in findings highlights the complex and multifactorial nature of female sexual function and focuses on the need for a comprehensive approach to management [2].

3.4. Management Strategies for Sexual Dysfunction Secondary to Hormonal Contraceptives

This section approaches the therapeutic possibilities for female sexual dysfunction described in the literature. In addition, some keys are given for the management of sexual dysfunction secondary to hormonal contraceptives (Figure 3).

First, when addressing a new sexual complaint, a thorough history using a biopsychosocial approach should be undertaken (Table 3) [18], including an assessment of any current or past psychiatric disorders; medication use and health problems; a history of emotional, physical, or sexual abuse; beliefs and attitudes regarding sex, menopause, and aging; and body image concerns. Particular attention should be paid to symptoms of depression, anxiety, and sleep problems, all of which are common during the menopause transition. Providers should inquire about alcohol or drug use, as substance use disorders are also associated with sexual dysfunction. Any health or sexual problems affecting the woman's sexual partner(s) should also be explored. Providers should inquire about relationship discord or communication issues, and if present, recommend therapy with a certified and specialized therapist [18]. A multidisciplinary approach to the management of female sexual dysfunction (FSD) is suggested, particularly when multiple contributing or complicating factors are identified, and this may consist of consultations with other professionals, such as a sex therapist, a pelvic floor physical therapist, and a sexual health specialist [2].

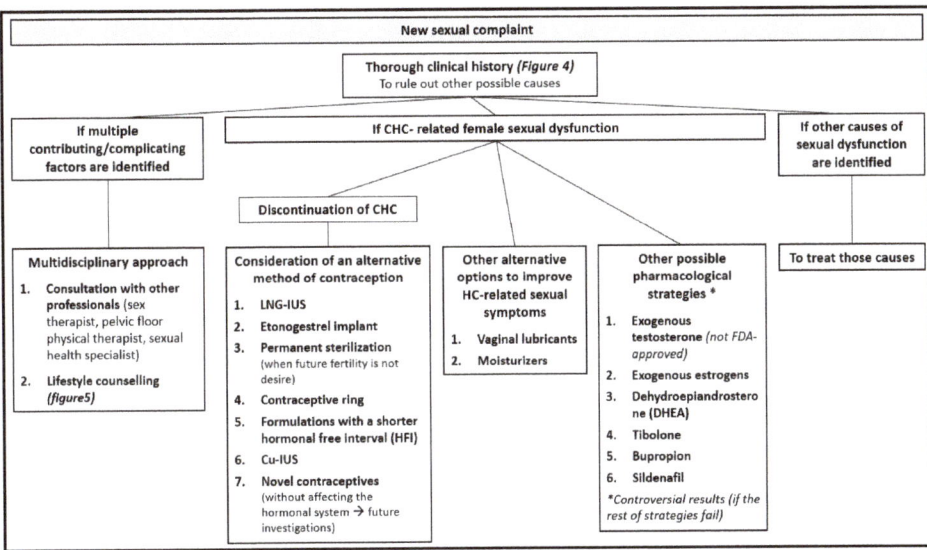

Figure 3. Management strategies for hormonal contraceptive (HC)-related sexual dysfunction.

Table 3. Main data to be collected in the clinical history in case of symptoms of sexual dysfunction.

Information that should be collected in the medical record by health providers in response to a complaint of sexual dysfunction:
1. Current or past psychiatric disorders.
2. Medication use and health problems.
3. History of emotional, physical, or sexual abuse.
4. Beliefs and attitudes regarding sex, menopause, and aging.
5. Body image concerns.
6. Symptoms of depression, anxiety, and sleep problems.
7. Alcohol or drug use and substance use disorders.
8. Health or sexual problems affecting the woman's sexual partner(s).
9. Relationship discord or communication issues.

Second, lifestyle counselling should be given by the health providers. General lifestyle counselling that may be useful for all types of female sexual dysfunction include recommending setting aside time for connecting with one's partner, increasing the woman's exposure to sexual stimuli such as erotic literature or films, encouraging the maintenance of a healthy weight, ensuring adequate physical activity and sleep, enhancing skills for coping with stress, and recommending books women can use for self-education (Table 4) [18].

Table 4. General lifestyle counselling.

1.	Setting aside time to connect with one's partner
2.	Increasing the woman's exposure to sexual stimuli: erotic literature or films
3.	Encouraging maintenance of a healthy weight
4.	Ensuring adequate physical activity and sleep
5.	Enhancing skills to cope with stress
6.	Recommending books women can use for self-education.

When choosing a new hormonal contraception method, health care providers (HCPs) should give information about all available methods in order to make a shared decision [34]. In the Contraceptive CHOICE Project, a prospective cohort study of 10,000 women 14–45 years who want to avoid pregnancy for at least one year and are initiating a new form of reversible contraception, 47% of women who had an interest in a CHC method selected a different method than the one they originally intended to use after receiving counselling about several CHC methods, including the pill, patch, and ring. Awareness of the decision-making factors that affect women's choices regarding methods of contraception may enable HCPs to make more informed recommendations that are targeted to the needs of each of their female patients [4]. The prescription of a contraceptive method is a great opportunity to clarify the multidimensional components of sexual health, including elements of anatomy and physiology of the sexual response [34].

Few clinical remedies or recommendations exist for women experiencing HC-related sexual side effects [54]. Unfortunately, no guidelines exist for the management of sexual dysfunction potentially associated with CHCs in reproductive-age women [2]. As such, when CHC-related female sexual dysfunction is suspected, the recommended therapy is discontinuation of a combined hormonal contraceptive, with consideration of an alternative method of contraception, such as LNG-IUS, a copper IUC, a etonogestrel implant, the permanent sterilization of either partner when future fertility is not desired, or a contraceptive ring (for women who prefer a CHC for cycle control and no contraceptive benefits) [2]. The ring appears to be a reasonable alternative to an oral CHC for women with sexual function concerns. Likewise, LARC methods also appear to be a reasonable alternative [2]. Nevertheless, switching to another combined oral contraceptive may provide some benefit, but there is no clear difference between androgenic or non-androgenic progestins [10]. In addition, the combination of dehydroepiandrosterone (DHEA) and an OC was not associated with improvements in sexual function, and it further negated the benefit of OCs on acne [2]. When COC-related female sexual dysfunction is suspected, another possible option could be to consider formulations with a shorter hormonal free interval (HFI). Formulations with a shorter HFI (24/4 and 26/2) have recently been developed with the aim of offering a reduction in hormone withdrawal-associated symptoms together with a more powerful ovarian suppression. Estradiol valerate/dienogest (E2V/DNG) is administered on a 26/2 regimen and has been shown to offer a high contraceptive efficacy, an improvement in hormone withdrawal-associated symptoms (including but not limited to headache and pelvic pain), and an improvement in sexual function [51,61]. In conclusion, the best contraceptive is one that fulfills women's needs with acceptable side effects and at an affordable price in different settings [32].

Other options to improve HC-related sexual dysfunction could be vaginal lubricants and moisturizers. They are the first-line treatment for vaginal dryness and consequent dyspareunia [2], side effects that are frequently associated with hormonal contraceptives, mainly with combined oral contraceptives. The majority of women participating in a daily study reported positive perceptions of lubricant use, including increased pleasure and comfort [62]. Sharing information on the high frequency of use and positive results experienced across age-groups may be helpful in counseling reproductive-age women about using lubricants [62].

Furthermore, concerning other possible strategies against sexual dysfunction, some studies show positive results on female sexual function with exogenous testosterone [2,18,29], exogenous estrogens [2,6], dehydroepiandrosterone (DHEA) [10,29], tibolone [29], bupropion, and sildenafil [18].

It appears that supraphysiological serum testosterone levels may be necessary to yield any benefit on sexual desire and arousal [18]. The use of compounded testosterone products for transdermal use is on the rise, but these products are not FDA-approved [18], and they can be associated with several side effects. Meanwhile, testosterone therapy in postmenopausal women has been associated with improvements in multiple dimensions of sexual function, including sexual desire, subjective arousal, vaginal blood flow, and frequency of orgasm [2]. Testosterone released from patches has also been described to produce positive effects on mood and sexual behavior and to increase bone mass significantly [63].

With regard to hormonal therapy with exogenous estrogens, results are controversial. On the one hand, exogenous estrogens have been shown to be an effective treatment for low libido and hypoactive sexual desire disorder [6], and, on the other hand, hormone therapy (estrogen with or without progesterone) does not appear to have a significant impact on sexual function, with the exception of vaginal estrogen in women with the genitourinary syndrome of menopause [18]; that is to say, hormonal therapy with estrogen is efficient with regard to genital atrophy, but it is not efficient in regard to sexual desire [29].

Furthermore, although dehydroepiandrosterone (DHEA) supplementation could have positive effects on the female libido [29] by restoring androgen levels in COC users, there is minimal evidence that this correlates with improved sexual functioning [10]. There is also evidence that bupropion and, to a lesser extent, sildenafil are effective for treating antidepressant-induced sexual dysfunction in women, although some conflicting evidence exists [18].

To conclude, even today, most of the contraceptives available on the market and those currently undergoing research and development interfere with ovulation or follicular development and also affect women's steroid production [32]. This mechanism of action is associated with several side effects, negative sexual effects included, that could be avoided by new contraceptives strategies. For that purpose, research conducted over the past few decades has provided more information on gamete physiology and interaction, offering new opportunities for the development of novel contraceptives that could act by interfering with the process of gamete interaction or with the chemo-attraction or chemo-repulsion of spermatozoa to the fertilization site without affecting the hormonal system [32].

4. Discussion

As discussed in the review above, hormonal contraception (HC) has made a difference in the control of female fertility since its approval by the FDA almost 60 years ago, and it is also widely used in the female population of child bearing age. Side effects, such as sexual dysfunction, may be sufficient reasons for the discontinuation of this contraceptive method. This represents an increase of the risk of unwanted pregnancy, with the possible worsening of women's wellbeing. However, female sexual function is complex and multifactorial and, despite an association between hormonal contraception and sexual dysfunction having been described in the past, the evidence on that topic is inconsistent.

Sexual problems are common, estimated to affect 22–43% of women worldwide [18], and influencing some types of female sexual dysfunction such as orgasm, sexual interest/arousal, and genito-pelvic pain. As a consequence of the multiple medications on sexual functioning, a specific category has been included in the new American DSM-5 classification system: Substance/ medication-induced sexual dysfunction) [18]. As said above, female sexual function is complex and multifactorial, and a biopsychosocial approach to sexual problems is recommended. It could be said that an HC can influence female sexual function in two different ways. On the one hand, an HC could have a negative influence on sexual function as a biologic factor, because HC use has been associated to hormonal changes. On the other hand, an HC could have a positive influence on sexual function, in psychological terms, since HC use has been associated with an improvement in mood symptoms and self-perception. Different options for hormonal contraception exist. There are three main groups: Combined hormonal contraception (pill, patch and vaginal ring); progestin-only contraceptives (POPs, DMPA, and implant); and intrauterine devices (LNG-IUDs). The hormonal composition of hormonal contraceptives is based on progestins alone or on a combination of progestogens and estrogens. Apparently, norgestimate and desogestrel, among progestogens, and 17β-estradiol (E2) and E2-valerate (E2V), among estrogens, have a profile less associated with side effects than the others in their respective groups.

The association between hormones and sexuality is multidimensional, as several hormones are important in the regulation of sexual behavior [29]. Hormonal contraceptives (HCs) seem to be responsible for a decrease of circulating androgen levels [1,2,29,35], baseline serum levels of estradiol [6,29,35], and baseline serum levels of progesterone [35], as well as the inhibition of oxytocin functioning [35]. However, the concentrations of the FSH and LH were similar in freely cycling women and in women using an HC [35]. These hormonal alterations can be translated into negative effects on the female sexual function, with reports of a decrease of the libido, increased sexual jealousy, and alterations on women pair-bonding behavior. It has been established that sexual desire, autoeroticism, and sexual fantasies of women depend on androgen levels [29]. However, the relevance of changes in androgen levels for an individual woman is unclear, and some women may be more sensitive to androgen level alteration than others [2]. Furthermore, while there is conflicting information concerning a link between progestins and libido, there is some evidence to suggest that estrogens play an essential role in female sexuality [6]. On the other hand, multiple lines of evidence suggest that the hypothalamic peptide oxytocin (OXT) is a key factor modulating pair-bonding behaviors, and it has been found to increase the intensity of orgasm and satisfaction after copulation. This mechanism was disturbed in those women using an HC, indicating that the partner-specific modulatory effects of OXT are antagonized by gonadal steroids. So, it could be said that HC use alters women's pair-bonding behavior, reduces neural response to the expectation of erotic stimuli, and increases sexual jealousy.

Despite an association between hormonal contraception and sexual function having been described, there are contradictory results between different studies in this respect. Some studies have found no change in sexual function with hormonal contraceptives (HCs) [2,3,6,10,42–46].

According to the studies reviewed, hormonal contraceptives have a series of non-contraceptive effects, which can be related to an improvement on different areas of female sexual function such as sexual desire, orgasm number and intensity, satisfaction, and arousal. All these effects contribute to the well-being of women and, consequently, to a possible improvement in the female sexual function.

By contrast, HCs could be associated with side effects that have an influence on female sexual function. Negative effects on some areas of female sexuality have been described with hormonal contraceptives, such as sexual desire [2,6,10,54], frequency of intercourse [2,54], arousal [2,54], pleasure [2,54], orgasm [2,54], sexual thoughts [54], interest, and enjoyment [6,54].

Combined oral contraceptives are widely studied, and most studies are based on COCs or used them as a comparative method of contraception. Nevertheless, other hormonal contraception methods have fewer studies about their influence on sexual function. There are mixed results with ring- and DMPA-related sexual side effects. The patch could be considered the most innocuous CHC regarding sexual side effects. The implant has been associated with negative sexual effects, such as a lack of interest in sex, a decreased libido, and a reduced sex drive. LNG-IUS have generally been associated with positive sexual effects, so it could be considered the most innocuous HC regarding sexual side effects. However, more studies are needed because of the inconsistency of current available data.

Finally, with regard to treatment options for sexual dysfunction, few clinical remedies or recommendations exist for women experiencing these sexual side effects [54]. Moreover, no clear guidelines exist for the management of sexual dysfunction potentially associated with CHCs in reproductive-age women [2]. First, when addressing a new sexual complaint, a thorough history using a biopsychosocial approach should be undertaken [18]. A multidisciplinary approach to the management of female sexual dysfunction (FSD) is suggested, particularly when multiple contributing or complicating factors are identified, and this may consist of consultations with other professionals, such as a sex therapist, a pelvic floor physical therapist, and a sexual health specialist [2]. Second, lifestyle counselling should be given by the health providers (Figure 3) [18]. When choosing a new hormonal contraception method, health care providers (HCPs) should give information about all available methods in order to make a shared decision [34]. When CHC-related female sexual dysfunction is suspected, the recommended therapy is the discontinuation of combined hormonal contraceptives with consideration of an alternative method of contraception, such as LNG-IUS, a copper IUC, an etonogestrel implant, the permanent sterilization of either partner when future fertility is not desired, or a contraceptive ring (for women who prefer CHCs for cycle control and non-contraceptive benefits) [2]. The ring appears to be a reasonable alternative to oral CHCs for women with sexual function concerns. Likewise, LARC methods appear to be a reasonable alternative too [2]. Other alternatives could be switching to another combined oral contraceptive [10] or formulations with a shorter hormonal free interval (HFI) [51,61]. Furthermore, with regard to other possible strategies against sexual dysfunction, some studies show positive results on female sexual function with exogenous testosterone [2,18,29], exogenous estrogens [2,6], dehydroepiandrosterone (DHEA) [10,29], tibolone [29], bupropion, and sildenafil [18]. Some alternative options to improve HC-related sexual dysfunction could be vaginal lubricants and moisturizers.

5. Conclusions

The results of the studies reviewed seem to indicate that hormonal contraception could influence different aspects of female sexual function. However, there are contradictory results between the different studies regarding the association between sexual dysfunction and hormonal contraceptives, so it could be firmly said that additional research is needed.

Meanwhile, it could be said that hormonal contraception has been associated with different alterations in sexual functioning. So, when addressing a new sexual complaint that is time-related with the beginning of hormonal contraception, health care providers should give information about other methods and try to switch them to a method less associated with sexual dysfunction. Vaginal rings and patches are possible options in case of women preferring combined hormonal contraception who report side effects with the pill.

To conclude, a multidisciplinary approach to the management of female sexual dysfunction is mandatory, and health care providers should give lifestyle counselling apart from proposing different treatment options. An adequate relationship with the patient, as well as the routine monitoring of possible sexual dysfunction, are essential in addressing these difficulties. Undoubtedly, the best contraceptive is one that fulfills the women's needs with acceptable side effects and agreed with the prescriber.

Author Contributions: Initial manuscripts selection (N.M.C.-E., R.d.A., J.I.d.l.I.-L.), additional review (A.L.M., B.B.-B.), writing of the first manuscript (N.M.C.-E., R.d.A., J.I.d.l.I.-L.) final review of the draft (A.L.M. and B.B.-B.).

Acknowledgments: In the name of the authors, we wanted to thank David González-Iglesias, translator of the Official College of Doctors of Salamanca, for his work and dedication.

Conflicts of Interest: AL Montejo has received consultancy fees or honoraria/research grants in the last five years from Boehringer Ingelheim, Forum Pharmaceuticals, Rovi, Servier, Lundbeck, Otsuka, Janssen Cilag, Pfizer, Roche, Instituto de Salud Carlos III and Junta de Castilla y León. Berta Bote has received fees to give lectures from Lundbeck and Janssen. Nerea M. Casado-Espada has received an economic award from Janssen in an oral communication contest. None of the other authors declare any conflict of interest.

References

1. Burrows, L.J.; Basha, M.; Goldstein, A.T. The Effects of Hormonal Contraceptives on Female Sexuality: A Review. *J. Sex. Med.* **2012**, *9*, 2213–2223. [CrossRef] [PubMed]
2. Casey, P.M.; MacLaughlin, K.L.; Faubion, S.S. Impact of Contraception on Female Sexual Function. *J. Women's Heal.* **2017**, *26*, 207–213. [CrossRef] [PubMed]
3. Champaneria, R.; D'Andrea, R.M.; Latthe, P.M. Hormonal contraception and pelvic floor function: a systematic review. *Int. Urogynecol. J.* **2016**, *27*, 709–722. [CrossRef] [PubMed]

4. Egarter, C.; Frey Tirri, B.; Bitzer, J.; Kaminskyy, V.; Oddens, B.J.; Prilepskaya, V.; Yeshaya, A.; Marintcheva-Petrova, M.; Weyers, S. Women's perceptions and reasons for choosing the pill, patch, or ring in the CHOICE study: A cross-sectional survey of contraceptive method selection after counseling. *BMC Womens. Health* **2013**, *13*, 1. [CrossRef] [PubMed]
5. Baird, D.T.; Castelo-Branco, C.; Collins, J.; Evers, J.L.H.; Glasier, A.; La Vecchia, C.; Leridon, H.; Mishell, D.R.; Wellings, K.; Arisi, E.; et al. Female contraception over 40. *Hum. Reprod. Update* **2009**, *15*, 599–612.
6. Boozalis, A.; Tutlam, N.T.; Chrisman Robbins, C.; Peipert, J.F. Sexual Desire and Hormonal Contraception. *Obstet. Gynecol.* **2016**, *127*, 563–572. [CrossRef] [PubMed]
7. Skouby, S.O. Contraceptive use and behavior in the 21st century: a comprehensive study across five European countries. *Eur. J. Contracept. Reprod. Heal. Care* **2010**, *15*, S42–S53. [CrossRef] [PubMed]
8. Oliveira Da Silva, M.; Albrecht, J.; Olsen, J.; Karro, H.; Temmerman, M.; Gissler, M.; Bloemenkamp, K.; Hannaford, P.; Fronteira, I. The Reproductive Health Report: The state of sexual and reproductive health within the European Union. *Eur. J. Contracept. Reprod. Heal. Care* **2011**, *16*, S1–S70.
9. Hall, K.S.; Trussell, J. Types of combined oral contraceptives used by US women. *Contraception* **2012**, *86*, 659–665. [CrossRef]
10. Black, A.; Guilbert, E.; Costescu, D.; Dunn, S.; Fisher, W.; Kives, S.; Mirosh, M.; Norman, W.V.; Pymar, H.; Reid, R.; et al. No. 329-Canadian Contraception Consensus Part 4 of 4 Chapter 9: Combined Hormonal Contraception. *J. Obstet. Gynaecol. Canada* **2017**, *39*, 229–268. [CrossRef]
11. Imprialos, K.P.; Stavropoulos, K.; Doumas, M.; Tziomalos, K.; Karagiannis, A.; Athyros, V.G. Sexual Dysfunction, Cardiovascular Risk and Effects of Pharmacotherapy. *Curr. Vasc. Pharmacol.* **2018**, *16*, 130–142. [CrossRef] [PubMed]
12. Montejo, A.L.; Montejo, L.; Navarro-Cremades, F. Sexual side-effects of antidepressant and antipsychotic drugs. *Curr. Opin. Psychiatry* **2015**, *28*, 418–423. [CrossRef] [PubMed]
13. Montejo, A.L.; Montejo, L.; Baldwin, D.S. The impact of severe mental disorders and psychotropic medications on sexual health and its implications for clinical management. *World Psychiatry* **2018**, *17*, 3–11. [CrossRef] [PubMed]
14. Montejo, A.L.; Majadas, S.; Rico-Villademoros, F.; Llorca, G.; De La Gándara, J.; Franco, M.; Martín-Carrasco, M.; Aguera, L.; Prieto, N.; Spanish Working Group for the Study of Psychotropic-Related Sexual Dysfunction. Frequency of sexual dysfunction in patients with a psychotic disorder receiving antipsychotics. *J. Sex. Med.* **2010**, *7*, 3404–3413. [CrossRef] [PubMed]
15. Montejo, A.L.; Calama, J.; Rico-Villademoros, F.; Montejo, L.; González-García, N.; Pérez, J. A Real-World Study on Antidepressant-Associated Sexual Dysfunction in 2144 Outpatients: The SALSEX I Study. *Arch. Sex. Behav.* **2019**, *48*, 923–933. [CrossRef] [PubMed]
16. Maiorino, M.I.; Bellastella, G.; Castaldo, F.; Petrizzo, M.; Giugliano, D.; Esposito, K. Sexual function in young women with type 1 diabetes: the METRO study. *J. Endocrinol. Invest.* **2017**, *40*, 169–177. [CrossRef] [PubMed]
17. Esposito, K.; Giugliano, D. Obesity, the metabolic syndrome, and sexual dysfunction. *Int. J. Impot. Res.* **2005**, *17*, 391–398. [CrossRef] [PubMed]
18. Thomas, H.N.; Thurston, R.C. A biopsychosocial approach to women's sexual function and dysfunction at midlife: A narrative review. *Maturitas* **2016**, *87*, 49–60. [CrossRef] [PubMed]
19. Hughes, H. Management of postpartum loss of libido. *J. Fam. Health Care* **2008**, *18*, 123–135. [PubMed]
20. FDA Office of Women's Health Birth Control Guide. Available online: https://www.fda.gov/media/99605/download (accessed on 5 January 2019).
21. Black, A.; Guilbert, E.; Costescu, D.; Dunn, S.; Fisher, W.; Kives, S.; Mirosh, M.; Norman, W.; Pymar, H.; Reid, R.; et al. Canadian Contraception Consensus (Part 3 of 4): Chapter 8-Progestin-Only Contraception. *J. Obstet. Gynaecol. Canada* **2016**, *38*, 279–300. [CrossRef]
22. Black, A.; Guilbert, E.; Costescu, D.; Dunn, S.; Fisher, W.; Kives, S.; Mirosh, M.; Norman, W.; Pymar, H.; Reid, R.; et al. Canadian Contraception Consensus (Part 3 of 4): Chapter 7-Intrauterine Contraception. *J. Obstet. Gynaecol. Canada* **2016**, *38*, 182–222. [CrossRef] [PubMed]
23. World Health Organization. *Recomendaciones sobre prácticas seleccionadas para el uso de anticonceptivos*; World Health Organization: Geneva, Switzerland, 2018; ISBN 978-92-4-356540-8.
24. Sánchez Borrego, R.; Martínez Pérez, Ó. *Guía práctica de anticoncepción oral basada en la evidencia*; Emisa: Madrid, Spain, 2003; ISBN 84-86917-66-2.

25. Roney, J.R.; Simmons, Z.L. Hormonal predictors of sexual motivation in natural menstrual cycles. *Horm. Behav.* **2013**, *63*, 636–645. [CrossRef] [PubMed]
26. Grøntvedt, T.V.; Grebe, N.M.; Kennair, L.E.O.; Gangestad, S.W. Estrogenic and progestogenic effects of hormonal contraceptives in relation to sexual behavior: insights into extended sexuality. *Evol. Hum. Behav.* **2017**, *38*, 283–292. [CrossRef]
27. Grebe, N.M.; Gangestad, S.W.; Garver-Apgar, C.E.; Thornhill, R. Women's luteal-phase sexual proceptivity and the functions of extended sexuality. *Psychol. Sci.* **2013**, *24*, 2106–2110. [CrossRef] [PubMed]
28. Raudrant, D.; Rabe, T. Progestogens with antiandrogenic properties. *Drugs* **2003**, *63*, 463–492. [CrossRef] [PubMed]
29. Bjelica, A.; Kapamadzija, A.; Maticki-Sekulic, M. Hormones and female sexuality. *Med. Pregl.* **2003**, *56*, 446–450. [CrossRef] [PubMed]
30. Sitruk-Ware, R. New progestagens for contraceptive use. *Hum. Reprod. Update* **2006**, *12*, 169–178. [CrossRef] [PubMed]
31. Espitia De La Hoz, F.J. O-08 Alteration of the Sexual Response Cycle in Women Using Combined Oral Contraceptives. *J. Sex. Med.* **2017**, *14*, e374. [CrossRef]
32. Bahamondes, L.; Bahamondes, M.V. New and emerging contraceptives: a state-of-the-art review. *Int. J. Womens. Health* **2014**, *6*, 221. [CrossRef]
33. Dennerstein, L.; Randolph, J.; Taffe, J.; Dudley, E.; Burger, H. Hormones, mood, sexuality, and the menopausal transition. *Fertil. Steril.* **2002**, *77*, 42–48. [CrossRef]
34. Benedetto, C.; Cagnacci, A.; De Seta, F.; Genazzani, A.R.; Guida, M.; Michieli, R.; Moscarini, M.; Primiero, F.; Russo, N. Counseling on vaginal delivery of contraceptive hormones: Implications for women's body knowledge and sexual health. *Gynecol. Endocrinol.* **2013**, *29*, 1015–1021.
35. Scheele, D.; Plota, J.; Stoffel-Wagner, B.; Maier, W.; Hurlemann, R. Hormonal contraceptives suppress oxytocin-induced brain reward responses to the partner's face. *Soc. Cogn. Affect. Neurosci.* **2016**, *11*, 767–774. [CrossRef] [PubMed]
36. American Psychiatric Association. *Diagnostic and Statistical Manual of Mental Disorders: DSM-5*, 5th ed.; American Psychiatric Association, Ed.; American Psychiatric Association: Washington, DC, USA, 2013; ISBN 9780890425558.
37. World Health Organization. *Defining Sexual Health: Report of a Technical Consultation on Sexual Health*; World Health Organization: Geneva, Switzerland, 2006.
38. Mercer, C.H.; Fenton, K.A.; Johnson, A.M.; Wellings, K.; Macdowall, W.; McManus, S.; Nanchahal, K.; Erens, B. Sexual function problems and help seeking behaviour in Britain: national probability sample survey. *BMJ* **2003**, *327*, 426–427. [CrossRef] [PubMed]
39. Sobecki, J.N.; Curlin, F.A.; Rasinski, K.A.; Lindau, S.T. What we don't talk about when we don't talk about sex: results of a national survey of U.S. obstetrician/gynecologists. *J. Sex. Med.* **2012**, *9*, 1285–1294. [CrossRef] [PubMed]
40. Sand, M.; Fisher, W.A. Women's Endorsement of Models of Female Sexual Response: The Nurses' Sexuality Study. *J. Sex. Med.* **2007**, *4*, 708–719. [CrossRef] [PubMed]
41. Wiegel, M.; Meston, C.; Rosen, R. The female sexual function index (FSFI): cross-validation and development of clinical cutoff scores. *J. Sex Marital Ther.* **2005**, *31*, 1–20. [CrossRef]
42. Davis, A.R.; Castaño, P.M. Oral contraceptives and libido in women. *Annu. Rev. Sex Res.* **2004**, *15*, 297–320.
43. Pastor, Z.; Holla, K.; Chmel, R. The influence of combined oral contraceptives on female sexual desire: a systematic review. *Eur. J. Contracept. Reprod. Health Care* **2013**, *18*, 27–43. [CrossRef]
44. Graham, C.A.; Bancroft, J.; Doll, H.A.; Greco, T.; Tanner, A. Does oral contraceptive-induced reduction in free testosterone adversely affect the sexuality or mood of women? *Psychoneuroendocrinology* **2007**, *32*, 246–255. [CrossRef]
45. Strufaldi, R.; Pompei, L.M.; Steiner, M.L.; Cunha, E.P.; Ferreira, J.A.S.; Peixoto, S.; Fernandes, C.E. Effects of two combined hormonal contraceptives with the same composition and different doses on female sexual function and plasma androgen levels. *Contraception* **2010**, *82*, 147–154. [CrossRef]
46. Elaut, E.; Buysse, A.; De Sutter, P.; Gerris, J.; De Cuypere, G.; T'Sjoen, G. Cycle-Related Changes in Mood, Sexual Desire, and Sexual Activity in Oral Contraception-Using and Nonhormonal-Contraception-Using Couples. *J. Sex Res.* **2016**, *53*, 125–136. [CrossRef] [PubMed]

47. Enzlin, P.; Weyers, S.; Janssens, D.; Poppe, W.; Eelen, C.; Pazmany, E.; Elaut, E.; Amy, J. Sexual Functioning in Women Using Levonorgestrel-Releasing Intrauterine Systems as Compared to Copper Intrauterine Devices. *J. Sex. Med.* **2012**, *9*, 1065–1073. [CrossRef]
48. Toorzani, Z.M.; Zahraei, R.H.; Ehsanpour, S.; Nasiri, M.; Shahidi, S.; Soleimani, B. A study on the relationship of sexual satisfaction and common contraceptive methods employed by the couples. *Iran. J. Nurs. Midwifery Res.* **2010**, *15*, 115–119. [PubMed]
49. Reed, B.; Harlow, S.; Legocki, L.; Helmuth, M.; Haefner, H.; Gillespie, B.; Sen, A. Oral contraceptive use and risk of vulvodynia: a population-based longitudinal study. *BJOG An Int. J. Obstet. Gynaecol.* **2013**, *120*, 1678–1684. [CrossRef] [PubMed]
50. Iliadou, A.; Milsom, I.; Pedersen, N.L.; Altman, D. Risk of urinary incontinence symptoms in oral contraceptive users: a national cohort study from the Swedish Twin Register. *Fertil. Steril.* **2009**, *92*, 428–433. [CrossRef] [PubMed]
51. Graziottin, A. The shorter, the better: A review of the evidence for a shorter contraceptive hormone-free interval. *Eur. J. Contracept. Reprod. Heal. Care* **2016**, *21*, 93–105. [CrossRef]
52. Guida, M.; Cibarelli, F.; Troisi, J.; Gallo, A.; Palumbo, A.R.; Di Spiezio Sardo, A. Sexual life impact evaluation of different hormonal contraceptives on the basis of their methods of administration. *Arch. Gynecol. Obstet.* **2014**, *290*, 1239–1247. [CrossRef] [PubMed]
53. Skrzypulec, V.; Drosdzol, A. Evaluation of quality of life and sexual functioning of women using levonorgestrel-releasing intrauterine contraceptive system–Mirena. *Coll. Antropol.* **2008**, *32*, 1059–1068.
54. Smith, N.K.; Jozkowski, K.N.; Sanders, S.A. Hormonal contraception and female pain, orgasm and sexual pleasure. *J. Sex. Med.* **2014**, *11*, 462–470. [CrossRef]
55. Li, D.; Wilcox, A.J.; Dunson, D.B. Benchmark pregnancy rates and the assessment of post-coital contraceptives: an update. *Contraception* **2015**, *91*, 344–349. [CrossRef]
56. Gracia, C.R.; Sammel, M.D.; Charlesworth, S.; Lin, H.; Barnhart, K.T.; Creinin, M.D. Sexual function in first-time contraceptive ring and contraceptive patch users. *Fertil. Steril.* **2010**, *93*, 21–28. [CrossRef] [PubMed]
57. Mohamed, A.M.M.; El-Sherbiny, W.S.M.; Mostafa, W.A.I. Combined contraceptive ring versus combined oral contraceptive (30-µg ethinylestradiol and 3-mg drospirenone). *Int. J. Gynaecol. Obstet.* **2011**, *114*, 145–148. [CrossRef] [PubMed]
58. Battaglia, C.; Morotti, E.; Persico, N.; Battaglia, B.; Busacchi, P.; Casadio, P.; Paradisi, R.; Venturoli, S. Clitoral vascularization and sexual behavior in young patients treated with drospirenone-ethinyl estradiol or contraceptive vaginal ring: a prospective, randomized, pilot study. *J. Sex. Med.* **2014**, *11*, 471–480. [CrossRef] [PubMed]
59. Guida, M.; Di Spiezio Sardo, A.; Bramante, S.; Sparice, S.; Acunzo, G.; Tommaselli, G.A.; Di Carlo, C.; Pellicano, M.; Greco, E.; Nappi, C. Effects of two types of hormonal contraception—oral versus intravaginal—on the sexual life of women and their partners. *Hum. Reprod.* **2005**, *20*, 1100–1106. [CrossRef] [PubMed]
60. Freeman, S. Nondaily hormonal contraception: considerations in contraceptive choice and patient counseling. *J. Am. Acad. Nurse Pract.* **2004**, *16*, 226–238. [CrossRef]
61. Nappi, R.E. Association of E2v/DNG as contraceptive choice for a better quality of life of women. *Minerva Ginecol.* **2012**, *64*, 41–52. [PubMed]
62. Jozkowski, K.N.; Herbenick, D.; Schick, V.; Reece, M.; Sanders, S.A.; Fortenberry, J.D. Women's perceptions about lubricant use and vaginal wetness during sexual activities. *J. Sex. Med.* **2013**, *10*, 484–492. [CrossRef]
63. Henzl, M.R.; Loomba, P.K. Transdermal delivery of sex steroids for hormone replacement therapy and contraception. A review of principles and practice. *J. Reprod. Med.* **2003**, *48*, 525–540.

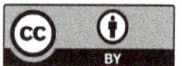

© 2019 by the authors. Licensee MDPI, Basel, Switzerland. This article is an open access article distributed under the terms and conditions of the Creative Commons Attribution (CC BY) license (http://creativecommons.org/licenses/by/4.0/).

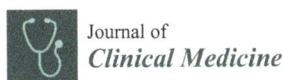

Review

Uncovering Female Child Sexual Offenders—Needs and Challenges for Practice and Research

Safiye Tozdan *, Peer Briken and Arne Dekker

Institute for Sex Research and Forensic Psychiatry, University Medical Center Hamburg–Eppendorf, 20251 Hamburg, Germany; briken@uke.de (P.B.); dekker@uke.de (A.D.)
* Correspondence: s.tozdan@uke.de

Received: 20 February 2019; Accepted: 21 March 2019; Published: 22 March 2019

Abstract: This article provides a short literature overview on female child sexual offenders (FCSO) focusing on the discrepancy between prevalence rates from different sources, characteristics of FCSO and their victims, as well as the societal "culture of denial" surrounding these women. FCSO are a powerful social taboo. Even professionals in the healthcare or justice system were shown to respond inappropriately in cases of child sexual abuse committed by women. As a result, offences of FCSO may be underreported and therefore difficult to research. The lack of scientific data on FSCO lowers the quality of child protection and treatment services. We therefore deem it particularly necessary for professionals in health care to break the social taboo that is FCSO and to further stimulate research on the topic of FCSO. We provide some general implications for professionals in health care systems as well as specific recommendations for researchers. We end with an overall conclusion.

Keywords: child sexual abuse; female perpetrator; mother-child incest; gender stereotypes; social taboo

1. Introduction

1.1. Background

Stereotypically, child sexual abuse implies the image of a male perpetrator sexually abusing a female child. However, due to an expanding research field since the 1980s [1], it is well established scientific knowledge today, that part of all child sexual offences are committed by women [2–6].

Although research data on female child sexual offenders (abbreviated female child sexual offenders (FCSO) in the following References [1,2,5,7–14]) is available and can be used for reviews and meta-analyses, there is still a noticeable gap of information on what is known about FCSO as opposed to male child sexual offenders [15]. Additionally, most of what is known resulted from studies with only small clinical samples of female offenders registered by the criminal system [16]. Consequently, the assessment and treatment of FCSO is insufficient [2].

Irrespective of the perpetrator's gender, child sexual abuse is an underreported crime [17]. One reason for the low level of knowledge about FCSO could be that FCSO are rarely registered in official statistics and are therefore difficult to reach for clinicians and researchers. One possible explanation for this phenomenon is that child sexual abuse committed by women seems to be a powerful social taboo [18]. Therefore, there is a marked resistance against the disclosure of FCSO [19] even among professionals in the health care and justice system [20]. In order to encourage the disclosure of FCSO, enhance the thematic research, and improve the quality of child protection and prevention, we deem it particularly necessary for clinicians and researchers in the field of sexual health to overcome this taboo.

1.2. Aim

This article is not a systematic review but is intended to provide a short narrative literature overview on the discrepancy between prevalence rates based on different sources (official reports vs. victimization surveys) and on the adult FCSO's characteristics (e.g., average age, socioeconomic status, mental health issues, victims). Secondly, we focus on FCSO as a social taboo that even percolates the health care and justice system. In order to overcome this social taboo, we provide some general implications for professionals in health care systems. In order to foster research activities on FCSO, we give specific recommendations for researchers in the field of sexual medicine.

2. Method

We explored the current literature on FCSO and mainly included reviews and studies on FCSO from 2000–2019 examining large and/or representative samples. We focused on data from countries sharing similar cultural and societal backgrounds. We included some additional studies that were published before the year 2000, but had an important impact on this research field and are still frequently cited. We excluded articles in which only juvenile FCSO or general female sexual offenders (with adult victims) were analyzed. Search terms included "female", "woman", or "mother" with "sexual child abuse", "child sexual offending", or "incest" as well as "social taboo" or "gender stereotypes". Searches were performed in PsychInfo, PubMed, KrimDok, and socINDEX. When necessary, additional references were used (e.g., Google).

3. Female Sexual Child Offenders

3.1. Prevalence of Female Child Sexual Offenders

Due to different methodologies and samples, prevalence reports of sexual child abuse committed by women vary within the literature. There are two main sources of information for estimating the prevalence of FCSO: Firstly, official reports (i.e., from police or court offices); secondly, victim reports. An overview of the results of different studies and reviews is shown in Tables 1 and 2.

Table 1. Prevalence rates (PR) for female child sexual offenders (FCSO) based on official reports.

Reference	Country	Year	Source of Information	Sample Size (Offenders)	PR for FCSO (%)
[21]	Australia	2005	Incidents reported in official statistics	1,294,000	1.7 [a]
[22]	Canada	2017	Accusations reported in official crime statistics	4703	3.7
[23]	USA	1991–1996	National Incident-Based Reporting System (incidents reported to law enforcement)	8539 (victims younger age 6) 12,260 (victims aged 6–12) 20,005 (victims aged 12–17)	12 6 3
[24]	Germany	2007–2014	Convictions reported in official crime statistics	14,069	1.4
[24]	Germany	2016	Inmates remanded in custody reported in official crime statistics	402	1.7

Studies included all met the definition of child sexual abuse as experiencing vaginal/anal penetration or attempted penetration with fingers, penis, objects and/or oral sex, attempted oral sex, unwanted sexual touching or fondling or any other kind of sexual interaction before the age of 17. [a] Only includes female relatives, no female strangers.

Table 2. Prevalence rates (PR) for female child sexual offenders (FCSO) based on victimization surveys.

Reference	Country	Year	Source of Information	Sample Size (Victims)	PR for FCSO (%)
[25]	USA	1996	National Incidence Study by the National Center on Child Abuse and Neglect (NCCAN)	300,200	12
[26]	USA	2009/10	Child protective system reports from the National Child Abuse and Neglect Data System (NCANDS)	66,765	20
[27]	UK	2008/09	Analyses of call records from ChildLine (free hotline for children in need)	12,268	17
[28]	UK	2005/06	Analyses of call records from ChildLine	6763 [a]	44 [b] (male victims) 5 (female victims)
[29]	USA	1995–1997	Cohort study among adult members of the Kaiser Permanent's Health Appraisal Centre in San Diego	1276 (male victims) 2310 (female victims)	20.8 2.1
[30]	UK	2007/08	Analyses of call records from ChildLine	1803 (male victims)	26 [c]
[15]	Ireland	2001	Retrospective data on adult accounts of childhood abuse from SAVI (population-based interview survey)	270 (male victims) 407 (female victims)	14.8 1.7
[31]	Germany	2011	Retrospective data from a population-based survey on child sexual abuse among 16–40 year olds	83 (male victims) 404 (female victims)	15.3 1.5

Studies included all met the definition of child sexual abuse as experiencing vaginal/anal penetration or attempted penetration with fingers, penis, objects and/or oral sex, attempted oral sex, unwanted sexually touching or foundling or any other. [a] To our knowledge, the data on ChildLine cited by Roberts [28] have not been published entirely elsewhere. Due to this, it was not possible to specify the sample size by gender. [b] PR specified by gender indicates the proportion of female perpetrators within gender groups. For instance, a PR of 44 for male victims indicates that 44% of all male victims reported a female perpetrator. [c] Only includes female relatives, no female strangers.

The comparison of prevalence rates based on official reports (Table 1) and those based on victimization surveys (Table 2) clearly demonstrate a great gap. Sexual offences against children committed by women appear to be underreported and not prosecuted adequately. Table 2 only includes studies with large sample sizes and/or those examined representative samples published from 2000 and onwards. Taking into account earlier studies on smaller and/or clinical samples, even higher prevalence rates for FCSO with male victims are reported. For instance, Fromuth and Buckhart [32] investigated male students from a midwestern (n = 253) and a southwestern (n = 329) American university. Thirty-eight males from the midwestern university reported that they were sexually abused as a child and 78% furthermore specified a female perpetrator. Forty-three males from the southwestern university had been sexually abused as children, of whom 78% reported a female perpetrator [32].

3.2. Characteristics of Female Child Sexual Offenders and Their Victims

Research so far indicates that FCSO are a rather heterogeneous population with different features [5,33–35]. However, some common characteristics of FCSO and their victims were found.

The average age of FCSO seems to range from 26–36 [5]. For instance, Faller [3,36] reported on a sample of 40 FCSO with a mean age of 26.1 years [36] and on another sample of 72 FCSO with a mean age of 28 years [3]; and Nathan and Ward [37] reported on 12 FCSO with a mean age of 30 years. The majority of FCSO in empirical research showed a rather low socioeconomic status [5,12,38] with little vocational qualifications [12,39,40]. According to Berner, Briken, and Hill [41], more than 50% of FCSO had experienced sexual and/or physical abuse themselves [41]. Indeed, many studies demonstrated FCSO as being mentally, sexually, and/or physically abused during childhood [12,38,42–45]. They often show mental health problems, particularly substance abuse [45], personality disorders (passive and/or dependent) with rather low self-esteem [46], and are frequently involved in abusive relationships during adulthood [38,47] or have an absence of intimate relationships [45]. FCSO further appear to be impulsive with low levels of emotional self-regulation [48].

Typically, FSCOs find their victims in their closer social circle [3,16,35,42,49,50]. Often they are their victims' caregivers, i.e., mothers, other relatives, or babysitters [3,16,38]. The prevalence rates shown in Table 2 indicate that FCSO appear to sexual abuse male victims more often than female victims. However, research results so far are not sufficiently reliably to predict who may be at higher risk to be abused by an adult woman: boys or girls [5]. Victims' age ranges from infants to adolescents [51,52].

3.3. Perception and Handling of Female Child Sexual Offenders

The discrepancy between official reports and victimization surveys on the prevalence of FCSO clearly demonstrates the under-recognition of women who behave in a sexually abusive manner. Official statistics only reflect those women who have had contact with the criminal justice or social service system. This indicates that reporting FCSO to the police or child welfare agencies seems to be a great obstacle. In fact, from the very beginning of scientific confrontation with FCSO in the 1930 [53], women who sexually abuse children have been a powerful social taboo [18]. Women are usually portrayed as victims and as being passive, innocent, and sexually submissive. Moreover, they are primarily normalized as the gatekeepers of sexuality [18]. In terms of anatomy, some have argued that women are receivers of sexuality which might make it difficult to imagine a woman as someone who sexually abuses others [54]. Instead, women are frequently seen as nurturers and protectors in positions of trust. They are thought of as mothers and those who provide care for others. Women who sexually abuse children undermine such normative labels and challenge traditional gender stereotypes that are firmly established in society [18].

3.3.1. Society

The way in which members of a society perceive and respond to certain events is significantly shaped by medial reports [55]. Research so far has shown that media's representation of sexual offenders is biased [56]. In an analysis of 29 newspaper articles published in Australian dailies, Landor and Eisenchlas [56] showed that male sexual offenders are strongly criticized in media reports, whereas female sexual offenders are usually described in a more sympathetic way. Furthermore, the articles on FCSO usually contain excuses to justify or lessen the seriousness of the women's abusive behavior [56]. Hayes and Baker [18] also analyzed the way in which the media reports on women who sexually abused children. The authors theorized that media reports tend to reinforce traditional gender stereotypes and therefore suppress the development of a public awareness of sexual offences committed by women. Examining 487 media reports from Australia and the United Kingdom, they found that the media mainly presents FCSO as aberrations and pariahs (in terms of outcasts), and thus do not contribute to an atmosphere supporting the safe and timely reporting of offences by victims [18].

Mackelprang and Becker [57] demonstrated that this unequal perception of men and women who sexually offend against children is in fact reflected in societal judgements. The authors asked 432 undergraduate students to judge teacher sexual offence vignettes (e.g., amount of time the offender should be incarcerated) that varied by offender's gender and attractiveness. For all outcome measures reflecting punitive judgements and attitudes towards the offender, female teachers who had had a sexual relationship with a student were evaluated more leniently and judged less punitively than male teachers who did the same. In addition, there has been an even greater tolerance for FCSO when they were described as attractive instead of unattractive. This effect was not observed for the vignettes on male child sexual offenders [57].

3.3.2. Professionals

Professionals in healthcare, criminal justice, and child protection systems were also shown to respond inappropriately in cases of child sexual abuse committed by women [58–62]. For instance, children's disclosure was brushed aside as fantasies [63] or abusive women gained further access to potential victims [64]. In 2010, Mellor and Deering [20] examined professional responses and attitudes toward FCSO. A total of 231 Australian psychiatrists, psychologists, probationary psychologists, and child protection workers were presented with a variation of vignettes describing women and men who had sexually offended against children. Afterwards they completed a questionnaire on their attitudes to women's offending behavior toward children. Compared to male-perpetrated child sexual abuse, female-perpetrated child sexual abuse was more likely to be rated leniently. This "indicates that a level of professional minimization towards female-perpetrated child sexual abuse exists" [20] (p. 433). Psychotherapists who treat young patients experiencing mother-incest-abuse initially often struggle with the idea of reporting these cases [65]. As Haliburn concluded, the frequency of mental health patients reporting histories of child sexual abuse does not surprise clinicians anymore. However, when the perpetrator is a woman, clinicians' reaction often is "shock and disbelief and a tendency to be dismissive" [65] (p. 423).

3.3.3. Victims and Offenders

As a consequence of FCSO being a social taboo, their victims often have difficulties in recognizing their experiences as sexually abusive [66] and feel intensely confused [67]. It is not unusual that FCSO disguise their abusive behavior as part of childlare activities [67]. This might in part be the reason why in fact even the offenders themselves have difficulties in recognizing their behavior as sexually abusive [68]. FCSO' victims are faced with serious issues regarding the disclosure of their abuse [69], thus hesitating more often to disclose the abuse than victims of male offenders [70]. It is particularly worth mentioning that victims of FCSO in early treatment stages even appear to lie to their therapists about their abuser's sex, claiming that they were perpetrated by a man [71]. These difficulties might be even worse when the female perpetrator is the own mother [72]. Usually shrouded in secrecy, Haliburn [65] called mother–child incest a "double betrayal", since both, the violation of trust as well as the exploitation of the child's affection and dependency needs to take place. Individuals who were sexually abused by their own mother were described as feeling additional shame and stigma [73].

4. Implications

Based on the outlined research, we propose some general implications for professionals in health care followed by more specific recommendations for researchers in the field of sexual health. As there are many possible clinical and research implications, we do not make any claim to comprehensiveness.

4.1. General Implications

Offences of FCSO are underreported and therefore FCSO are difficult to study. The resulting knowledge gap about FSCOs reduces the quality of child protection and treatment services. We therefore deem it particularly necessary for health care professionals to overcome the social taboo that is FCSO.

As mentioned, there seems to be a marked resistance in the general public and the health care system to detect FCSO [19]. Historically, the same kind of resistance was documented for the acceptance and awareness of men who sexually abuse children [74]. Thus, in accordance with Mellor and Deering [20], we state that the overall awareness and appropriate attitude towards FCSO have to be improved in health care, criminal justice, and child protection systems. Since a structured training as proposed by Mellor and Deering [20] may strain the organizational capacities of most institutions, we recommend an increased engagement of the issues concerning FCSO in internal conferences and discussions. This may lead to a more open discussion of FCSO among colleagues and therefore to a stronger representation of the issue in the professional's mind. Consequently, this should help to uncover the abusive behavior for both victims and offenders.

As media portrayals of FCSO and their victims are generally inadequate [18], instructions for journalists concerning the appropriate attitude towards FCSO are also deemed necessary.

The tendency to deny and minimize, leads to FCSO being a hidden phenomenon, undeniably difficult to uncover (cf. References [18,75–80]). We therefore advise professionals in both clinical practice and scientific research to consciously challenge and control their own underlying mechanisms of denial when confronted with cases of FCSO.

Since it is assumed that victims of FCSO and even FCSO themselves have difficulties to recognize the women's behavior as sexually abusive [18], we deem an active approach towards FCSO in order to meet their needs is most appropriate. Therefore, we propose education and information within health care, justice, and other systems. For instance, wherever undetected FCSO and/or their victims might occur (e.g., pediatrician practices, youth welfare offices, kindergarten, schools, counselling for victims of sexual offending, women's house), an educational brochure could be distributed to adults. It might briefly and simply inform the reader about the fact that women are also capable of sexually abusing children including contact details for both FCSO and victims. By this, a network including members of different professions within health care, justice, and other systems might be built so that regular communication and information between different systems regarding the issues of FCSO can be established.

Furthermore, we find it important that FCSO are also recognized by the general public, making public outreach necessary. Where great campaigns and activities for public outreach are difficult to implement, we suggest rather simple ways to contribute to public awareness of FCSO. Media reports can be considered to have an impact on social discourses [81] and to play a crucial role in the way society perceives and responds to women who sexually abuse children and therefore undermine traditional gender stereotypes [55]. Professionals in the health care system are sometimes being consulted as experts for child sexual abuse, child sexual offenders, or any other related topic for newspaper articles or television reports. In these situations, we believe in the professional's responsibility to address child sexual abuse by women as an existing problem which can be just as harmful for the victims as child sexual abuse by men can be. In time, the topic may affect and receive more attention in broader circles of the general public and be discussed beyond the professional fields.

4.2. Implications for Researchers

FCSO are usually only investigated when they are registered in the judicial system (i.e., when they were reported to the police by victims or others). As described earlier, women who sexually offended against children remain undetected very often due to several reasons [70]. We therefore encourage researchers to attempt additional and more active approaches to recruit FCSO for their examinations. For instance, as research results indicate that FCSO are young women between mid-twenties and mid-thirties, online surveys may be an appropriate tool to investigate this population. Online surveys are a highly economic way to reach out for participants who are inhibited due to several barriers such as women who sexually abuse children and furthermore provide a high level of identity protection. Both of which should be helpful when trying to recruit FCSO. Additionally, online surveys are highly suitable to reach women who are at risk to sexually abuse children but did not yet offend against a child. Besides, researchers already investigated female sexual offenders on the internet concluding that they use the internet to connect with like-minded women [82,83].

When creating the survey, we recommend simple language due to the relatively low socioeconomic status of FCSO [5]. As many FCSO reported on being abused in their childhood [41] and having mental health problems, such as depression [84] and alcohol abuse [45], researchers are advised to distribute their study link in internet forums and self-help groups on the internet for victims of child abuse, depressive patients and alcohol abusers.

Additionally, we suggest that researchers should not only include FCSO in their online surveys but also those women who are solely at risk to offend against children and did not yet offend against children. Differentiation between women who have a sexual interest in children can be made, e.g., those who have a pedophilic interest as motive vs. those who have other motives for offending against children or those who are willing to be in treatment vs. those who do not want to be in treatment. These differentiations may lead to different subgroups with varying characteristics implying different research questions and assumptions. This would be in alignment with research on men who are sexually interested in children [85–87].

Finally, if the conditions regarding institutional capacity and financial management are met, qualitative interviews with FCSO or those women who are at risk to sexually offend against children would be valuable to ascertain more details of FCSO' characteristics, their offence behavior, and their specific underlying mechanisms of denial and minimization.

5. Conclusions

General public and professionals both reinforce and maintain traditional gender stereotypes which appear to be barriers to the detection of FCSO [80]. The "culture of denial" surrounding women who are sexually offensive [67] conceals their acts as "silent crimes" [88]. It is likely that the diverting prevalence rates based on different sources (official reports vs. victimization surveys) are related to this biased perception and inappropriate handling of FCSO. As a result, FCSO are underreported and difficult to study which leads to insufficient scientific knowledge. The lack of research data on FSCOs lowers the quality of child protection and treatment services. The fact that even professionals in the judicial and health system appear to be part of this collective repression clearly demonstrates that there is a particular responsibility for researchers and clinicians in the field of sexual health to be aware of their own underlying mechanisms and inner processes of denial. It is important to pursue an active approach towards FCSO. Overcoming the social taboo of FCSO is obligatory, especially in the light of the harsh consequences for victims of FCSO [89]. Moving beyond traditional gender stereotypes seems to be necessary to get over the confusion that women considered so far as caregivers, guardians, and defenders (cf. Reference [90]) are able to be just as sexually abusive to children as men.

Author Contributions: Conceptualization, S.T., P.B., A.D.; Methodology, S.T., P.B., A.D.; Software, not applicable; Validation, S.T., P.B., A.D.; Formal Analysis, not applicable; Investigation, S.T.; Resources, P.B., A.D.; Data Curation, not applicable; Writing-Original Draft Preparation, S.T.; Writing-Review & Editing, S.T., P.B., A.D.; Visualization, S.T.; Supervision, P.B.; Project Administration, P.B.; Funding Acquisition, P.B., A.D.

Funding: Research is funded by the German Federal Ministry of Education and Research (Bundesministerium für Bildung und Forschung, BMBF, 01SR1602).

Conflicts of Interest: The authors declare no conflict of interest.

References

1. Stathopoulos, M. *The Exception that Proves the Rule: Female Sex Offending and the Gendered Nature of Sexual Violence*. ACSSA Research Summary, 5th ed.; Australian Institute of Family Studies: Melbourne, Australia, 2014.
2. Cortoni, F.; Hanson, R.K.; Coache, M.E. The recidivism rates of female sexual offenders are low: A meta-analysis. *Sex Abuse* **2010**, *22*, 387–401. [CrossRef]
3. Faller, K.C. A clinical sample of women who have sexually abused children. *J. Child Sexual Abuse* **1995**, *4*, 13–30. [CrossRef]
4. Finkelhor, D.; Hotaling, G.; Lewis, I.A.; Smith, C. Sexual abuse in a national survey of adult men and women-Prevalence, characteristics, and risk-factors. *Child Abuse Neglect.* **1990**, *14*, 19–28. [CrossRef]
5. Gannon, T.A.; Rose, M.R. Female child sexual offenders: Towards integrating theory and practice. *Aggress. Violent Behav.* **2008**, *13*, 442–461. [CrossRef]
6. Peter, T. Exploring taboos comparing male- and female-perpetrated child sexual abuse. *J. Interpers. Violence* **2009**, *24*, 1111–1128. [CrossRef] [PubMed]
7. Becker, J.V.; Hall, S.R.; Stinson, J.D. Female sexual offenders: Clinical, legal and policy issues. *J. Forensic Psychol. P.* **2001**, *1*, 29–50. [CrossRef]
8. Clements, H.; Dawson, D.L.; das Nair, R. Female perpetrated sexual abuse: a review of victim and professional perspectives. *J. Sex. Aggress.* **2014**, *20*, 197–215. [CrossRef]
9. Cortoni, F.; Babchishin, K.M.; Rat, C. The proportion of sexual offenders who are female is higher than thought: A meta-analysis. *Crim. Justice Behav.* **2017**, *44*, 145–162. [CrossRef]
10. Grayston, A.D.; De Luca, R.V. Female perpetrators of child sexual abuse: A review of the clinical and empirical literature. *Aggress. Violent Behav.* **1999**, *4*, 93–106. [CrossRef]
11. Johansson-Love, J.; Fremouw, W. A critique of the female sexual perpetrator research. *Aggress. Violent Behav.* **2006**, *11*, 12–26. [CrossRef]
12. Nathan, P.; Ward, T. Females who sexually abuse children: Assessment and treatment issues. *Psychiatr. Psychol. Law* **2001**, *8*, 44–45. [CrossRef]

13. Tsopelas, C.; Spyridoula, T.; Athanasios, D. Review on female sexual offenders: Findings about profile and personality. *Int. J. Law Psychiatry* **2011**, *34*, 122–126. [CrossRef] [PubMed]
14. Wakefield, H.; Underwager, R. Female child sexual abusers: A critical review of the literature. *Am. J. Forensic Psychol.* **1991**, *9*, 45–69.
15. Bourke, A.; Doherty, S.; McBride, O.; Morgan, K.; McGee, H. Female perpetrators of child sexual abuse: characteristics of the offender and victim. *Psychol. Crime Law* **2014**, *20*, 769–780. [CrossRef]
16. Vandiver, D.M.; Walker, J.T. Female sex offenders: An overview and analysis of 40 cases. *Crim. Justice Rev.* **2002**, *27*, 284–300. [CrossRef]
17. Dreßing, H.; Dölling, D.; Hermann, D.; Kruse, A.; Schmitt, E.; Bannenberg, B.; Salize, H.J. Sexueller Missbrauch von Kindern [Child sexual abuse]. *PSYCH up2date* **2018**, *12*, 79–94.
18. Hayes, S.; Baker, B. Female Sex Offenders and Pariah Femininities: Rewriting the Sexual Scripts. *J. Criminol.* **2014**, *1*, 1–8. [CrossRef]
19. Kramer, S.; Bowman, B. Accounting for the "invisibility" of the female paedophile: An expert-based perspective from South Africa. *Psychol. Sexualit.* **2011**, *2*, 244–258. [CrossRef]
20. Mellor, D.; Deering, R. Professional response and attitudes toward female-perpetrated child sexual abuse: A study of psychologists, psychiatrists, probationary psychologists and child protection workers. *Psychol. Crime Law* **2010**, *16*, 415–438. [CrossRef]
21. Richards, K. Misperceptions about child sexual offenders. *Trends Issues Crime Crim. Justice* **2011**, *429*, 1–8.
22. Savage, L. Female offenders in Canada, 2017. *Juristat* **2019**, *1*, 1–20.
23. Snyder, H.N. *Sexual Assault of Young Children as Reported to Law Enforcement: Victim, Incident, and Offender Characteristics*; DIANE Publishing: Washington, DC, USA, 2000.
24. German Federal Statistical Office. *Lange reihen zur Strafverfolgungsstatistik–II.2 Verurteilte nach ausgewählten Straftaten, Geschlecht und Altersgruppen (Deutschland) [Criminal prosecution statistics–II.2 convicts among offences, sex, and age groups (Germany)]*.; Statistisches Bundesamt: Wiesbaden, Germany, 2016.
25. Boroughs, D. Female sexual abusers of children. *Child. Youth Serv. Rev* **2004**, *26*, 481–487. [CrossRef]
26. McLeod, D.A.; Craft, M.L. Female sexual offenders in child sexual abuse cases: National trends associated with child protective services systems entry, exit, utilization, and socioeconomics. *J. Publ. Child Welfare* **2015**, *9*, 399–416. [CrossRef]
27. NSPCC. ChildLine Case Notes. 2009. Children Talking to ChildLine About Sexual Abuse. Available online: https://www.scribd.com/document/39443061/Childline-Child-Abuse-Report# (accessed on 20 March 2019).
28. Roberts, S.M. Experiencing Sexual Victimisation in Childhood: Meaning and Impact—The Perspectives of Child Sexual Abusers. Ph.D. Thesis, Swansea University, Swansea, UK, 2017.
29. Dube, S.R.; Anda, R.F.; Whitfield, C.L.; Brown, D.W.; Felitti, V.J.; Dong, M.; Giles, W.H. Long-term consequences of childhood sexual abuse by gender of victim. *Am. J. Prev. Med.* **2005**, *28*, 430–438. [CrossRef]
30. NSPCC. ChildLine Case Notes. 2009. What Boys Talk About to ChildLine. Available online: http://assets.mesmac.co.uk/images/what-boys-talk-about-to-childline.pdf?mtime=20151109131208 (accessed on 20 March 2019).
31. Stadler, L.; Bieneck, S.; Pfeiffer, C. *Forschungsbericht Nr. 118. Repräsentativbefragung sexueller Missbrauch 2011*; Kriminologisches Forschungsinstitut Niedersachsen e.V: Hannover, Germany, 2012.
32. Fromuth, M.; Burkhart, B. Long-term psychological correlates of childhood sexual abuse in two samples of college men. *Child Abuse Negl.* **1989**, *13*, 533–542. [CrossRef]
33. Miccio-Fonseca, L.C. Adult and adolescent female sex offenders: Experiences compared to other female and male sex offenders. *J. Psychol. Hum. Sex.* **2000**, *11*, 75–88. [CrossRef]
34. Sandler, J.C.; Freeman, N.J. Typology of female sex offenders: A test of Vandiver and Kercher. *Sex. Abuse* **2007**, *19*, 73–89. [CrossRef]
35. Vandiver, D.M.; Kercher, G. Offender and victim characteristics of registered female sexual offenders in Texas: A proposed typology of female sexual offenders. *Sex. Abuse* **2004**, *16*, 121–137. [CrossRef]
36. Faller, K.C. Women who sexually abuse children. *Violence Vict.* **1987**, *2*, 263–276. [CrossRef]
37. Nathan, P.; Ward, T. Female sex offenders: Clinical and demographic features. *J. Sex. Aggress.* **2002**, *8*, 5–21. [CrossRef]
38. Lewis, C.F.; Stanley, C.R. Women accused of sexual offenses. *Behav. Sci. Law* **2000**, *18*, 73–81. [CrossRef]

39. Matravers, A. Understanding women sex offenders. In *Criminology in Cambridge: Newsletter of the Institute of Criminology*; Institute of Criminology: Cambridge, UK, 2005; pp. 10–13.
40. Tardif, M.; Auclair, N.; Jacob, M.; Carpentier, J. Sexual abuse perpetrated by adult and juvenile females: An ultimate attempt to resolve a conflict associated with maternal identity. *Child. Abuse Neglect* **2005**, *29*, 153–167. [CrossRef]
41. Berner, W.; Briken, P.; Hill, A. Female Sexual Offenders. In *Sex Offenders—Identification, Risk Assessment, Treatment, and Legal Issues*; Saleh, F.M., Grudzinskas, A.J., Bradford, J.M., Brodsky, D.J., Eds.; Oxford University Press: Oxford, UK, 2009.
42. Fromuth, M.E.; Conn, V.E. Hidden perpetrators: Sexual molestation in a nonclinical sample of college women. *J. Interpers. Violence* **1997**, *12*, 456–465. [CrossRef]
43. Green, A.H.; Kaplan, M.S. Psychiatric impairment and childhood victimization experiences in female child molesters. *J. Am. Acad. Child Adolesc. Psychiatry* **1994**, *33*, 954–961. [CrossRef]
44. McCarty, L.M. Mother–child incest: Characteristics of the offender. *Child Welfare* **1986**, *65*, 447–458.
45. Center for Sex Offender Management; U.S. Department of Justice. Female Sex Offenders. 2007. Available online: http://www.csom.org/pubs/female_sex_offenders_brief.pdf (accessed on 20 March 2019).
46. Hunter, J.A.; Mathews, R. Sexual deviance in females. In *Sexual Deviance: Theory, Assessment, and Treatment*; Laws, D.R., O'Donohue, W.T., Eds.; Guilford Press: New York, NY, USA, 1997; pp. 465–480.
47. Matthews, J.K. Working with female sexual abusers. In *Female Sexual Abuse of Children*; Elliott, M., Ed.; Guilford Press: New York, NY, USA, 1993; pp. 57–73.
48. Miller, L. Sexual offenses against children: Patterns and motives. *Aggress. Violent Behav.* **2013**, *18*, 506–519. [CrossRef]
49. Hunter, J.A.; Lexier, L.J.; Goodwin, D.W.; Browne, P.A.; Dennis, C. Psychosexual, attitudinal, and developmental characteristics of juvenile female perpetrators in a residential treatment setting. *J. Child Fam. Stud.* **1993**, *2*, 317–326. [CrossRef]
50. Kercher, G.; McShane, M. The prevalence of child sexual abuse victimization in an adult sample of Texas residents. *Child Abuse Neglect* **1984**, *8*, 495–502. [CrossRef]
51. Briggs, F.; Hawkins, R. Protecting boys from the risk of sexual abuse. *Early Child Dev. Care* **1995**, *110*, 19–32. [CrossRef]
52. Ogilvie, B.; Daniluk, J. Common themes in the experiences of mother–daughter incest survivors: Implications for counseling. *J. Couns. Dev.* **1995**, *73*, 598–602. [CrossRef]
53. Bender, L.; Blau, A. The reaction of children to sexual relations with adults. *Am. J. Orthopsychiatry* **1937**, *7*, 500–518. [CrossRef]
54. Jennings, K. Female child molesters: A review of literature. In *Female Sexual Abuse of Children*; Elliott, M., Ed.; Guilford Press: New York, NY, USA, 1994; pp. 219–234.
55. Berrington, E.; Honkatukia, P. An evil monster and a poor thing: Female violence in the media. *J. Scand. Stud. Criminol. Crime. Prev.* **2002**, *3*, 50–72. [CrossRef]
56. Landor, R.; Eisenchlas, S. "Coming clean" on duty of care: Australian print media's representation of male versus female sex offenders in institutional contexts. *Sex. Cult.* **2012**, *16*, 486–502. [CrossRef]
57. Mackelprang, E.; Becker, J.V. Beauty and the eye of the beholder: Gender and attractiveness affect judgements in teacher sex offense cases. *Sex. Abuse* **2017**, *29*, 375–395. [CrossRef]
58. Bunting, L. Dealing with a problem that doesn't exist? Professional responses to female perpetrated child sexual abuse. *Child Abuse Rev.* **2007**, *16*, 252–267. [CrossRef]
59. Deering, R.; Mellor, D. Sentencing of male and female sex offenders: Australian study. *Psychiatr. Psychol. Law* **2009**, *16*, 394–412. [CrossRef]
60. Hislop, J. *Female Sex Offenders: What Therapists, Law Enforcement and Child Protective Services Need to Know*; Issues Pres: Ravensdale, Ireland, 2001.
61. Mayer, A. *Women Sex Offenders: Treatment and Dynamics*; Learning Publications Inc.: Holmes Beach, FL, USA, 1992.
62. Saradjian, J. *Women Who Sexually Abuse Children: From Research to Clinical Practice*; Wiley: Chichester, UK, 1996.
63. Wilkins, R. Women who sexually abuse children: Doctors need to become sensitised to the possibility. *BMJ* **1990**, *300*, 1153–1159. [CrossRef]
64. Freel, M. *Women Who Sexually Abuse Children*; Social Work Monograph: Norwich, UK, 1995.

65. Haliburn, J. Mother-child incest, psychosis, and the dynamics of relatedness. *J. Trauma Dissociation* **2017**, *18*, 409–426. [CrossRef] [PubMed]
66. Hayes, S. *Sex, Love and Abuse: Discourses of Domestic Violence and Sexual Assault*; Palgrave Macmillan: Bassingstoke, UK, 2014.
67. Denov, M.S. *Perspectives on Female Sex Offending: A Culture of Denial*; Ashgate: Aldershot, UK, 2004.
68. Elliott, M. *Female Sexual Abuse of Children–The Ultimate Taboo*; Longman: Harlow, UK, 1993.
69. Goldhill, R. What was she thinking? Women who sexually offend against children–implications for probation practice. *Probat. J.* **2013**, *60*, 415–424. [CrossRef]
70. Davidson, J. *Child Sexual Abuse: Media Representations and Government Reactions*; Routledge-Cavendish: Abingdon, UK, 2008.
71. Bunting, L. *Females Who Sexually Offend Against Children: Responses of the Child Protection and Criminal Justice Systems*; Executive summary; NSPCC: London, UK, 2005.
72. Peter, T. Mad, bad, or victim? Making sense of mother-daughter sexual abuse. *Fem. Criminol.* **2006**, *1*, 283–302. [CrossRef]
73. Courtois, C.A. *Healing the Incest Wound: Adult Survivors in Therapy*, 2nd ed.; Norton: New York, NY, USA, 2010.
74. Jenkins, P. *Moral Panic: Changing Concepts of the Child Molester in Modern America*; Yale University Press: New Haven, CT, USA, 1998.
75. Amendt, G. *Wie Mütter ihre Söhne sehen*; Ikaru: Bremen, Germany, 1993.
76. Gavin, H. "Mummy wouldn't do that": The perception and construction of the female child sex abuse. In *Grotesque feminities: Evil, women and the feminine*; Barrett, M., Porter, T., Eds.; The Inter-Disciplinary Press: Oxford, UK, 2006.
77. Heyne, C. *Täterinnen-Offene und versteckte Aggression von Frauen [Female Offenders—Women's Visible and Hidden Aggressions]*; Kreuz-Verlag: Zurich, Switzerland, 1993.
78. Robinson, S. From victim to offender: Female offenders of child sexual abuse. *Eur. J. Crim. Pol. Res.* **1998**, *6*, 59–73. [CrossRef]
79. Cortoni, F.; Gannon, T.A. Understanding female sexual offenders. In *Theories of Sexual Offending*; Ward, T., Beech, A.R., Eds.; Wiley-Blackwell: Chichester, UK, 2017; pp. 453–471.
80. Denov, M.S. The myth of innocence: Sexual scripts and the recognition of child sexual abuse by female perpetrators. *J. Sex Res.* **2003**, *40*, 303–314. [CrossRef]
81. Kuhlmann, C. Journalismus als Moderation gesellschaftlicher Diskurse [Journalism as moderation of social discourses]. In *Handbuch Journalismustheorien [Handbook Theories of Journalism]*; Löffelholz, M., Rothenberger, L., Eds.; Springer: Wiesbaden, Germany, 2016; pp. 403–416.
82. Elliott, I.A.; Ashfield, S. The use of online technology in the modus operandi of female sex offenders. *J. Sex. Aggress.* **2011**, *17*, 92–104. [CrossRef]
83. Lawson, L. Female sex offenders' relationship experiences. *Violence Vict.* **2008**, *23*, 331–343. [CrossRef]
84. Muskens, M.; Bogaerts, S.; Van Casteren, M.; Labrijn, S. Adult female sexual offending: A comparison between co-offenders and solo offenders in a Dutch sample. *J. Sex. Aggress.* **2011**, *17*, 46–60. [CrossRef]
85. Tozdan, S.; Kalt, A.; Dekker, A.; Keller, L.B.; Thiel, S.; Müller, J.L.; Briken, P. Why information matters—A randomized controlled trial on the consequences of suggesting that pedophilia is immutable. *Int. J. Offender Ther. Comp. Criminol.* **2016**, *62*, 1241–1261. [CrossRef]
86. Tozdan, S.; Briken, P. The earlier, the worse? Age of onset of sexual interest in children. *J. Sex. Med.* **2015**, *12*, 1602–1608. [CrossRef]
87. Tozdan, S.; Jakob, C.; Schuhmann, P.; Budde, M.; Briken, P. Spezifische Selbstwirksamkeit zur Beeinflussung des sexuellen Interesses an Kindern (SSIK): Konstruktion und Validierung eines Messinstruments [Specific self-efficacy for modifying sexual interest in children (SSIC): Construction and validation of a measuring instrument]. *Psychother. Psychosom. Med. Psychol.* **2015**, *65*, 345–352.
88. Eastwood, C. The experiences of child complainants of sexual abuse in the criminal justice system. *Trends Issues Crime Crim. Justice* **2003**, *250*, 1–6.

89. Denov, M.S. The Long-Term Effects of Child Sexual Abuse by Female Perpetrators: A Qualitative Study of Male and Female Victims. *J. Interpers. Violence* **2004**, *19*, 1137–1156. [CrossRef]
90. Schippers, M. Recovering the feminine other: Masculinity, femininity, and gender hegemony. *Theory Soc.* **2007**, *36*, 85–102. [CrossRef]

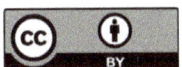

© 2019 by the authors. Licensee MDPI, Basel, Switzerland. This article is an open access article distributed under the terms and conditions of the Creative Commons Attribution (CC BY) license (http://creativecommons.org/licenses/by/4.0/).

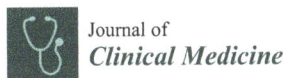

Review

Serotonergic, Dopaminergic, and Noradrenergic Modulation of Erotic Stimulus Processing in the Male Human Brain

Heiko Graf [1,*], Kathrin Malejko [1], Coraline Danielle Metzger [2,3,4], Martin Walter [5,6], Georg Grön [1] and Birgit Abler [1]

1. Department of Psychiatry and Psychotherapy III, Ulm University, 89075 Ulm, Germany; kathrin.malejko@uni-ulm.de (K.M.); georg.groen@uni-ulm.de (G.G.); birgit.abler@uni-ulm.de (B.A.)
2. Department of Psychiatry, Otto von Guericke University, 39120 Magdeburg, Germany; coraline.metzger@med.ovgu.de
3. Institute of Cognitive Neurology and Dementia Research (IKND), Otto von Guericke University, 39106 Magdeburg, Germany
4. German Center for Neurodegenerative Diseases (DZNE), 39120 Magdeburg, Germany
5. Department of Psychiatry, Eberhard Karls University, 72074 Tuebingen, Germany; martin.walter@uni-tuebingen.de
6. Leibniz Institute for Neurobiology, 39120 Magdeburg, Germany
* Correspondence: heiko.graf@uni-ulm.de; Tel.: +49-731-500-61401; Fax: +49-731-500-61402

Received: 8 February 2019; Accepted: 12 March 2019; Published: 14 March 2019

Abstract: Human sexual behavior is mediated by a complex interplay of cerebral and spinal centers, as well as hormonal, peripheral, and autonomic functions. Neuroimaging studies identified central neural signatures of human sexual responses comprising neural emotional, motivational, autonomic, and cognitive components. However, empirical evidence regarding the neuromodulation of these neural signatures of human sexual responses was scarce for decades. Pharmacological functional magnetic resonance imaging (fMRI) provides a valuable tool to examine the interaction between neuromodulator systems and functional network anatomy relevant for human sexual behavior. In addition, this approach enables the examination of potential neural mechanisms regarding treatment-related sexual dysfunction under psychopharmacological agents. In this article, we introduce common neurobiological concepts regarding cerebral sexual responses based on neuroimaging findings and we discuss challenges and findings regarding investigating the neuromodulation of neural sexual stimulus processing. In particular, we summarize findings from our research program investigating how neural correlates of sexual stimulus processing are modulated by serotonergic, dopaminergic, and noradrenergic antidepressant medication in healthy males.

Keywords: erotic stimulus processing; serotonin; noradrenaline; dopamine; fMRI; healthy; human

1. Introduction

Human sexual behavior is mediated by the integration of endocrine, vascular, peripheral, and central nervous mechanisms. The brain is considered as the "master organ" of sexual functioning [1] and is involved in all successive steps of human sexual behavior [2]. Electrophysiological and behavioral studies provided considerable insights into human sexual function, but underlying neural substrates were largely unknown until functional neuroimaging methods were widely introduced into neuroscientific research. Since then, the basic principles of neural processing of sexual stimulation were described in several studies [2–4]. However, empirical evidence regarding the effects of neuromodulators on these neural mediators was scarce.

Pharmacological functional magnetic resonance imaging (pharmaco-fMRI) provides a valuable tool to examine modulatory effects of different neurotransmitter systems on neural signatures of sexual function. Apart from clarifying these basic principles and the complex interaction between neuromodulators and functional network anatomy of sexual behavior, investigations with pharmaco-fMRI also have the potential to elucidate the neural correlates of treatment-related sexual dysfunction.

Various psychiatric disorders are commonly accompanied by sexual dysfunction, and have an immediate impact on subjective well-being and quality of life [5,6]. Of note, sexual dysfunction also occurs as a frequent side effect of psychopharmacological treatment and considerably compromises adherence to therapy. Clinical observational studies suggest that about 40% of patients with psychopharmacological antidepressant treatment discontinue their medication due to treatment-related sexual dysfunction [7]. Thus, the crucial implication of sexual dysfunction as a disease- and treatment-related symptom motivated the investigation of the underlying neural mechanisms.

In this review, we introduce common concepts of sexual behavior and evidence regarding neural substrates of sexual responses. We shortly discuss the challenges investigating the neuromodulation of neural sexual stimulus processing by pharmaco-fMRI. In particular, we summarize our research program that focused on how these neural correlates were modulated by serotonergic, dopaminergic, and noradrenergic antidepressant medication in healthy male subjects.

2. Conceptualizing Sexual Behavior and Neural Responses

Despite its debut already in the 1960s, the most commonly used model to conceptualize sexual activity is still the sexual response cycle by Masters and Johnson [8]. The term "sexual response" denotes the set of behaviors and functions related to sexual stimulation and the pursuit of a sexual goal. Based on their observations, Masters and Johnson [8] defined four different phases of sexual responses that refer to the sequence of physical and emotional changes during sexual arousal and activity. They distinguished a period of sexual desire and arousal, followed by a plateau, culminating in orgasm and ending in a refraction period. Kaplan proposed a slightly modified triphasic model comprising sexual desire, excitement, and orgasm [9]. However, these models were criticized for the linear sequence of the phases that may, for example, not be entirely transferable to female sexual responses.

Neuroimaging techniques such as positron emission tomography (PET) or functional magnetic resonance imaging (fMRI) made valuable contributions to identify underlying neural correlates of sexual responses. As outlined and summarized by Reference [10], the behavioral and neurofunctional principles underlying the sexual response cycle largely overlap with those related to other primary rewards such as food [10]. Analogous to concepts related to other rewards, Georgiadis and Kringelbach [10] suggested that sexual responses may be characterized by terms of motivation–consummation–satiety or wanting–liking–inhibition. Linking psychological with physiological and neurofunctional processes in more detail, a meta-analysis of functional imaging studies on sexual arousal conceptualized the neurophenomenological model of sexual arousal [2]. The model suggests a cognitive component, comprising the appraisal of and the attention to a subsequent sexual stimulus, which is represented by neural reactivity within the orbitofrontal cortex (OFC), the inferior temporal cortices, the inferior and superior parietal lobules, premotor and supplementary motor areas, and within the cerebellum. An emotional component representing sexual pleasure and hedonic qualities of sexual arousal as a primary reward is suggested to be mediated by neural activations of the amygdala, the insula, and primary and secondary somatosensory cortices. Neural processes comprising goal-directed behavior and the perceived urge to express overt sexual behavior are represented by activations within the anterior cingulate cortex (ACC), the claustrum, the posterior parietal cortex, the hypothalamus, the substantia nigra, and the ventral striatum. The autonomic/neuroendocrine component is thought to be mediated by activations within the ACC, the anterior insula, the putamen, and hypothalamus, and is supposed to lead subjects to a state of physiological readiness for sexual behavior [2,3,11].

A more recent meta-analysis [12] distinguished brain networks underlying psychosexual and physiosexual arousal. Hereby, the psychosexual network was suggested to include the lateral prefrontal cortex and the hippocampus (cognitive and memory-guided evaluations), the occipitotemporal cortex, superior parietal lobules (sensory processing), the amygdala and the thalamus (relevance detection and affective evaluation), the hypothalamus (autonomic responses), basal ganglia (sexual urge), and the anterior insula (awareness of sexual arousal). Physiosexual processes were conceptualized within a network comprising the subgenual anterior cingulate cortex (sgACC; autonomic and corresponding emotion regulation), the anterior midcingulate cortex (aMCC; initiation of copulatory behavior), the putamen and claustrum (sexual urge), the anterior insula (awareness of rising sexual desire and engendered bodily reactions), the insular cortex (somatosensory information), and the operculum (monitoring bodily changes during sexual arousal). Of note, the putamen and the claustrum were identified as brain regions that connect both psychosexual und physiosexual networks, with potentially dissociable functions. While the putamen is thought to orchestrate the integration of sensorimotor information in the context of sexual desire, the putamen might be responsible for cross-modal processing between and within the networks of sexual arousal.

Most of these studies summarized neural sexual responses that were investigated using visual stimuli. However, slightly divergent patterns of brain activations were reported due to different stimulus content (e.g., sexual intensity), presentation mode (visual static images versus dynamic video sequences), or design type (block versus event-related design) [13]. While sexual motivation and wanting is reliably induced by visual sexual stimulation, genital stimulation is usually required to enter the consummatory plateau [4] of the sexual response cycle. Indeed, the use of other types of stimulus material (e.g., haptic or acoustic) is limited by the circumstances of neuroimaging methods, like noise and motion sensitivity. A few studies simultaneously recorded fMRI blood oxygenation level dependent (BOLD) signals elicited by visual stimuli and the corresponding time course of penile tumescence to investigate neural substrates of orgasm and erection. Neural activations within the ACC, the insula, amygdala, hypothalamus, and secondary somatosensory cortices were considered to be associated with penile erection [14,15]. Neural activations in mid-anterior and medial subregions of the OFC were suggested to relate specifically to orgasm [16]. Only few neuroimaging studies investigated sexual inhibition/refraction; however, these were mainly in subjects with low sexual desire. These studies indicate that sexual inhibition is mediated by prefrontal hyperactivity [17,18]. Accordingly, volitional inhibition of sexual arousal in healthy subjects was indeed accompanied by increased activations within the superior parietal, the ventrolateral prefrontal [19], and the inferior frontal cortex [20]. Moreover, it was suggested that both intended and unintended sexual inhibition are related to an exaggerated activity within the neural network of sexual interest that may, however, prevent a shift to the neural sexual consummation network [4]. Investigating neural responses a few minutes after ejaculation, one fMRI study linked activation of the amygdala, the temporal lobes, and the septal area specifically to sexual satiety [21].

3. Neuromodulation of Sexual Responses

Despite these valuable insights arising from neuroimaging studies into potentially underlying neural correlates of sexual responses, modulatory effects of neurotransmitter systems or monoaminergic drugs like antidepressants on these neural substrates are largely unknown. Most of the evidence regarding the neuromodulation of sexual functions stems from animal studies (e.g., References [22,23]) or clinical observations in patients during the treatment with psychoactive drugs (e.g., References [7,24–26]). Understanding the underlying mechanisms is indeed of great relevance considering the high prevalence of psychopharmacologically related sexual dysfunction, quite likely arising from central nervous rather than peripheral mechanisms [27].

Apart from sexual hormones and neuropeptides, central monoamines and catecholamines that are commonly modulated by psychopharmacological agents exert a pivotal role in the neuromodulation of sexual behavior. Here, we concentrate on dopamine, serotonin, and noradrenaline as the most commonly altered neuromodulator systems in psychopharmacotherapy. While an elevated central dopaminergic neurotransmission was observed to be accompanied by increased sexual interest, serotonergic agents are associated with an opposite pattern of behavior [27–29]. Considering the overlap of behavioral and neurofunctional principles of sexual functioning with other primary rewards [10], the favorable effects of dopamine on sexual behavior seem plausible. Accordingly, the antidepressant and selective noradrenaline and dopamine reuptake inhibitor (SSNDRI) bupropion is associated with subjectively improved sexual functioning, such as the ability to achieve and maintain an erection and orgasm, along with increased sexual satisfaction [30]. Moreover, dopamine-agonist treatment in Parkinson's disease is frequently accompanied by the clinical observation of hypersexuality [31]. In contrast, up to 70% of patients with schizophrenia report sexual dysfunction under treatment with antidopaminergic antipsychotics like haloperidol [32]. Apart from hyperprolactinemia due to dopamine D_2-receptor blockage in the tuberoinfundibular pathway [33], the inhibitory effects of dopamine antagonists on the mesolimbic/mesocortical reward system are considered as a crucial mechanism underlying antipsychotic related sexual dysfunction [34].

The considerable impact of the neuromodulator serotonin in mediating sexual activity was recognized by the rising prevalence of sexual dysfunction during antidepressant medication, in particular with selective serotonin reuptake inhibitors (SSRIs) [35]. Although the stimulation of some specific serotonin receptor subtypes, e.g., $5-HT_{2c}$- or $5-HT_{1A}$-receptors, may facilitate erection or ejaculation, primary central serotonergic effects are thought to be inhibitory. These effects are presumably mediated via decreased dopamine release in mesolimbic regions [28,36] and by suppressing spinal ejaculatory centers [37]. Accordingly, up to 80% of patients treated with the SSRI sertraline report sexual dysfunction and, in particular in young patients, antidepressant-related decrease in sexual function is one of the most relevant side effects [24,38]. Apart from the immediate negative impact on the quality of life [39,40], antidepressant-related sexual dysfunction is also one of the major reasons that lead to non-adherence to treatment [41], especially after remission of depressive symptoms. Since early discontinuation compared to the recommended maintenance therapy over several months is related to increased rates of relapse [42], the side effect compromises the overall success of antidepressant treatment.

Compared to serotonin, the contribution of the neuromodulator noradrenaline in mediating sexual responses is less well understood. Clinical observations assume a favorable effect of selective noradrenaline reuptake inhibitors (SNRIs) on sexual functions compared to SSRIs based on lower rates of sexual dysfunction under SNRIs [24,43,44]. In line with this, actual sexual activity is related with an increase in plasma noradrenaline levels during orgasm with a subsequent rapid decline [45]. However, the limited available data regarding the effects of SNRIs on sexual functioning compromise definite conclusions [24].

4. Challenges

The conclusions regarding the effects of monoaminergic psychopharmaceuticals on sexual functions are mainly based on clinical observations and may be confounded by the disease itself. Most studies did not assess baseline sexual function before the initiation of medication. However, up to 75% of patients with major depression report sexual dysfunction prior to antidepressant treatment, in particular decreased sexual interest [46,47]. Thus, the mechanisms related to sexual dysfunction under monoaminergic agents have also to be investigated in healthy subjects to exclude confounds by the disease itself. Moreover, to meet clinical conditions as much as possible, but also to reach steady-state conditions, multi-dose trials over several days rather than single-dose applications are required to investigate neural correlates of sexual responses under antidepressants. Another limitation often arises from the study design, especially when two agents are compared with each other or relative to placebo in two different study groups. These study designs limit the capability to differentiate effects of group from those of medication, even when randomization was applied to minimize between-group effects. Also, between-group designs usually require larger sample sizes to reduce putative and systematic effects of group. Thus, apart from placebo-controlled investigations in healthy subjects under subchronic administration of study medication, repeated measures within one group (within-subject and cross-over) may represent the most desirable study design to investigate psychopharmacological effects on neural responses of sexual behavior.

5. Serotonergic, Dopaminergic, and Noradrenergic Neuromodulation of Sexual Responses

One of the first studies investigating sexual dysfunction under monoaminergic agents and underlying neural correlates was conducted in 2009 [48] in male patients with major depression. Neural activations under visual erotic stimulation in nine patients taking SSRIs (six took paroxetine and three fluoxetine) and in 10 patients taking mirtazapine, which blocks central adrenergic and serotonin receptors, were compared to 10 healthy controls. This study demonstrated decreased neural activation within the ACC, the OFC, the insula, and the caudate nucleus in the SSRI-group compared to controls. These brain regions with attenuated responses were related to attentional and motivational components of the sexual response cycle. Neural activations in the group treated with mirtazapine were relatively lower than in controls but still elevated compared to those treated with SSRIs. Sexual dysfunction as assessed by questionnaires was significantly more frequent in depressed patients compared to controls, but did not differ between the two treatment groups. This study provided first evidence for the potential underlying neural correlates of sexual dysfunction in depression while under antidepressant treatment. However, the study design was not in the position to distinguish effects of disease from treatment-related effects on sexual functions.

We, therefore, investigated a sample of 18 healthy heterosexual males using fMRI and a randomized placebo-controlled within-subject cross-over study design. Participants were investigated after subchronic administration of the SSRI paroxetine, the SSNDRI bupropion, and placebo. Each treatment was applied for seven days separated by a wash-out time of at least 14 days [49]. During fMRI, we used a dynamic visual erotic stimulus paradigm consisting of erotic and non-erotic video clips. Erotic video clips depicted sexual interactions between one man or two women (petting, oral sex, and vaginal intercourse) extracted from commercial adult films. Non-erotic video clips showed men and women in emotionally neutral interactions. Subjective behavioral changes in sexual interest, sexual arousal, the ability to achieve orgasm, the ability to achieve and maintain an erection, and overall sexual satisfaction during drug administration were assessed by the Massachusetts General Hospital Sexual Functioning Questionnaire (MGH-SFQ) [50]. We demonstrated significantly attenuated neural activations within the sgACC, the pgACC, the aMCC, the pMCC, the nucleus accumbens, the midbrain, and the amygdala under the SSRI during visual erotic stimulation. In line with these neural alterations under the SSRI, we found a decrease in subjective sexual functions under paroxetine compared to placebo. In particular, we observed a significant decrease in subjective sexual arousal and the ability to achieve an orgasm under the SSRI compared to placebo.

Neural activations within the anterior but also rather rostral subdivisions of the ACC were previously found to be modulated by SSRIs during emotional aversive stimuli [51]. Within the context of sexual behaviour, neural activations within the ACC are associated with autonomic components of sexual responses [2,3]. Moreover, neural activity within the pgACC is related to the interaction of subjective sexual intensity and its hedonic and emotional value [52]. The results, therefore, suggested an altered neural reactivity within brain regions linked to autonomic and emotional components of sexual responses under SSRIs. In particular, attenuated neural activations within the pMCC under the SSRI were correlated with paroxetine blood-serum levels and with detrimental overall subjective functions under this antidepressant. In addition, by demonstrating attenuated neural activations within the nucleus accumbens under the SSRI, we found evidence for a diminished neural motivational component of sexual responses. This attenuation may relate to the close interaction and opposing effects between dopaminergic and serotonergic systems [53–55]. Increasing levels of serotonin as seen under SSRIs seem to dampen the functioning of the dopaminergic reward system [54,56]. To further examine whether the SSRI-related attenuation of the dopaminergic reward system and, in particular, within the nucleus accumbens might be mediated by other brain regions as observed in secondary rewards [57], we applied a psychophysiological interaction approach [58]. Indeed, we observed a significantly elevated negative reciprocal interaction between the anteroventral prefrontal cortex (avPFC) and the nucleus accumbens under the SSRI that was also associated with impulsivity as a personality trait. Thus, an increase in PFC activation may mediate the dampening effects of SSRIs on the human reward system and associated functions, e.g., sexual satisfaction.

In line with the opposing effects of serotonin and dopamine on reward-related functions and neural activity, we observed slightly enhanced and prolonged neural activations within the pMCC and within subcortical regions such as the midbrain, the amygdala, and the thalamus under the SSNDRI bupropion compared to placebo. Subjective sexual functions were indeed unimpaired under this agent in accordance to clinical studies, suggesting bupropion as a treatment alternative in patients with SSRI-related sexual dysfunction [59]. The dopaminergic agents also reveal favourable effects on sexual functions as compared to SSRIs [59–62]. The elevated neural activation pattern as found in our study and, in particular, within the ventral striatum and the midbrain as dopaminergic reward-related brain regions may represent a neural correlate of increased responsiveness to sexual stimuli arising from the dopaminergic properties of bupropion. Moreover, with concomitant activations within the amygdala that were previously related to perceived sexual arousal and to orgasmic pleasure [63], and neural activations within the thalamus and cortical regions such as the MCC, we observed activations within a neural network referred to as the salience network, which integrates homeostatic autonomic functions, emotion, and reward processing [64] (see Figure 1).

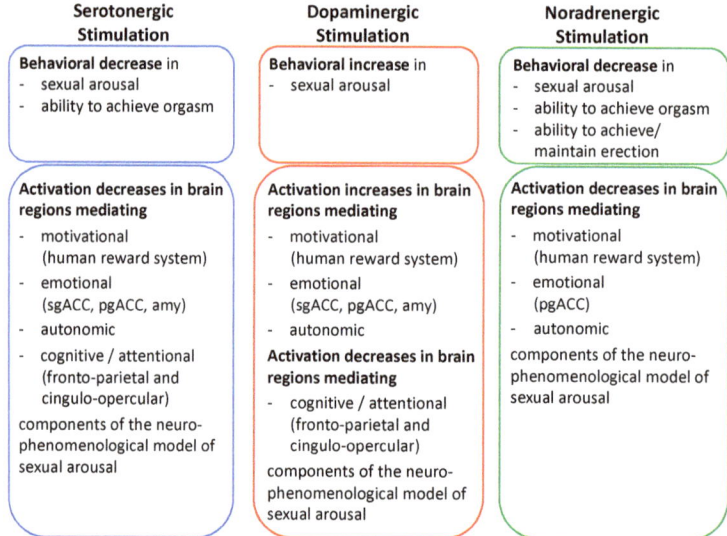

Figure 1. Implications of subchronic steady state serotonergic, noradrenergic, and dopaminergic stimulation on subjective sexual functions and neural responses to erotic stimulation in healthy subjects. For further information on the neurophenomenological model of sexual arousal, see Stoléru et al. [2]. SgACC = subgenual anterior cingulate cortex, pgACC = pregenual anterior cingulate cortex, amy = amygdala.

Apart from these diverging effects of the neuromodulators serotonin and dopamine, a unidirectional neural activation was found under both the SSRI and the SSNDRI within the aMCC and, thus, in a brain region associated with attentional top-down control [65]. However, the video-clip task limited the specific investigation of attentional components of sexual responses. We, therefore, investigated the same sample of 18 healthy male subjects with fMRI under the two antidepressants paroxetine and bupropion compared to placebo. During fMRI, we now used an established visual erotic picture task [52,66] consisting of erotic and non-erotic pictures of positive emotional content taken from the International Affective Picture System (IAPS) [67]. Of note, half of the stimuli of each condition (erotic, non-erotic) were announced. The implementation of these anticipatory periods allowed the reliable investigation of attentional processes [68]. In general, anticipation is regarded as preceding attention to an upcoming predicted stimulus [69,70] and numerous studies showed neural parallels between anticipatory and attentional processes [68,71]. Under both serotonergic and dopaminergic antidepressants, we revealed attenuated neural activations within the fronto-parietal and cingulo-opercular neural network, essential for task initiation and adjustment, as well as for the maintenance of attention [65]. Accordingly, these network alterations were accompanied by unidirectional detrimental effects on the behavioral level under both agents in terms of prolonged reactions in a divided attention task.

Beneficial effects of increasing dopaminergic neurotransmission on attention and prefrontal cortical functions were conceptualized as an inverted u-shaped curve [72], whereby either too low or too high levels of dopamine [73] led to a worsening of prefrontal cortex functioning. Thus, one may argue that an increase in dopaminergic neurotransmission in healthy subjects as induced by the SSNDRI bupropion may have increased the responsivity of the neural attention network beyond the optimum and led to detrimental attentional functioning on a behavioral level. A similar response pattern was shown for increases in noradrenergic neurotransmission and other cognitive functions such as error monitoring [74]. In addition, it is of note that an increase in dopaminergic neurotransmission in prefrontal regions is not only described for bupropion but also for paroxetine via indirect pathways [75,76], supporting our observation regarding similar attention network alterations. In line with this, detrimental sustained attention was also found in other studies under SSRI administration in healthy subjects [77,78].

Apart from the serotonergic and dopaminergic antidepressants, we further investigated neural effects of noradrenergic antidepressants. Within a randomized placebo-controlled within-subject cross-over design, 19 healthy heterosexual male subjects were investigated after subchronic administration of the selective noradrenaline reuptake inhibitor (SNRI) reboxetine and the second-generation antipsychotic amisulpride. During fMRI, we again used the dynamic erotic video-clip task. Noradrenergic agents and, in particular, reboxetine were thought to exert less detrimental effects on sexual functioning compared to serotonergic agents [24,79]. However, this assumption was mainly derived from investigations in depressive patients that demonstrated greater improvement in sexual satisfaction, in the ability to become sexually excited [80], and in achieving orgasm [43] under reboxetine. In contrast to these beneficial effects on sexual functions, we observed a significant decrease in overall subjective sexual function under the noradrenergic agent reboxetine compared to placebo and amisulpride in healthy subjects. In particular sexual arousal, the ability to achieve orgasm and penile erection [81] decreased. These results were, however, in line with other previous clinical reports of prolonged orgasm [82], erectile dysfunction [83], and anorgasmia [43] under this drug. On the neural level, we revealed diminished neural activations within the caudate nucleus under reboxetine compared to placebo that were significantly associated with the decreased sexual interest under this agent. With regard to erotic stimulation, caudate nucleus activation was linked to goal-directed behavior and reward [84]. Whereas ventral parts of the striatum are commonly associated with the expectation and the receipt of incentives, dorsal striatal/caudate nucleus activation was associated with motivational rather than reward processing [85]. Thus, our findings may support the notion that an increase in noradrenergic neurotransmission might have detrimental effects on motivational components of sexual responses along with diminished subjective sexual functioning.

It is of note that we did not find significant neural alterations during visual erotic stimulation and in subjective sexual functions under the antipsychotic drug amisulpride compared to placebo. The antipsychotic drug amisulpride has high and selective affinity to postsynaptic D_2- und D_3-receptors [86–88] and it is known for its capacity to induce sexual dysfunction mainly due to the blockage of dopamine D_2-receptors [33] with secondary increases of prolactin levels [34]. The lack of significant alterations in neural visual erotic stimulus processing along with unchanged subjective sexual functions in our study was most likely due to the low dosage of 200 mg/day amisulpride for seven days. Antipsychotic effects of amisulpride were reported for high dosages from about 400 to 600 mg/day due to reliable D_2-receptor occupancy [86]. In contrast, lower dosages (50 to 200 mg/day) as used in our study are thought to primarily block presynaptic dopamine autoreceptors with the consequence of mild pro-dopaminergic effects [86,89,90] that may have left sexual functions and corresponding neural correlates unimpaired in our sample of healthy male subjects.

To further investigate neural responses to visual erotic stimulus processing including preceding attention and their modulation by noradrenergic agents, we also applied the abovementioned erotic picture paradigm with anticipatory periods [91]. Notably, upon static rather than previously applied dynamic visual erotic stimulation, we observed additional treatment effects of the noradrenergic agent reboxetine compared to placebo during visual erotic stimulation by diminished neural activations not only within the caudate nucleus, but also within the ventral striatum/nucleus accumbens, the pgACC, the aMCC, and the OFC. In addition, decreases in subjective sexual arousal correlated with attenuated neural activations within the posterior insula, a region that is repeatedly associated with sexual arousal and penile response [14,84]. Thus, our results support the notion of detrimental effects of noradrenergic agents on emotional, motivational, and autonomic neural components of sexual responses, along with decreased subjective sexual function (see Figure 1). In addition, they also underpin the implication regarding stimulus presentation mode in investigating neural substrates of erotic stimulus processing considering that treatment effects of noradrenergic agents were found within a broader neural network during static rather than dynamic visual erotic stimulation.

Similar to the investigation by erotic video stimulation, we also found no significant neural alteration under amisulpride compared to placebo. Moreover, in contrast to serotonergic and predominantly dopaminergic antidepressants, neither the noradrenergic agent reboxetine nor the antipsychotic amisulpride led to neural alterations during the anticipation of erotic stimuli, in line with unimpaired attentional functions on a behavioral level in this study. However, it is of note that major nodes of the neural network altered by the noradrenergic agent reboxetine compared to placebo such as the ventral striatum, the pgACC, aMCC, and the OFC highly resemble those brain regions that were also modulated by serotonergic agents upon erotic video stimulation in our previous investigation.

While it remains speculative, one may argue that either monoaminergic modulation ends up via similar neural pathways and presumably also on a molecular level. Interactions of both the serotonergic and noradrenergic system with dopaminergic projections were extensively studied [54,92], and a modulation of one system will invariably influence the transmission of the other. Here, the human reward system may represent a major or common final pathway. The specific increase in serotonergic and noradrenergic turnover under paroxetine and reboxetine, respectively, dampened the neural activity within the dopaminergic human reward system and, in particular, within the nucleus accumbens. However, this attenuation is potentially restricted to the processing of specific rewards or reinforcers such as sexual stimuli or primary rewards, considering that the serotonergic and noradrenergic attenuation of neural activity within the nucleus accumbens was not evident when processing monetary rewards as secondary reinforcers [93,94].

6. Perspectives

Our project using pharmacological and task-based fMRI identified neuromodulatory effects of monoamines and catecholamines on neural sexual responses and potential neural proxies for the development of sexual dysfunction under antidepressants. Insights from this methodological approach mainly concern basic research; however, some aspects might be transferred to clinical practices. Considering that task-based fMRI may not be easily implemented in clinical routines due to its complexity and dependency on a subject's motivation and performance, resting-state fMRI may provide a valuable alternative. Accordingly, we investigated healthy subjects using resting-state fMRI [95] and demonstrated that more impaired subjective sexual function under serotonergic agents was predicted by low baseline functional connectivities under placebo. In particular, functional connectivities of the sublenticular extended amygdala with midbrain, pgACC, and the insula revealed a predictive potential for the development of SSRI-related decreases in sexual functioning. Although these results await empirical replication in larger samples, they may support the idea of a potentially valuable contribution of imaging techniques in the prediction of pharmaco-related sexual dysfunction within the context of personalized medicine.

It is of note that the investigations presented were exclusively conducted in healthy male subjects and the conclusions drawn may not be transferable to females. Within the past years, gender and sex aspects were widely recognized in scientific research and, with regard to sexual responses, sex differences are proposed to not only occur on behavioral and downstream peripheral, but also on the neural level. Relative to men, meta-analyses suggest a less consistent and decreased neurofunctional activation in subcortical regions in women during sexual arousal [96,97]. In addition, female sex hormones appear to play a crucial role in mediating particularly cortical activations in response to sexual stimulation [97–99]. Moreover, there is evidence for an interaction between sex hormones and the dominant neurotransmitters such as serotonin and dopamine [100]. These observations suggest a divergent monoaminergic neuromodulation of erotic stimulus processing in females. Consequently, the investigation of females under different levels of monoaminergic or catecholaminergic neurotransmitter levels in combination with different hormonal states is highly encouraged as a future research topic.

7. Conclusions

Within a broader research program, we investigated healthy male subjects under visual erotic stimulation by fMRI and different antidepressant medication to disentangle effects of monoaminergic and catecholaminergic neuromodulatory substances on neural substrates of sexual responses. After increasing serotonergic neurotransmission, we observed attenuated neural activations within cerebral networks previously related to motivational, emotional, and autonomic components of sexual behavior along with diminished subjective sexual functions. Psychophysiological interaction analyses revealed that the dampening of the motivational component and, in particular, human reward system activation was presumably mediated by an increase in prefrontal cortex activation as a potential correlate of increased cognitive control under serotonergic agents. Of note, neural motivational and emotional components, as well as subjective sexual functions, were either unaffected or even increased under dopaminergic stimulation. Apart from these divergent effects on erotic stimulus processing, both serotonergic and dopaminergic stimulation diminished neural attention network activation during the anticipation of visual sexual stimuli, along with a decrease in behavioral measures of attention. Investigating the noradrenergic neuromodulation of neural substrates of erotic stimulus processing revealed similar neural alterations as serotonergic agents, and showed again attenuation of neural emotional and motivation components along with a decrease in subjective sexual functions. However, neural activations during the anticipation of sexual stimuli and behavioral attentional functioning were not altered by a noradrenergic agent. Thus, our results provided evidence for the neuromodulatory effects of serotonergic, noradrenergic, and dopaminergic agents on neural substrates of erotic stimulus processing. Considering the overlay of neuromodulatory effects of serotonergic and noradrenergic neurotransmission, this may suggest that both monoaminergic modulations end up via similar neural pathways and presumably affect dopaminergic projections within the human reward system. Notably, the dampening of the human reward system by both serotonergic and noradrenergic agents was, however, restricted to the processing of visual sexual stimuli as primary reinforcers and was not evident during processing of monetary rewards as secondary reinforcers.

From a basic research perspective, we demonstrate that modulations in sexual functioning on the subjective behavioral level are indeed closely linked to cerebral networks that mediate motivational, emotional, autonomic, and attentional components of the sexual response. Our data emphasize the hypothesis that altered cerebral reactivity rather than peripheral effects might be the key to explain side effects of monoaminergic substances on sexual functioning.

Author Contributions: Conceptualization, H.G., M.W., G.G. and B.A.; writing—original draft preparation, H.G., G.G. and B.A.; writing—review and editing, H.G., K.M., C.D.M, G.G. and B.A.; visualization, H.G.; supervision, H.G., G.G. and B.A.; project administration, H.G.

Acknowledgments: We thank C. Hiemke and his stuff at the University of Mainz, Germany, Department of Psychiatry and Psychotherapy, for measuring drug serum levels in our research project.

Conflicts of Interest: The authors declare no potential (including financial) conflicts of interests related to this work.

References

1. McKenna, K. The brain is the master organ in sexual function: Central nervous system control of male and female sexual function. *Int. J. Impot. Res.* **1999**, *1*, 48–55. [CrossRef]
2. Stoléru, S.; Fonteille, V.; Cornélis, C.; Joyal, C.; Moulier, V. Functional neuroimaging studies of sexual arousal and orgasm in healthy men and women: A review and meta-analysis. *Neurosci. Biobehav. Rev.* **2012**, *36*, 1481–1509. [CrossRef]
3. Redouté, J.; Stoléru, S.; Grégoire, M.C.; Costes, N.; Cinotti, L.; Lavenne, F.; Le Bars, D.; Forest, M.G.; Pujol, J.F. Brain processing of visual sexual stimuli in human males. *Hum. Brain Mapp.* **2000**, *11*, 162–177. [CrossRef]
4. Georgiadis, J.R.; Kringelbach, M.L.; Pfaus, J.G. Sex for fun: A synthesis of human and animal neurobiology. *Nat. Rev. Urol.* **2012**, *9*, 486–498. [CrossRef] [PubMed]
5. Bossini, L.; Fortini, V.; Casolaro, I.; Caterini, C.; Koukouna, D.; Cecchini, F.; Benbow, J.; Fagiolini, A. Sexual dysfunctions, psychiatric diseases and quality of life: A review. *Psychiatr. Pol.* **2014**, *48*, 715–726. [PubMed]
6. Waldinger, M.D. Psychiatric disorders and sexual dysfunction. *Handb. Clin. Neurol.* **2015**, *130*, 469–489. [PubMed]
7. Montejo, A.L.; Llorca, G.; Izquierdo, J.A.; Rico-Villademoros, F. Incidence of sexual dysfunction associated with antidepressant agents: A prospective multicenter study of 1022 outpatients. Spanish Working Group for the Study of Psychotropic-Related Sexual Dysfunction. *J. Clin. Psychiatry* **2001**, *62*, 10–21. [PubMed]
8. Masters, W.J.; Johnson, V.E. *Human Sexual Response*, 1st ed.; Brown, Little: Boston, MA, USA, 1966; ISBN 9781483198064.
9. Kaplan, H.S. *Disorders of Sexual Desire and Other New Concepts and Techniques in sex Therapy/Helen Singer Kaplan*; Kaplan, H.S., Ed.; New Sex Therapy; Brunner/Mazel: New York, NY, USA, 1979; ISBN 0876302126.
10. Georgiadis, J.R.; Kringelbach, M.L. The human sexual response cycle: Brain imaging evidence linking sex to other pleasures. *Prog. Neurobiol.* **2012**, *98*, 49–81. [CrossRef] [PubMed]
11. Stoléru, S.; Gregoire, M.C.; Gerard, D.; Decety, J.; Lafarge, E.; Cinotti, L.; Lavenne, F.; Le Bars, D.; Vernet-Maury, E.; Rada, H.; et al. Neuroanatomical correlates of visually evoked sexual arousal in human males. *Arch. Sex. Behav.* **1999**, *28*, 1–21. [CrossRef]
12. Poeppl, T.B.; Langguth, B.; Laird, A.R.; Eickhoff, S.B. The functional neuroanatomy of male psychosexual and physiosexual arousal: A quantitative meta-analysis. *Hum. Brain Mapp.* **2014**, *35*, 1404–1421. [CrossRef]
13. Bühler, M.; Vollstädt-Klein, S.; Klemen, J.; Smolka, M.N. Does erotic stimulus presentation design affect brain activation patterns? Event-related vs. blocked fMRI designs. *Behav. Brain Funct.* **2008**, *4*, 30. [CrossRef]
14. Ferretti, A.; Caulo, M.; Del Gratta, C.; Di Matteo, R.; Merla, A.; Montorsi, F.; Pizzella, V.; Pompa, P.; Rigatti, P.; Rossini, P.M.; et al. Dynamics of male sexual arousal: Distinct components of brain activation revealed by fMRI. *Neuroimage* **2005**, *26*, 1086–1096. [CrossRef]
15. Cera, N.; di Pierro, E.D.; Sepede, G.; Gambi, F.; Perrucci, M.G.; Merla, A.; Tartaro, A.; del Gratta, C.; Galatioto Paradiso, G.; Vicentini, C.; et al. The Role of Left Superior Parietal Lobe in Male Sexual Behavior: Dynamics of Distinct Components Revealed by fMRI. *J. Sex. Med.* **2012**, *9*, 1602–1612. [CrossRef]
16. Georgiadis, J.R.; Kortekaas, R.; Kuipers, R.; Nieuwenburg, A.; Pruim, J.; Reinders, A.A.T.S.; Holstege, G. Regional cerebral blood flow changes associated with clitorally induced orgasm in healthy women. *Eur. J. Neurosci.* **2006**, *24*, 3305–3316. [CrossRef]
17. Gizewski, E.R.; Krause, E.; Karama, S.; Baars, A.; Senf, W.; Forsting, M. There are differences in cerebral activation between females in distinct menstrual phases during viewing of erotic stimuli: A fMRI study. *Exp. Brain Res.* **2006**, *174*, 101–108. [CrossRef]

18. Arnow, B.A.; Millheiser, L.; Garrett, A.; Lake Polan, M.; Glover, G.H.; Hill, K.R.; Lightbody, A.; Watson, C.; Banner, L.; Smart, T.; et al. Women with hypoactive sexual desire disorder compared to normal females: A functional magnetic resonance imaging study. *Neuroscience* **2009**, *158*, 484–502. [CrossRef]
19. Beauregard, M.; Lévesque, J.; Bourgouin, P. Neural Correlates of Conscious Self-Regulation of Emotion. *J. Neurosci.* **2001**, *21*, RC165. [CrossRef]
20. Rodriguez, G.; Sack, A.T.; Dewitte, M.; Schuhmann, T. Inhibit My Disinhibition: The Role of the Inferior Frontal Cortex in Sexual Inhibition and the Modulatory Influence of Sexual Excitation Proneness. *Front. Hum. Neurosci.* **2018**, *12*, 300. [CrossRef]
21. Mallick, H.N.; Tandon, S.; Jagannathan, N.R.; Gulia, K.K.; Kumar, V.M. Brain areas activated after ejaculation in healthy young human subjects. *Indian J. Physiol. Pharmacol.* **2007**, *51*, 81–85.
22. Brackett, N.L.; Iuvone, P.M.; Edwards, D.A. Midbrain lesions, dopamine and male sexual behavior. *Behav. Brain Res.* **1986**, *20*, 231–240. [CrossRef]
23. Zahran, A.R.; Simmerman, N.; Carrier, S.; Vachon, P. Erectile dysfunction occurs following substantia nigra lesions in the rat. *Int. J. Impot. Res.* **2001**, *13*, 255–260. [CrossRef]
24. La Torre, A.; Giupponi, G.; Duffy, D.; Conca, A. Sexual dysfunction related to psychotropic drugs: A critical review—Part I: Antidepressants. *Pharmacopsychiatry* **2013**, *46*, 191–199. [CrossRef]
25. La Torre, A.; Conca, A.; Duffy, D.; Giupponi, G.; Pompili, M.; Grözinger, M. Sexual dysfunction related to psychotropic drugs: A critical review part II: Antipsychotics. *Pharmacopsychiatry* **2013**, *46*, 201–208. [CrossRef]
26. La Torre, A.; Giupponi, G.; Duffy, D.M.; Pompili, M.; Grözinger, M.; Kapfhammer, H.P.; Conca, A. Sexual dysfunction related to psychotropic drugs: A critical review part III: Mood stabilizers and anxiolytic drugs. *Pharmacopsychiatry* **2014**, *47*, 1–6. [CrossRef]
27. Pfaus, J.G. Pathways of sexual desire. *J. Sex. Med.* **2009**, *6*, 1506–1533. [CrossRef]
28. Hull, E.M.; Muschamp, J.W.; Sato, S. Dopamine and serotonin: Influences on male sexual behavior. *Physiol. Behav.* **2004**, *83*, 291–307. [CrossRef]
29. Clayton, A.H. The pathophysiology of hypoactive sexual desire disorder in women. *Int. J. Gynecol. Obstet.* **2010**, *110*, 7–11. [CrossRef]
30. Modell, J.G.; May, R.S.; Katholi, C.R. Effect of bupropion-sr on orgasmic dysfunction in nondepressed subjects: A pilot study. *J. Sex Marital Ther.* **2000**, *26*, 231–240.
31. Voon, V.; Fernagut, P.O.; Wickens, J.; Baunez, C.; Rodriguez, M.; Pavon, N.; Juncos, J.L.; Obeso, J.A.; Bezard, E. Chronic dopaminergic stimulation in Parkinson's disease: From dyskinesias to impulse control disorders. *Lancet Neurol.* **2009**, *8*, 1140–1149. [CrossRef]
32. Dossenbach, M.; Dyachkova, Y.; Pirildar, S.; Anders, M.; Khalil, A.; Araszkiewicz, A.; Shakhnovich, T.; Akram, A.; Pecenak, J.; McBride, M.; et al. Effects of atypical and typical antipsychotic treatments on sexual function in patients with schizophrenia: 12-month results from the Intercontinental Schizophrenia Outpatient Health Outcomes (IC-SOHO) study. *Eur. Psychiatry* **2006**, *21*, 251–258. [CrossRef]
33. Haddad, P.M.; Sharma, S.G. Adverse effects of atypical antipsychotics: Differential risk and clinical implications. *CNS Drugs* **2007**, *21*, 911–936. [CrossRef]
34. Park, Y.W.; Kim, Y.; Lee, J.H. Antipsychotic-induced sexual dysfunction and its management. *World J. Mens. Health* **2012**, *30*, 153–159. [CrossRef]
35. Montejo, A.L.; Calama, J.; Rico-Villademoros, F.; Montejo, L.; Gonzalez-Garcia, N.; Perez, J. A Real-World Study on Antidepressant-Associated Sexual Dysfunction in 2144 Outpatients: The SALSEX I Study. *Arch. Sex. Behav.* **2019**, 1–11. [CrossRef]
36. Santana, Y.; Montejo, A.L.; Martin, J.; LLorca, G.; Bueno, G.; Blazquez, J.L. Understanding the Mechanism of Antidepressant-Related Sexual Dysfunction: Inhibition of Tyrosine Hydroxylase in Dopaminergic Neurons after Treatment with Paroxetine but Not with Agomelatine in Male Rats. *J. Clin. Med.* **2019**, *8*, 133. [CrossRef]
37. Allard, J.; Truitt, W.A.; McKenna, K.E.; Coolen, L.M. Spinal cord control of ejaculation. *World J. Urol.* **2005**, *23*, 119–126. [CrossRef]
38. Serretti, A.; Chiesa, A. Treatment-emergent sexual dysfunction related to antidepressants: A meta-analysis. *J. Clin. Psychopharmacol.* **2009**, *29*, 259–266. [CrossRef]
39. Williams, V.S.L.; Baldwin, D.S.; Hogue, S.L.; Fehnel, S.E.; Hollis, K.A.; Edin, H.M. Estimating the Prevalence and Impact of Antidepressant-Induced Sexual Dysfunction in 2 European Countries A Cross-Sectional Patient Survey. *J. Clin. Psychiatry* **2006**, *67*, 204–210. [CrossRef]

40. Williams, V.S.L.; Edin, H.M.; Hogue, S.L.; Fehnel, S.E.; Baldwin, D.S. Prevalence and impact of antidepressant-associated sexual dysfunction in three European countries: Replication in a cross-sectional patient survey. *J. Psychopharmacol.* **2010**, *24*, 489–496. [CrossRef]
41. Clayton, A.; Kornstein, S.; Prakash, A.; Mallinckrodt, C.; Wohlreich, M. Changes in sexual functioning associated with duloxetine, escitalopram, and placebo in the treatment of patients with major depressive disorder. *J. Sex. Med.* **2007**, *4*, 917–929. [CrossRef]
42. Berwian, I.M.; Walter, H.; Seifritz, E.; Huys, Q.J.M. Predicting relapse after antidepressant withdrawal—A systematic review. *Psychol. Med.* **2016**, *47*, 426–437. [CrossRef]
43. Langworth, S.; Bodlund, O.; Agren, H. Efficacy and tolerability of reboxetine compared with citalopram: A double-blind study in patients with major depressive disorder. *J. Clin. Psychopharmacol.* **2006**, *26*, 121–127. [CrossRef] [PubMed]
44. Clayton, A.H.; Zajecka, J.; Ferguson, J.M.; Filipiak-Reisner, J.K.; Brown, M.T.; Schwartz, G.E. Lack of sexual dysfunction with the selective noradrenaline reuptake inhibitor reboxetine during treatment for major depressive disorder. *Int. Clin. Psychopharmacol.* **2003**, *18*, 151–156.
45. Krüger, T.H.C.; Haake, P.; Chereath, D.; Knapp, W.; Janssen, O.E.; Exton, M.S.; Schedlowski, M.; Hartmann, U. Specificity of the neuroendocrine response to orgasm during sexual arousal in men. *J. Endocrinol.* **2003**, *177*, 57–64. [CrossRef]
46. Mihailescu, C.; Mihailesku, A. Sexual dysfunction in a group of depressed female patients. Conference abstract, 21st ECNP Congress, Barcelona, Spain. *Eur. Neuropsychopharmacol.* **2008**, *18*, 341–342. [CrossRef]
47. Thakurta, R.; Singh, O.; Bhattacharya, A.; Mallick, A.; Ray, P.; Sen, S.; Das, R. Nature of Sexual Dysfunctions in Major Depressive Disorder and its Impact on Quality of Life. *Indian J. Psychol. Med.* **2012**, *34*, 365–370.
48. Kim, W.; Jin, B.R.; Yang, W.S.; Lee, K.U.; Juh, R.H.; Ahn, K.J.; Chung, Y.A.; Chae, J.H. Treatment with selective serotonin reuptake inhibitors and mirtapazine results in differential brain activation by visual erotic stimuli in patients with major depressive disorder. *Psychiatry Investig.* **2009**, *6*, 85–95. [CrossRef]
49. Abler, B.; Seeringer, A.; Hartmann, A.; Grön, G.; Metzger, C.; Walter, M.; Stingl, J. Neural Correlates of Antidepressant-Related Sexual Dysfunction: A Placebo-Controlled fMRI Study on Healthy Males Under Subchronic Paroxetine and Bupropion. *Neuropsychopharmacology* **2011**, *36*, 1837–1847. [CrossRef]
50. Labbate, L.A.; Lare, S.B. Sexual dysfunction in male psychiatric outpatients: Validity of the Massachusetts General Hospital sexual functioning questionnaire. *Psychother. Psychosom.* **2001**, *70*, 221–225. [CrossRef]
51. Simmons, A.N.; Arce, E.; Lovero, K.L.; Stein, M.B.; Paulus, M.P. Subchronic SSRI administration reduces insula response during affective anticipation in healthy volunteers. *Int. J. Neuropsychopharmacol.* **2009**, *12*, 1009–1020. [CrossRef]
52. Walter, M.; Bermpohl, F.; Mouras, H.; Schiltz, K.; Tempelmann, C.; Rotte, M.; Heinze, H.J.; Bogerts, B.; Northoff, G. Distinguishing specific sexual and general emotional effects in fMRI-Subcortical and cortical arousal during erotic picture viewing. *Neuroimage* **2008**, *40*, 1482–1492. [CrossRef]
53. Hayes, D.J.; Greenshaw, A.J. 5-HT receptors and reward-related behaviour: A review. *Neurosci. Biobehav. Rev.* **2011**, *35*, 1419–1449. [CrossRef] [PubMed]
54. Kranz, G.S.; Kasper, S.; Lanzenberger, R. Reward and the serotonergic system. *Neuroscience* **2010**, *166*, 1023–1035. [CrossRef] [PubMed]
55. Seo, D.; Patrick, C.J.; Kennealy, P.J. Role of serotonin and dopamine system interactions in the neurobiology of impulsive aggression and its comorbidity with other clinical disorders. *Aggress. Violent Behav.* **2008**, *13*, 383–395. [CrossRef] [PubMed]
56. Boureau, Y.L.; Dayan, P. Opponency revisited: Competition and cooperation between dopamine and serotonin. *Neuropsychopharmacology* **2011**, *36*, 74–97. [CrossRef] [PubMed]
57. Diekhof, E.K.; Gruber, O. When Desire Collides with Reason: Functional Interactions between Anteroventral Prefrontal Cortex and Nucleus Accumbens Underlie the Human Ability to Resist Impulsive Desires. *J. Neurosci.* **2010**, *30*, 1488–1493. [CrossRef]
58. Abler, B.; Gron, G.; Hartmann, A.; Metzger, C.; Walter, M. Modulation of Frontostriatal Interaction Aligns with Reduced Primary Reward Processing under Serotonergic Drugs. *J. Neurosci.* **2012**, *32*, 1329–1335. [CrossRef]
59. Coleman, C.C.; King, B.R.; Bolden-Watson, C.; Book, M.J.; Taylor Segraves, R.; Richard, N.; Ascher, J.; Batey, S.; Jamerson, B.; Metz, A. A placebo-controlled comparison of the effects on sexual functioning of bupropion sustained release and fluoxetine. *Clin. Ther.* **2001**, *23*, 1040–1058. [CrossRef]

60. Coleman, C.C.; Cunningham, L.A.; Foster, V.J.; Batey, S.R.; Donahue, R.M.J.; Houser, T.L.; Ascher, J.A. Sexual dysfunction associated with the treatment of depression: A placebo-controlled comparison of bupropion sustained release and sertraline treatment. *Ann. Clin. Psychiatry* **1999**, *11*, 205–215. [CrossRef]
61. Croft, H.; Settle, E.; Houser, T.; Batey, S.R.; Donahue, R.M.J.; Ascher, J.A. A placebo-controlled comparison of the antidepressant efficacy and effects on sexual functioning of sustained-release bupropion and sertraline. *Clin. Ther.* **1999**, *21*, 643–658. [CrossRef]
62. Segraves, R.T.; Kavoussi, R.; Hughes, A.R.; Batey, S.R.; Johnston, J.A.; Donahue, R.; Ascher, J.A. Evaluation of sexual functioning depressed outpatients: A double-blind comparison of sustained-release bupropion and sertraline treatment. *J. Clin. Psychopharmacol.* **2000**, *20*, 122–128. [CrossRef]
63. Georgiadis, J.R.; Farrell, M.J.; Boessen, R.; Denton, D.A.; Gavrilescu, M.; Kortekaas, R.; Renken, R.J.; Hoogduin, J.M.; Egan, G.F. Dynamic subcortical blood flow during male sexual activity with ecological validity: A perfusion fMRI study. *Neuroimage* **2010**, *50*, 208–216. [CrossRef] [PubMed]
64. Seeley, W.W.; Menon, V.; Schatzberg, A.F.; Keller, J.; Glover, G.H.; Kenna, H.; Reiss, A.L.; Greicius, M.D. Dissociable Intrinsic Connectivity Networks for Salience Processing and Executive Control. *J. Neurosci.* **2007**, *27*, 2349–2356. [CrossRef]
65. Dosenbach, N.U.F.; Fair, D.A.; Cohen, A.L.; Schlaggar, B.L.; Petersen, S.E. A dual-networks architecture of top-down control. *Trends Cogn. Sci.* **2008**, *12*, 99–105. [CrossRef]
66. Walter, M.; Witzel, J.; Wiebking, C.; Gubka, U.; Rotte, M.; Schiltz, K.; Bermpohl, F.; Tempelmann, C.; Bogerts, B.; Heinze, H.J.; et al. Pedophilia is Linked to Reduced Activation in Hypothalamus and Lateral Prefrontal Cortex During Visual Erotic Stimulation. *Biol. Psychiatry* **2007**, *62*, 698–701. [CrossRef]
67. Lang, P.; Bradley, M.; Cuthbert, B. *International Affective Picture System (IAPS): Digitized Photographs, Instruction Manual and Affective Ratings*; Technical Report; University of Florida: Gainesville, FL, USA, 2005; A-6.
68. Walter, M.; Matthiä, C.; Wiebking, C.; Rotte, M.; Tempelmann, C.; Bogerts, B.; Heinze, H.J.; Northoff, G. Preceding attention and the dorsomedial prefrontal cortex: Process specificity versus domain dependence. *Hum. Brain Mapp.* **2009**, *30*, 312–326. [CrossRef] [PubMed]
69. Bermpohl, F.; Pascual-Leone, A.; Amedi, A.; Merabet, L.B.; Fregni, F.; Gaab, N.; Alsop, D.; Schlaug, G.; Northoff, G. Dissociable networks for the expectancy and perception of emotional stimuli in the human brain. *Neuroimage* **2006**, *30*, 588–600. [CrossRef] [PubMed]
70. Herwig, U.; Abler, B.; Walter, H.; Erk, S. Expecting unpleasant stimuli—An fMRI study. *Psychiatry Res. Neuroimaging* **2007**, *154*, 1–12. [CrossRef]
71. Corbetta, M.; Shulman, G.L. Control of goal-directed and stimulus-driven attention in the brain. *Nat. Rev. Neurosci.* **2002**, *3*, 201–215. [CrossRef]
72. Arnsten, A.F.T. Catecholamine influences on dorsolateral prefrontal cortical networks. *Biol. Psychiatry* **2011**, *69*, 89–99. [CrossRef] [PubMed]
73. Dreher, J.C.; Guigon, E.; Burnod, Y. A model of prefrontal cortex dopaminergic modulation during the delayed alternation task. *J. Cogn. Neurosci.* **2002**, *14*, 853–865. [CrossRef]
74. Graf, H.; Abler, B.; Freudenmann, R.; Beschoner, P.; Schaeffeler, E.; Spitzer, M.; Schwab, M.; Grn, G. Neural correlates of error monitoring modulated by atomoxetine in healthy volunteers. *Biol. Psychiatry* **2011**, *69*, 890–897. [CrossRef] [PubMed]
75. Lavergne, F.; Jay, T.M. A new strategy for antidepressant prescription. *Front. Neurosci.* **2010**, *4*, 192. [CrossRef] [PubMed]
76. Owen, J.C.E.; Whitton, P.S. Effects of amantadine and budipine on antidepressant drug-evoked changes in extracellular dopamine in the frontal cortex of freely moving rats. *Brain Res.* **2006**, *1117*, 206–212. [CrossRef] [PubMed]
77. Riedel, W.J.; Eikmans, K.; Heldens, A.; Schmitt, J.A.J. Specific serotonergic reuptake inhibition impairs vigilance performance acutely and after subchronic treatment. *J. Psychopharmacol.* **2005**, *19*, 12–20. [CrossRef] [PubMed]
78. Wingen, M.; Kuypers, K.P.C.; van de Ven, V.; Formisano, E.; Ramaekers, J.G. Sustained attention and serotonin: A pharmaco-fMRI study. *Hum. Psychopharmacol.* **2008**, *23*, 221–230. [CrossRef]
79. Whiskey, E.; Taylor, D. A review of the adverse effects and safety of noradrenergic antidepressants. *J. Psychopharmacol.* **2013**, *27*, 732–739. [CrossRef] [PubMed]
80. Baldwin, D.; Bridgman, K.; Buis, C. Resolution of sexual dysfunction during double-blind treatment of major depression with reboxetine or paroxetine. *J. Psychopharmacol.* **2006**, *20*, 91–96. [CrossRef]

81. Graf, H.; Wiegers, M.; Metzger, C.D.; Walter, M.; Grön, G.; Abler, B. Erotic stimulus processing under amisulpride and reboxetine: A placebo-controlled fMRI study in healthy subjects. *Int. J. Neuropsychopharmacol.* **2015**, *18*. [CrossRef]
82. Haberfellner, E.M. Sexual dysfunction caused by reboxetine. *Pharmacopsychiatry* **2002**, *35*, 77–78. [CrossRef]
83. Sivrioglu, E.Y.; Topaloglu, V.C.; Sarandol, A.; Akkaya, C.; Eker, S.S.; Kirli, S. Reboxetine induced erectile dysfunction and spontaneous ejaculation during defecation and micturition. *Prog. Neuro-Psychopharmacol. Biol. Psychiatry* **2007**, *31*, 548–550. [CrossRef]
84. Arnow, B.A.; Desmond, J.E.; Banner, L.L.; Glover, G.H.; Solomon, A.; Polan, M.L.; Lue, T.F.; Atlas, S.W. Brain activation and sexual arousal in healthy, heterosexual males. *Brain* **2002**, *125*, 1014–1023. [CrossRef]
85. Miller, E.M.; Shankar, M.U.; Knutson, B.; McClure, S.M. Dissociating motivation from reward in human striatal activity. *J. Cogn. Neurosci.* **2014**, *26*, 1075–1084. [CrossRef]
86. Perrault, G.; Depoortere, R.; Morel, E.; Sanger, D.J.; Scatton, B. Psychopharmacological profile of amisulpride: An antipsychotic drug with presynaptic D2/D3 dopamine receptor antagonist activity and limbic selectivity. *J. Pharmacol. Exp. Ther.* **1997**, *280*, 73–782.
87. Castelli, M.P.; Mocci, I.; Sanna, A.M.; Gessa, G.L.; Pani, L. (-)S amisulpride binds with high affinity to cloned dopamine D3 and D2 receptors. *Eur. J. Pharmacol.* **2001**, *432*, 143–147. [CrossRef]
88. Härtter, S.; Hüwel, S.; Lohmann, T.; Abou El Ela, A.; Langguth, P.; Hiemke, C.; Galla, H.J. How Does the Benzamide Antipsychotic Amisulpride get into the Brain?—An in Vitro Approach Comparing Amisulpride with Clozapine. *Neuropsychopharmacology* **2003**, *28*, 1916–1922. [CrossRef]
89. Smeraldi, E. Amisulpride versus fluoxetine in patients with dysthymia or major depression in partial remission. A double-blind, comparative study. *J. Affect. Disord.* **1998**, *48*, 47–56. [CrossRef]
90. Montgomery, S.A. Dopaminergic deficit and the role of amisulpride in the treatment of mood disorders. *Int. Clin. Psychopharmacol.* **2002**, *17*, 9–15.
91. Graf, H.; Wiegers, M.; Metzger, C.D.; Walter, M.; Grön, G.; Abler, B. Noradrenergic modulation of neural erotic stimulus perception. *Eur. Neuropsychopharmacol.* **2017**, *27*, 845–853. [CrossRef]
92. El Mansari, M.; Guiard, B.P.; Chernoloz, O.; Ghanbari, R.; Katz, N.; Blier, P. Relevance of norepinephrine-dopamine interactions in the treatment of major depressive disorder. *CNS Neurosci. Ther.* **2010**, *16*, e1–e17. [CrossRef]
93. Graf, H.; Metzger, C.D.; Walter, M.; Abler, B. Serotonergic antidepressants decrease hedonic signals but leave learning signals in the nucleus accumbens unaffected. *Neuroreport* **2016**, *27*, 18–22. [CrossRef]
94. Graf, H.; Wiegers, M.; Metzger, C.D.; Walter, M.; Abler, B. Differential Noradrenergic Modulation of Monetary Reward and Visual Erotic Stimulus Processing. *Front. Psychiatry* **2018**, *9*, 346. [CrossRef]
95. Metzger, C.D.; Walter, M.; Graf, H.; Abler, B. SSRI-related modulation of sexual functioning is predicted by pre-treatment resting state functional connectivity in healthy men. *Arch. Sex. Behav.* **2013**, *42*, 935–947. [CrossRef]
96. Rupp, H.A.; Wallen, K. Sex differences in response to visual sexual stimuli: A review. *Arch. Sex. Behav.* **2008**, *37*, 206–218. [CrossRef]
97. Poeppl, T.B.; Langguth, B.; Rupprecht, R.; Safron, A.; Bzdok, D.; Laird, A.R.; Eickhoff, S.B. The neural basis of sex differences in sexual behavior: A quantitative meta-analysis. *Front. Neuroendocrinol.* **2016**, *43*, 28–43. [CrossRef]
98. Abler, B.; Kumpfmüller, D.; Grön, G.; Walter, M.; Stingl, J.; Seeringer, A. Neural Correlates of Erotic Stimulation under Different Levels of Female Sexual Hormones. *PLoS ONE* **2013**, *8*, e54447. [CrossRef]
99. Bonenberger, M.; Groschwitz, R.C.; Kumpfmueller, D.; Groen, G.; Plener, P.L.; Abler, B. It's all about money: Oral contraception alters neural reward processing. *Neuroreport* **2013**, *24*, 951–955. [CrossRef]
100. Barth, C.; Villringer, A.; Sacher, J. Sex hormones affect neurotransmitters and shape the adult female brain during hormonal transition periods. *Front. Neurosci.* **2015**, *9*, 37. [CrossRef]

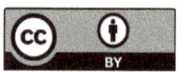

© 2019 by the authors. Licensee MDPI, Basel, Switzerland. This article is an open access article distributed under the terms and conditions of the Creative Commons Attribution (CC BY) license (http://creativecommons.org/licenses/by/4.0/).

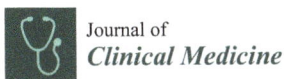

Review

Online Porn Addiction: What We Know and What We Don't—A Systematic Review

Rubén de Alarcón [1], Javier I. de la Iglesia [1], Nerea M. Casado [1] and Angel L. Montejo [1,2,*]

[1] Psychiatry Service, Hospital Clínico Universitario de Salamanca, Institute of Biomedical Research of Salamanca (IBSAL), 37007 Salamanca, Spain; ruperghost@gmail.com (R.d.A.); javidelaiglesia.jdli@gmail.com (J.I.d.l.I.); nmcasado91@gmail.com (N.M.C.)
[2] University of Salamanca, EUEF, 37007 Salamanca, Spain
* Correspondence: amontejo@usal.es; Tel.: +34-639754620

Received: 27 November 2018; Accepted: 10 January 2019; Published: 15 January 2019

Abstract: In the last few years, there has been a wave of articles related to behavioral addictions; some of them have a focus on online pornography addiction. However, despite all efforts, we are still unable to profile when engaging in this behavior becomes pathological. Common problems include: sample bias, the search for diagnostic instrumentals, opposing approximations to the matter, and the fact that this entity may be encompassed inside a greater pathology (i.e., sex addiction) that may present itself with very diverse symptomatology. Behavioral addictions form a largely unexplored field of study, and usually exhibit a problematic consumption model: loss of control, impairment, and risky use. Hypersexual disorder fits this model and may be composed of several sexual behaviors, like problematic use of online pornography (POPU). Online pornography use is on the rise, with a potential for addiction considering the "triple A" influence (accessibility, affordability, anonymity). This problematic use might have adverse effects in sexual development and sexual functioning, especially among the young population. We aim to gather existing knowledge on problematic online pornography use as a pathological entity. Here we try to summarize what we know about this entity and outline some areas worthy of further research.

Keywords: online pornography; addiction; cybersex; internet; compulsive sexual behavior; hypersexuality

1. Introduction

With the inclusion of "Gambling Disorder" in the "Substance Use and Addictive Disorders" chapter of the DSM-5 [1], the APA publicly acknowledged the phenomenon of behavioral addiction. Furthermore, "Internet Gaming Disorder" was placed in Section 3—conditions for further study.

This represents the ongoing paradigm shift in the field of addictions that relates to addictive behavior, and paves the way for new research in the light of cultural changes caused by the new technologies.

There is apparently an existing common neurobiological [2] and environmental [3] ground between the varying addictive disorders, including both substance abuse and addictive behavior; this can manifest as an overlapping of both entities [4].

Phenomenologically, behaviorally addicted individuals frequently exhibit a problematic consumption model: impaired control (e.g., craving, unsuccessful attempts to reduce the behavior), impairment (e.g., narrowing of interests, neglect of other areas of life), and risky use (persisting intake despite awareness of damaging psychological effects). Whether these behaviors also meet physiological criteria relating to addiction (tolerance, withdrawal) is more debatable [4–6].

Hypersexual disorder is sometimes considered one of those behavioral addictions. It is used as an umbrella construct that encompasses various problematic behaviors (excessive masturbation, cybersex, pornography use, telephone sex, sexual behavior with consenting adults, strip club visitations, etc.) [7]. Its prevalence rates range from 3% to 6%, though it is difficult to determine since there is not a formal definition of the disorder [8,9].

The lack of robust scientific data makes its research, conceptualization, and assessment difficult, leading to a variety of proposals to explain it, but is usually associated with significant distress, feelings of shame and psychosocial dysfunction [8], as well as other addictive behaviors [10] and it warrants direct examination.

Concurrently, the rise of the new technologies has also opened up a pool of problematic addictive behavior, mainly Internet Addiction. This addiction may focus on a specific application on the internet (gaming, shopping, betting, cybersex . . .) [11] with potential for risk-addictive behavior; in this case, it would act as a channel for concrete manifestations of said behavior [4,12]. This means inevitable escalation, providing new outlets for established addicts as well as tempting people (due to increased privacy, or opportunity) who would not have previously engaged in these behaviors.

Online pornography use, also known as Internet pornography use or cybersex, may be one of those Internet-specific behaviors with a risk for addiction. It corresponds to the use of Internet to engage in various gratifying sexual activities [13], among which stands the use of pornography [13,14] which is the most popular activity [15–17] with an infinite number of sexual scenarios accessible [13,18–20]. Continued use in this fashion sometimes derives in financial, legal, occupational, and relationship trouble [6,21] or personal problems, with diverse negative consequences. Feelings of loss of control and persistent use despite these adverse results constitute "online sexual compulsivity" [22] or Problematic Online Pornography Use (POPU). This problematic consumption model benefits from the "Triple A" factors [23].

Due to this model, pornography-related masturbation may be more frequent nowadays, but this is not necessarily a sign of pathology [21]. We know that a considerable proportion of young male population access Internet for pornography consumption [24,25]; in fact, it is one of their key sources for sexual health [26]. Some have expressed concern about this, addressing the time gap between when porn material is consumed for the first time ever, and an actual first sexual experience; specifically, how the former can have an impact on sexual development [27] like abnormally low sexual desire when consuming online pornography [28] and erectile dysfunction, which has spiked dramatically among young men in the past few years when compared to a couple decades ago [29–33].

We systematically reviewed the existing literature on the subject of POPU to try and summarize the various recent advances made in terms of epidemiology, clinical manifestations, neurobiological evidence that supports this model of problematic use, its diagnostic conceptualization in relation to hypersexual disorder, its proposed assessment instruments and treatment strategies.

2. Methods

We performed the systematic review following PRISMA guidelines (Figure 1). Given the relatively new body of evidence regarding this subject, we conducted our review with no specific time-delimitation. Priority was placed upon literature reviews and articles published via a newest to oldest methodology, preferentially for already published reviews on the subject. PubMed and Cochrane were the main databases used, though a number of articles were compiled through cross-referencing.

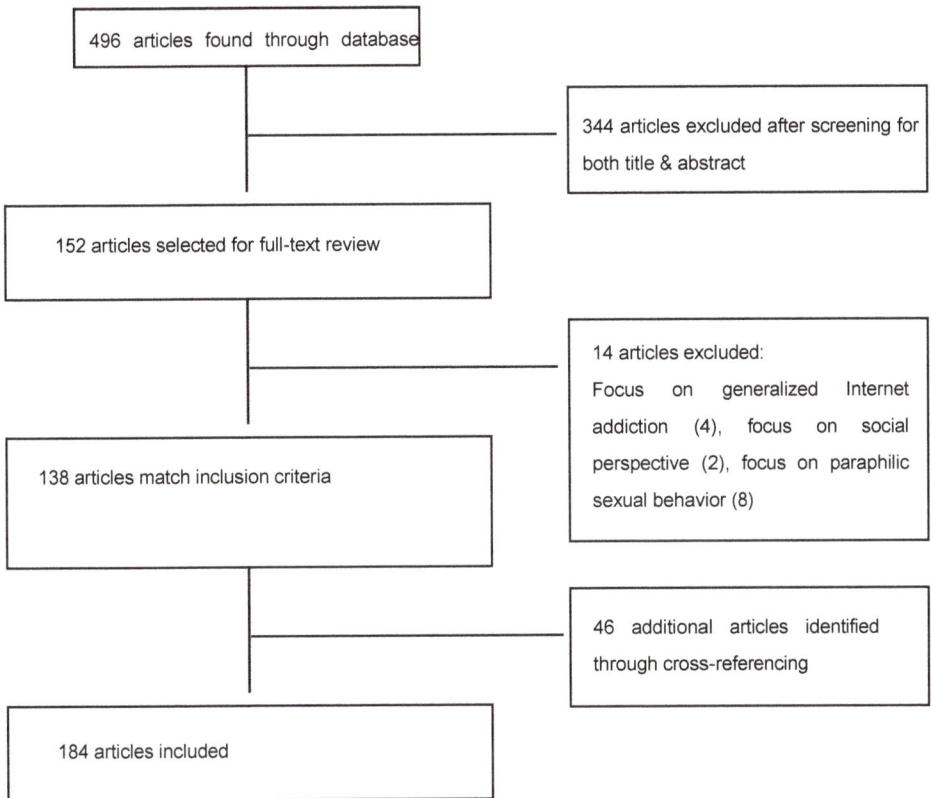

Figure 1. PRISMA flow diagram.

Since our focus was mainly online pornography and addictive sexual behavior, we excluded those articles that had only a peripheral association with it in our search: those with a focus on generalized Internet addiction, those centered on the pornographic equivalent of varying paraphilias, and those that approached the subject from a social perspective.

The following search terms and their derivatives were used in multiple combinations: cybersex, porn* (to allow for both "pornography" and "pornographic"), addict* (to allow for both "addiction" and "addictive"), online, internet, sex, compulsive sex, hypersexuality. The reference management tool Zotero was used to build a database of all articles considered.

3. Results

3.1. Epidemiology

Pornography consumption in the general population proves difficult to be adequately measured, especially since the rise of the Internet and the "triple A" factors which have allowed for both privacy and ease of access. Wright's study about the use of pornography in U.S. male population using the General Social Survey (GSS) [34], and Price's study (which expands upon Wright's by distinguishing among age, cohort, and period effects) [35] constitute some of the few, if not the only ones, existing sources that track pornography use in the general population. They show the overall increasing consumption of pornography over the years, especially among male population in contrast to females. This is particularly prevalent among young adults, and it steadily decreases with age.

Some interesting facts about pornography consumption tendencies stand out. One of them is that the 1963 and 1972 male cohort showed only a very small decline on their usage from the year 1999 onwards, suggesting that porn consumption among these groups has remained relatively constant since [35]. The other one is that 1999 is also the year the tendency for women aged 18 to 26 to consume pornography became three times as likely than the ones aged 45 to 53, instead of just two times as likely as it used to be up until that point [35]. These two facts could be related to changing tendencies in pornography consumption motivated by technology (switching from the offline to the online model of consumption), but it is impossible to know for sure since the original data does not account for differences in both offline and online variants when tracking pornography usage.

As for POPU, there is no clear and reliable data in the literature reviewed that can offer a solid estimation of its prevalence. Adding up to the already mentioned motives for lack of data on general pornography consumption, part of it might stem from the perceived taboo nature of the topic at hand by possible participants, the wide range of assessment tools used by researchers, and the lack of consensus on what actually constitutes a pathological usage of pornography, which are all issues also reviewed further into this paper.

The vast majority of studies pertaining POPU or hypersexual behavior prevalence use convenience samples to measure it, usually finding, despite population differences, that very few users consider this habit an addiction, and even when they do, even fewer consider that this could have a negative effect on them. Some examples:

(1) A study assessing behavioral addictions among substance users, found that only 9.80% out of 51 participants considered they had an addiction to sex or pornography [36].
(2) A Swedish study that recruited a sample of 1913 participants through a web questionnaire, 7.6% reported some Internet sexual problem and 4.5% indicated feeling 'addicted' to Internet for love and sexual purposes, and that this was a 'big problem' [17].
(3) A Spanish study with a sample of 1557 college students found that 8.6% was in a potential risk of developing a pathological usage of online pornography, but that the actual pathological user prevalence was 0.7% [37].

The only study with a representative sample to date is an Australian one, with a sample of 20,094 participants; 1.2% of the women surveyed considered themselves addicted, whereas for the men it was 4.4% [38]. Similar findings also apply to hypersexual behavior outside of pornography [39].

Predictors for problematic sexual behavior and pornography use are, across populations: being a man, young age, religiousness, frequent Internet use, negative mood states, and being prone to sexual boredom, and novelty seeking [17,37,40,41]. Some of this risk factors are also shared by hypersexual behavior patients [39,42].

3.2. Ethiopathogenical and Diagnostic Conceptualization

Conceptualizing pathological behaviors continues to be a challenge today. While several attempts have been made regarding hypersexual behavior, the lack of robust data as of now explains the fact that there's no consensus on this matter [9]. POPU comprises a very specific set of sexual behaviors that involve technology. Due to problematic technology use (especially online technology) being relatively recent, we need first to talk about hypersexual behavior not related to technology in order to understand the place of online pornography in it.

Sexuality as a behavior is vastly heterogeneous, and its potential pathological side has been studied for centuries [43]. Therefore, it represents a challenge to models trying to adequately define it, since it can incorporate practices ranging from solitary fantasizing to sexual violence [21]. It is also difficult to define what constitutes an actual dysfunction and manage to avoid the possible misuse of that definition to stigmatize and pathologize individuals [44]. For example, some set the limit between normal and pathological sexual behavior at more than seven orgasms in a week [43] (p. 381), but this approach focusing on quantity can be dangerous, since what constitutes normal and pathological behavior can vastly vary between individuals. This lack of uniformity and consistency in its classification may hinder future research on investigating hypersexual behavior [45] and ignore the quality aspects that focus on the negative emotions associated with it [46,47]. There have been proposals to redeem this issue using certain tools, already developed as part of the hypersexual disorder proposal used in the DSM-5 field trial [43,47].

Hypersexuality generally acts as an umbrella construct [7]. Its nomenclature is still a matter of debate to this day, and it is frequent to encounter several terms that refer to the same concept: compulsive sexual behavior, sex addiction, sexual impulsivity, hypersexual behavior or hypersexual disorder. Some authors, while recognizing the value of the terms "addiction" and "compulsivity", prefer to draw attention to the issue of control and its possible loss or compromise as the primary concern about this behavior, thus referring to it as "out of control sexual behavior" [45,48,49].

Although definitions are not uniform, they usually focus on the frequency or intensity of symptoms [46] of otherwise normal urges and fantasies, that would result in dysfunction. This differentiates it from paraphilic sexual behavior, though the need for a better clarification of possible differences, similarities, and overlap between the two types still persists [45].

Usually included in hypersexual behavior are excessive masturbation and various sexual related behaviors, like dependence on anonymous sexual encounters, repetitive promiscuity, internet pornography, telephone sex, and visiting strip clubs [43,44,49–51]. Bancroft particularly thought that, in using Internet, both masturbation and these sexual activities could blend themselves, stating that men "use it as an almost limitless extension of their out of control masturbatory behavior".

While the possibility to diagnose hypersexual behavior was always available with "sexual disorder not otherwise specified" in the DSM [1], Kafka [43] tried to propose it as a diagnostic entity for the DSM-5. He presented a set of criteria for it, as part of the sexual disorders chapter. These proposed models included hypersexual behavior as: (1) sexually motivated, (2) a behavioral addiction, (3) part of the obsessive-compulsive spectrum disorder, (4) part of the impulsivity-spectrum disorders, and (5) an "out of control" excessive sexual behavior. This proposal was ultimately rejected due to several reasons; the main was said to be absence of consolidated epidemiological and neuroimaging data regarding this behavior [52,53], but also its potential for forensic abuse, a not specific enough set of diagnostic criteria, and potential politic and social ramifications of pathologizing an integral area of behavior to human life [54]. It is interesting to compare it to the other two previous set of criteria present in the reviewed literature, those of Patrick Carnes and Aviel Goodman [9]. All three share the concepts of loss of control, excessive time spent on sexual behavior and negative consequences to self/others, but diverge on the other elements. This reflects in broad strokes the lack of consensus in conceptualizing hypersexual behavior across the years. Currently, the main options propose hypersexual behavior either as an impulse control disorder or a behavioral addiction [55].

From an impulse control disorder perspective, hypersexual behavior is generally referred to as Compulsive Sexual Behavior (CSB). Coleman [56] is a proponent of this theory. While he includes paraphilic behavior under this term [57], and they may coexist in some cases, he distinctly differentiates it from nonparaphilic CSB, which is what we want to focus on in this review. Interestingly, nonparaphilic hypersexual behavior is usually as frequent, if not more, than some paraphilias [43,58].

However, more recent definitions of CSB usually refer to multiple sexual behaviors that can be compulsive: the most commonly reported being masturbation, being followed by compulsive use of pornography, and promiscuity, compulsive cruising, and multiple relationships (22–76%) [9,59,60].

While there are definite overlaps between hypersexuality and conditions such as obsessive-compulsive disorder (OCD) and other impulse control disorders [61], there are also some notable differences pointed out: for example, OCD behaviors do not involve reward, unlike sexual behavior. Moreover, while engaging in compulsions might result in temporary relief for OCD patients [62], hypersexual behavior is usually associated by guilt and regret after committing the act [63]. Also, the impulsivity that can sometimes dominate the patient's behavior is incompatible with the careful planning that is sometimes required in CSB (for example, in regards to a sexual encounter) [64].

Goodman thinks that addiction disorders lie at the intersection of compulsive disorders (which involve anxiety reduction) and impulsive disorders (which involve gratification), with the symptoms being underpinned by neurobiological mechanisms (serotoninergic, dopaminergic, noradrenergic, and opioid systems) [65]. Stein agrees with a model combining several ethiopathogenical mechanisms and proposes an A-B-C model (affective dysregulation, behavioral addiction, and cognitive dyscontrol) to study this entity [61].

From an addictive behavior standpoint, hypersexual behavior relies on sharing core aspects of addiction. These aspects, according to the DSM-5 [1], refer to the mentioned problematic consumption model applied to hypersexual behavior, both offline and online [6,66,67]. Evidence of tolerance and withdrawal in these patients might probably be key in characterizing this entity as an addictive disorder [45]. Problematic use of cybersex is also often conceptualized as a behavioral addiction [13,68].

The term "addiction" applying to this entity is still subject to great debate. Zitzman considers that the resistance to use the term addiction is "more a reflection of cultural sexual liberality and permissiveness than any lack of symptomatic and diagnostic correspondence with other forms of addiction" [69]. However, the term needs to be used with caution, since it can be interpreted as a justification for an irresponsible search for gratification and hedonist pleasure, and blame the disruptive consequences on it.

There has long been a debate between Patrick Carnes and Eli Coleman over the diagnostics of hypersexual behavior. Coleman has considered hypersexuality to be driven by the need to reduce some type of anxiety, not by sexual desire [56] having classified it in seven subtypes (one of them being use of online pornography) [57], while Carnes (who defined addiction as "a pathological relationship with a mood altering experience") finds similitudes to other behavioral addictions like gambling, focusing on the loss of control and continued behavior despite negative consequences [70].

A thorough review of the literature by Kraus [71], concluded that despite these similitudes, significant gaps in the concept's understanding complicate its classification as an addiction. The main concerns are aimed towards quantity of large-scale prevalence, longitudinal and clinical data (defining main symptoms and its diagnostic limits), supported by neuropsychological, neurobiological, and genetic data, as well as some information regarding possible treatment screening and prevention, and points to digital technology in hypersexual behavior as a key point for future research.

The rise of the Internet increases the possibilities for sexual interactions, and not just online pornography (webcamming, casual sex websites). Even whether Internet use represents a conduit for other types of repetitive behavior (e.g., sexual behavior or gambling) or constitutes a different entity in its own right is still debated [72]. Nevertheless, if the case is the former, the previous evidence and considerations could very well apply to its online counterpart.

There is currently a need for empirically derived criteria that takes into account unique factors characterizing online (versus offline) sexual behaviors, since most of them do not have an offline version that can be compared to [73]. So far, there have been mentions of new phenomena when dealing with online sexual behavior, like the presence of online dissociation [74], which causes to "be mentally and emotionally detached when engaged, with compromised time and depersonalization". This dissociation has already been described in relation to other online activities [75], which supports the notion that cybersex problematic use could be related to both internet and sex addiction [76].

Finally, we have to mention that a diagnostic entity called "compulsive sexual behavior disorder" is being included in the upcoming definitive edition of ICD-11, in the "impulse control disorders" chapter [77]. The definition can be consulted at https://icd.who.int/dev11/l-m/en#/http%3a%2f%2fid.who.int%2ficd%2fentity%2f1630268048.

The inclusion of this category in the ICD-11 may be a response to the relevance of this issue and attest to its clinical utility, whereas the growing but yet inconclusive data prevents us from properly categorizing it as a mental health disorder [72]. It is believed to provide a better tool (yet in refinement process) for addressing the needs of treatment seeking patients and the possible guilt associated [78], and also may reflect the ongoing debates regarding the most appropriate classification of CSB and its limited amount of data in some areas [55,71] (Table 1). This inclusion could be the first step towards recognizing this issue and expanding on it, one key point being undoubtedly its online pornography subtype.

Table 1. DSM-5 and ICD-11 approaches to classifying hypersexual behavior.

	DSM-5	ICD-11
Goal	Provide common research and clinical language for mental health problems	Reflect issues of clinical utility in a broad range of settings, global applicability, and scientific validity [79]
Conceptualization of hypersexual disorder	Addiction model	Impulse control model
Available diagnosis	No current hypersexual disorder diagnosis, due to insufficient evidence to categorize it as addiction	Compulsive sexual behavior disorder

3.3. Clinical Manifestations

Clinical manifestations of POPU can be summed up in three key points:

- Erectile dysfunction: while some studies have found little evidence of the association between pornography use and sexual dysfunction [33], others propose that the rise in pornography use may be the key factor explaining the sharp rise in erectile dysfunction among young people [80]. In one study, 60% of patients who suffered sexual dysfunction with a real partner, characteristically did not have this problem with pornography [8]. Some argue that causation between pornography use and sexual dysfunction is difficult to establish, since true controls not exposed to pornography are rare to find [81] and have proposed a possible research design in this regard.
- Psychosexual dissatisfaction: pornography use has been associated with sexual dissatisfaction and sexual dysfunction, for both males and females [82], being more critical of one's body or their partner's, increased performance pressure and less actual sex [83], having more sexual partners and engaging in paid sex behavior [34]. This impact is especially noted in relationships when it is one sided [84], in a very similar way to marijuana use, sharing key factors like higher secrecy [85]. These studies are based on regular non-pathological pornography use, but online pornography may not have harmful effects by itself, only when it has become an addiction [24]. This can explain the relationship between the use of female-centric pornography and more positive outcomes for women [86].
- Comorbidities: hypersexual behavior has been associated with anxiety disorder, followed by mood disorder, substance use disorder and sexual dysfunction [87]. These findings also apply to POPU [88], also being associated with smoking, drinking alcohol or coffee, substance abuse [41] and problematic video-game use [89,90].

Having some very specific pornographic content interests has been associated with an increase in reported problems [17]. It has been debated if these clinical features are the consequence of direct cybersex abuse or due to the subjects actually perceiving themselves as addicts [91].

3.4. Neurobiological Evidence Supporting Addiction Model

Collecting evidence about POPU is an arduous process; main data on this subject is still limited by small sample sizes, solely male heterosexual samples and cross-sectional designs [71], with not enough neuroimaging and neuropsychological studies [4], probably due to conceptual, financial and logistic obstacles. In addition, while substance addiction can be observed and modeled in experimental animals, we cannot do this with a candidate behavioral addiction; this may limit our study of its neurobiological underpinnings [72]. Current knowledge gaps regarding the research of hypersexual behavior, as well as possible approaches for addressing them, are expertly covered and summarized in Kraus' article [71]. Most of the studies found in our research pertain hypersexual behavior, with pornography being only one of its accounted accessories.

This evidence is based on an evolving understanding of the neural process among addiction-related neuroplasticity changes. Dopamine levels play an important part in this sexual reward stimuli, as observed already in frontotemporal dementia and pro-dopaminergic medication in Parkinson's disease being linked with sexual behavior [92,93].

The addictive process with online pornography may be amplified by the accelerated novelty and the "supranormal stimulus" (term coined by Nobel prize winner Nikolaas Tinbergen) that constitutes Internet pornography [94]. This phenomenon would supposedly make artificial stimuli (in this case, pornography in the way it is mostly consumed today, its online form) override an evolutionarily developed genetic response. The theory is that they potentially activate our natural reward system at higher levels than what ancestors typically encountered as our brains evolved, making it liable to switch into an addictive mode [2]. If we consider online porn from this perspective, we can start seeing similarities to regular substance addicts.

Major brain changes observed across substance addicts lay the groundwork for the future research of addictive behaviors [95], including:

1. Sensitization [96]
2. Desensitization [97]
3. Dysfunctional prefrontal circuits (hypofrontality) [98]
4. Malfunctioning stress system [99]

These brain changes observed in addicts have been linked with patients with hypersexual behavior or pornography users through approximately 40 studies of different types: magnetic resonance imaging, electroencephalography (EEG), neuroendocrine, and neuropsychological.

For example, there are clear differences in brain activity between patients who have compulsive sexual behavior and controls, which mirror those of drug addicts. When exposed to sexual images, hypersexual subjects have shown differences between liking (in line with controls) and wanting (sexual desire), which was greater [8,100]. In other words, in these subjects there is more desire only for the specific sexual cue, but not generalized sexual desire. This points us to the sexual cue itself being then perceived as a reward [46].

Evidence of this neural activity signaling desire is particularly prominent in the prefrontal cortex [101] and the amygdala [102,103], being evidence of sensitization. Activation in these brain regions is reminiscent of financial reward [104] and it may carry a similar impact. Moreover, there are higher EEG readings in these users, as well as the diminished desire for sex with a partner, but not for masturbation to pornography [105], something that reflects also on the difference in erection quality [8]. This can be considered a sign of desensitization. However, Steele's study contains several methodological flaws to consider (subject heterogeneity, a lack of screening for mental disorders or addictions, the absence of a control group, and the use of questionnaires not validated for porn use) [106]. A study by Prause [107], this time with a control group, replicated these very findings. The role of cue reactivity and craving in the development of cybersex addiction have been corroborated in heterosexual female [108] and homosexual male samples [109].

This attentional bias to sexual cues is predominant in early hypersexual individuals [110], but a repeated exposure to them shows in turn desensitization [111,112]. This means a downregulation of reward systems, possibly mediated by the greater dorsal cingulate [107,113,114]. Since the dorsal cingulate is involved in anticipating rewards and responding to new events, a decrease in its activity after repeated exposure points us to the development of habituation to previous stimuli. This results in a dysfunctional enhanced preference for sexual novelty [115], which may manifest as attempts to overcome said habituation and desensitization through the search for more (new) pornography as a means of sexual satisfaction, choosing this behavior instead of actual sex [20].

These attempts at novelty seeking may be mediated through ventral striatal reactivity [116] and the amygdala [117]. It is known that the viewing of pornography in frequent users has also been associated with greater neural activity [99], especially in the ventral striatum [116,118] which plays a major role in anticipating rewards [119].

However, connectivity between ventral striatum and prefrontal cortex is decreased [103,113]; a decrease in connectivity between prefrontal cortex and the amygdala has also been observed [117]. In addition, hypersexual subjects have shown reduced functional connectivity between caudate and temporal cortex lobes, as well as gray matter deficit in these areas [120]. All of these alterations could explain the inability to control sexual behavior impulses.

Moreover, hypersexual subjects showed an increased volume of the amygdala [117], in contrast to those with a chronic exposure to a substance, which show a decreased amygdala volume [121]; this difference could be explained by the possible neurotoxic effect of the substance. In hypersexual subjects, increased activity and volume may reflect overlapping with addiction processes (particularly supporting incentive motivation theories) or be the consequence to chronic social stress mechanisms, such as the behavioral addiction itself [122].

These users also have shown a dysfunctional stress response, mainly mediated through the hypothalamus–pituitary–adrenal axis [122] in a way that mirror those alterations seen in substance addicts. These alterations may be the result of epigenetic changes on classic inflammatory mediators driving addictions, like corticotropin-releasing-factor (CRF) [123]. This epigenetic regulation hypothesis considers both hedonic and anhedonic behavioral outcomes are at least partially affected by dopaminergic genes, and possibly other candidate neurotransmitter-related gene polymorphisms [124]. There is also evidence of higher tumor necrosis factor (TNF) in sex addicts, with a strong correlation between TNF levels and high scores in hypersexuality rating scales [125].

3.5. Neuropsychological Evidence

In regard to the manifestations of these alterations in sexual behavior, most neuropsychological studies show some kind of indirect or direct consequence in executive function [126,127], possibly as a consequence of prefrontal cortex alterations [128]. When applied to online pornography, it contributes to its development and maintenance [129,130].

The specifics of this poorer executive functioning include: impulsivity [131,132], cognitive rigidity that impedes learning processes or the ability to shift attention [120,133,134], poor judgment and decision making [130,135], interference of working memory capacity [130], deficits in emotion regulation, and excessive preoccupation with sex [136]. These findings are reminiscent of other behavioral addictions (such as pathological gambling) and the behavior in substance dependencies [137]. Some studies directly contradict these findings [58], but there may be some limitations in methodology (for example, small sample size).

Approaching the factors that play a role in the development of hypersexual behavior and cybersex, there are a number of them. We can think of cue-reactivity, positive reinforcement and associative learning [104,109,136,138,139] as the core mechanisms of porn addiction development. However, there may be factors of underlying vulnerability [140], like: (1) the role of sexual gratification and dysfunctional coping in some predisposed individuals [40,141–143] whether it is a consequence of trait impulsivity [144,145] or state impulsivity [146], and (2) approach/avoidance tendencies [147–149].

3.6. Prognosis

Most of the studies referenced use subjects with a long-term exposure to online pornography [34,81,113,114], so its clinical manifestations appear to be a direct and proportional consequence of engaging in this maladaptive behavior. We mentioned difficulty in obtaining controls to establish causation, but some case reports suggest that reducing or abandoning this behavior may cause improvement in pornography-induced sexual dysfunction and psychosexual dissatisfaction [79,80] and even full recovery; this would imply that the previously mentioned brain alterations are somewhat reversible.

3.7. Assessment Tools

Several screening instruments exist for addressing CSB and POPU. They all rely on the responder's honesty and integrity; perhaps even more so than regular psychiatry screening tests, since sexual practices are the most humbling due to their private nature.

For hypersexuality, there are over 20 screening questionnaires and clinical interviews. Some of the most notable include the Sexual Addiction Screening Test (SAST) proposed by Carnes [150], and its later revised version SAST-R [151], the Compulsive Sexual Behavior Inventory (CSBI) [152,153] and the Hypersexual Disorder Screening Inventory (HDSI) [154]. The HDSI was originally used for the clinical screening of the DSM-5 field proposal of hypersexual disorder. While further explorations of the empirical implications regarding criteria and the refinements of cutoff scores are needed, it currently holds the strongest psychometric support and is the best valid instrument in measuring hypersexual disorder [151].

As for online pornography, the most used screening tool is the Internet Sex-screening test (ISST) [155]. It assesses five distinct dimensions (online sexual compulsivity, online sexual behavior-social, online sexual behavior-isolated, online sexual spending and interest in online sexual behavior) through 25 dichotomic (yes/no) questions. However, its psychometric properties haven only been mildly analyzed, with a more robust validation in Spanish [156] that has served as a blueprint for posterior studies [157].

Other notable instruments are the problematic pornography use scale (PPUS) [158] which measures four facets of POPU (including: distress and functional problems, excessive use, control difficulties and use for escape/avoidance of negative emotions), the short internet addiction test adapted to online sexual activities (s-IAT-sex) [159], a 12-item questionnaire measuring two dimensions of POPU, and the cyber-pornography use inventory (CPUI-9) [160].

The CPUI-9 evaluates three dimensions: (1) access efforts, (2) perceived compulsivity, and (3) emotional distress. At first considered to have convincing psychometric properties [9], this inventory has more recently proved to be unreliable: the inclusion of the "emotional distress" dimension address levels of shame and guilt, which do not belong in an addiction assessment and thus skews the scores upward [161]. Applying the inventory without this dimension appears to accurately reflect to some extent compulsive pornography use.

One of the most recent is the pornographic problematic consumption scale (PPCS) [162], based on Griffith six-component addiction model [163], though it does not measure addiction, only problematic use of pornography with strong psychometric properties.

Other measures of POPU that are not designed to measure online pornography use but have been validated using online pornography users [9], include the Pornography Consumption Inventory (PCI) [164,165], the Compulsive Pornography Consumption Scale (CPCS) [166] and the Pornography Craving Questionnaire (PCQ) [167] which can assess contextual triggers among different types of pornography user.

There are also tools for assessing pornography users' readiness to abandon the behavior through self-initiated strategies [168] and an assessment of treatment outcome in doing so [169], identifying in particular three potential relapse motivations: (a) sexual arousal/boredom/opportunity, (b) intoxication/locations/easy access, and (c) negative emotions.

3.8. Treatment

Given that still many questions remain regarding the conceptualization, assessment, and causes of hypersexual behavior and POPU, there have been relatively few attempts to research possible treatment options. In published studies, sample sizes are usually small and too homogeneous, clinical controls are lacking, and the research methods are scattered, unverifiable, and not replicable [170].

Usually, combining psychosocial, cognitive–behavioral, psychodynamic, and pharmacologic methods is considered most efficient in treatment of sexual addiction, but this non-specific approach reflects the lack of knowledge about the subject [9].

3.8.1. Pharmacological Approaches

The studies have centered on paroxetine and naltrexone thus far. One case series involving paroxetine on POPU helped to decrease the anxiety levels, but eventually failed to reduce the behavior by itself [171]. Additionally, using SSRIs to create sexual dysfunction through their side effects is apparently not effective, and according to clinical experience are useful only in patients with comorbid psychiatric disorders [172].

Four case reports involving naltrexone to treat POPU have been described. Previous findings have suggested that naltrexone could be a potential treatment for behavioral addictions and hypersexual disorder [173,174], theoretically reducing cravings and urges by blocking the euphoria associated with the behavior. While there is not yet a randomized controlled trial with naltrexone in these subjects, there are four case reports. Results obtained in reducing pornography use varied from good [175–177] to moderate [178]; at least in one of them the patient also received sertraline, so it is unclear how much can be attributed to naltrexone [176].

3.8.2. Psychotherapeutic Approaches

Undoubtedly, psychotherapy can be an important tool in fully comprehending and changing a behavior. While cognitive-behavioral therapy (CBT) is considered by many clinicians to be useful in treating hypersexual disorder [179], a study that involved problematic online pornography users failed to achieve a reduction of the behavior [180], even if the severity of comorbid depressive symptoms and general quality of life was improved. This brings up the interest notion that merely reducing pornography use may not represent the most important treatment goal [170]. Other approaches using CBT to treat POPU have been made, but reoccurring methodological problems in this area prevent us from extracting reliable conclusions [181,182].

Psychodynamic psychotherapy and others like family therapy, couples' therapy, and psychosocial treatments modeled after 12 step programs may prove vital when addressing themes of shame and guilt and restoring trust among the users' closest relationships [170,172]. The only randomized controlled trial that exists with problematic online pornography users focuses on Acceptance and Commitment Therapy (ACT) [183], an improvement from their 2010 case series [184], which was the first experimental study to specifically address POPU. The study showed effective results but it is hard to extrapolate since the sample was again too small and focused on a very specific population.

The reported success with CBT, conjoint therapy and ACT might rely on the fact that are based on mindfulness and acceptance frameworks; depending on the context, increasing pornography use acceptance may be equally or more important than reducing its use [170].

4. Discussion

It seems that POPU is not only one subtype of hypersexual disorder, but currently the most prevalent since it also frequently involves masturbation. Although this is difficult to accurately determine given the anonymity and accessibility factors that make pornography use today so pervasive, we can at least confirm that the patron of consumption for pornography has changed for roughly the last decade. It would not be absurd to assume its online variant has had a significant impact on its consumers, and that the triple A factors enhance the potential risk for POPU and other sexual behaviors.

As we mentioned, anonymity is a key risk factor for this sexual behavior to develop into a problem. We need to keep in mind that statistics regarding this problem are obviously limited to people of legal age to engage in sexual activity, online or otherwise; but it does not escape us that sexual activity rarely starts after this threshold, and there is a likely chance that minors still in the process of sexual neurodevelopment are a particularly vulnerable population. The truth is that a stronger consensus on what pathological sexual behavior constitutes, both offline and online, is necessary to adequately measure it in a representative manner and confirm how much of a problem it is in today's society.

As far as we know, a number of recent studies support this entity as an addiction with important clinical manifestations such as sexual dysfunction and psychosexual dissatisfaction. Most of the existing work is based off on similar research done on substance addicts, based on the hypothesis of online pornography as a 'supranormal stimulus' akin to an actual substance that, through continued consumption, can spark an addictive disorder. However, concepts like tolerance and abstinence are not yet clearly established enough to merit the labeling of addiction, and thus constitute a crucial part of future research. For the moment, a diagnostic entity encompassing out of control sexual behavior has been included in the ICD-11 due to its current clinical relevance, and it will surely be of use to address patients with these symptoms that ask clinicians for help.

A variety of assessment tools exist to help the average clinician with diagnostic approaches, but delimiting what is truly pathological and not in accurate manner is still an ongoing problem. So far, a crucial part of the three sets of criteria proposed by Carnes, Goodman, and Kafka include core concepts of loss of control, excessive time spent on sexual behavior and negative consequences to self and others. In some manner or other, they are also present in the majority of screening tools reviewed.

They may be an adequate structure in which to build upon. Other elements, that are considered with varying degrees of importance, probably signal us to take individual factors into account. Devising an assessment tool that retains some level of flexibility while also being significant for determining what is problematic is surely another of the current challenges that we face, and will probably go in hand with further neurobiological research that help us better understand when a specific dimension of common human life shifts from normal behavior to a disorder.

As for treatment strategies, the main goal currently focuses on reducing pornography consumption or abandoning it altogether, since clinical manifestations appear to be reversible. The way to achieve this varies accordingly to the patient and might also require some individual flexibility in the strategies utilized, with a mindfulness and acceptance-based psychotherapy being equally or more important than a pharmacological approach in some cases.

Funding: This research received no external funding.

Conflicts of Interest: Rubén de Alarcón, Javier I. de la Iglesia, and Nerea M. Casado declare no conflict of interest. A.L. Montejo has received consultancy fees or honoraria/research grants in the last five years from Boehringer Ingelheim, Forum Pharmaceuticals, Rovi, Servier, Lundbeck, Otsuka, Janssen Cilag, Pfizer, Roche, Instituto de Salud Carlos III, and Junta de Castilla y León.

References

1. American Psychiatry Association. *Manual Diagnóstico y Estadístico de los Trastornos Mentales*, 5th ed.; Panamericana: Madrid, España, 2014; pp. 585–589. ISBN 978-84-9835-810-0.
2. Love, T.; Laier, C.; Brand, M.; Hatch, L.; Hajela, R. Neuroscience of Internet Pornography Addiction: A Review and Update. *Behav. Sci. (Basel)* **2015**, *5*, 388–433. [CrossRef] [PubMed]
3. Elmquist, J.; Shorey, R.C.; Anderson, S.; Stuart, G.L. A preliminary investigation of the relationship between early maladaptive schemas and compulsive sexual behaviors in a substance-dependent population. *J. Subst. Use* **2016**, *21*, 349–354. [CrossRef] [PubMed]
4. Chamberlain, S.R.; Lochner, C.; Stein, D.J.; Goudriaan, A.E.; van Holst, R.J.; Zohar, J.; Grant, J.E. Behavioural addiction-A rising tide? *Eur. Neuropsychopharmacol.* **2016**, *26*, 841–855. [CrossRef] [PubMed]
5. Blum, K.; Badgaiyan, R.D.; Gold, M.S. Hypersexuality Addiction and Withdrawal: Phenomenology, Neurogenetics and Epigenetics. *Cureus* **2015**, *7*, e348. [CrossRef] [PubMed]
6. Duffy, A.; Dawson, D.L.; Nair, R. das Pornography Addiction in Adults: A Systematic Review of Definitions and Reported Impact. *J. Sex. Med.* **2016**, *13*, 760–777. [CrossRef] [PubMed]
7. Karila, L.; Wéry, A.; Weinstein, A.; Cottencin, O.; Petit, A.; Reynaud, M.; Billieux, J. Sexual addiction or hypersexual disorder: Different terms for the same problem? A review of the literature. *Curr. Pharm. Des.* **2014**, *20*, 4012–4020. [CrossRef] [PubMed]

8. Voon, V.; Mole, T.B.; Banca, P.; Porter, L.; Morris, L.; Mitchell, S.; Lapa, T.R.; Karr, J.; Harrison, N.A.; Potenza, M.N.; et al. Neural correlates of sexual cue reactivity in individuals with and without compulsive sexual behaviours. *PLoS ONE* **2014**, *9*, e102419. [CrossRef]
9. Wéry, A.; Billieux, J. Problematic cybersex: Conceptualization, assessment, and treatment. *Addict. Behav.* **2017**, *64*, 238–246. [CrossRef]
10. Garcia, F.D.; Thibaut, F. Sexual addictions. *Am. J. Drug Alcohol Abuse* **2010**, *36*, 254–260. [CrossRef]
11. Davis, R.A. A cognitive-behavioral model of pathological Internet use. *Comput. Hum. Behav.* **2001**, *17*, 187–195. [CrossRef]
12. Ioannidis, K.; Treder, M.S.; Chamberlain, S.R.; Kiraly, F.; Redden, S.A.; Stein, D.J.; Lochner, C.; Grant, J.E. Problematic internet use as an age-related multifaceted problem: Evidence from a two-site survey. *Addict. Behav.* **2018**, *81*, 157–166. [CrossRef] [PubMed]
13. Cooper, A.; Delmonico, D.L.; Griffin-Shelley, E.; Mathy, R.M. Online Sexual Activity: An Examination of Potentially Problematic Behaviors. *Sex. Addict. Compuls.* **2004**, *11*, 129–143. [CrossRef]
14. Döring, N.M. The internet's impact on sexuality: A critical review of 15 years of research. *Comput. Hum. Behav.* **2009**, *25*, 1089–1101. [CrossRef]
15. Fisher, W.A.; Barak, A. Internet Pornography: A Social Psychological Perspective on Internet Sexuality. *J. Sex. Res.* **2001**, *38*, 312–323. [CrossRef]
16. Janssen, E.; Carpenter, D.; Graham, C.A. Selecting films for sex research: Gender differences in erotic film preference. *Arch. Sex. Behav.* **2003**, *32*, 243–251. [CrossRef] [PubMed]
17. Ross, M.W.; Månsson, S.-A.; Daneback, K. Prevalence, severity, and correlates of problematic sexual Internet use in Swedish men and women. *Arch. Sex. Behav.* **2012**, *41*, 459–466. [CrossRef] [PubMed]
18. Riemersma, J.; Sytsma, M. A New Generation of Sexual Addiction. *Sex. Addict. Compuls.* **2013**, *20*, 306–322. [CrossRef]
19. Beyens, I.; Eggermont, S. Prevalence and Predictors of Text-Based and Visually Explicit Cybersex among Adolescents. *Young* **2014**, *22*, 43–65. [CrossRef]
20. Rosenberg, H.; Kraus, S. The relationship of "passionate attachment" for pornography with sexual compulsivity, frequency of use, and craving for pornography. *Addict. Behav.* **2014**, *39*, 1012–1017. [CrossRef]
21. Keane, H. Technological change and sexual disorder. *Addiction* **2016**, *111*, 2108–2109. [CrossRef]
22. Cooper, A. Sexuality and the Internet: Surfing into the New Millennium. *CyberPsychol. Behav.* **1998**, *1*, 187–193. [CrossRef]
23. Cooper, A.; Scherer, C.R.; Boies, S.C.; Gordon, B.L. Sexuality on the Internet: From sexual exploration to pathological expression. *Prof. Psychol. Res. Pract.* **1999**, *30*, 154–164. [CrossRef]
24. Harper, C.; Hodgins, D.C. Examining Correlates of Problematic Internet Pornography Use Among University Students. *J. Behav. Addict.* **2016**, *5*, 179–191. [CrossRef] [PubMed]
25. Pornhub Insights: 2017 Year in Review. Available online: https://www.pornhub.com/insights/2017-year-in-review (accessed on 15 April 2018).
26. Litras, A.; Latreille, S.; Temple-Smith, M. Dr Google, porn and friend-of-a-friend: Where are young men really getting their sexual health information? *Sex. Health* **2015**, *12*, 488–494. [CrossRef] [PubMed]
27. Zimbardo, P.; Wilson, G.; Coulombe, N. How Porn Is Messing with Your Manhood. Available online: https://www.skeptic.com/reading_room/how-porn-is-messing-with-your-manhood/ (accessed on 25 March 2018).
28. Pizzol, D.; Bertoldo, A.; Foresta, C. Adolescents and web porn: A new era of sexuality. *Int. J. Adolesc. Med. Health* **2016**, *28*, 169–173. [CrossRef] [PubMed]
29. Prins, J.; Blanker, M.H.; Bohnen, A.M.; Thomas, S.; Bosch, J.L.H.R. Prevalence of erectile dysfunction: A systematic review of population-based studies. *Int. J. Impot. Res.* **2002**, *14*, 422–432. [CrossRef] [PubMed]
30. Mialon, A.; Berchtold, A.; Michaud, P.-A.; Gmel, G.; Suris, J.-C. Sexual dysfunctions among young men: Prevalence and associated factors. *J. Adolesc. Health* **2012**, *51*, 25–31. [CrossRef]
31. O'Sullivan, L.F.; Brotto, L.A.; Byers, E.S.; Majerovich, J.A.; Wuest, J.A. Prevalence and characteristics of sexual functioning among sexually experienced middle to late adolescents. *J. Sex. Med.* **2014**, *11*, 630–641. [CrossRef]
32. Wilcox, S.L.; Redmond, S.; Hassan, A.M. Sexual functioning in military personnel: Preliminary estimates and predictors. *J. Sex. Med.* **2014**, *11*, 2537–2545. [CrossRef]

33. Landripet, I.; Štulhofer, A. Is Pornography Use Associated with Sexual Difficulties and Dysfunctions among Younger Heterosexual Men? *J. Sex. Med.* **2015**, *12*, 1136–1139. [CrossRef]
34. Wright, P.J. U.S. males and pornography, 1973–2010: Consumption, predictors, correlates. *J. Sex. Res.* **2013**, *50*, 60–71. [CrossRef] [PubMed]
35. Price, J.; Patterson, R.; Regnerus, M.; Walley, J. How Much More XXX is Generation X Consuming? Evidence of Changing Attitudes and Behaviors Related to Pornography Since 1973. *J. Sex Res.* **2015**, *53*, 1–9. [CrossRef] [PubMed]
36. Najavits, L.; Lung, J.; Froias, A.; Paull, N.; Bailey, G. A study of multiple behavioral addictions in a substance abuse sample. *Subst. Use Misuse* **2014**, *49*, 479–484. [CrossRef] [PubMed]
37. Ballester-Arnal, R.; Castro Calvo, J.; Gil-Llario, M.D.; Gil-Julia, B. Cybersex Addiction: A Study on Spanish College Students. *J. Sex. Marital Ther.* **2017**, *43*, 567–585. [CrossRef] [PubMed]
38. Rissel, C.; Richters, J.; de Visser, R.O.; McKee, A.; Yeung, A.; Caruana, T. A Profile of Pornography Users in Australia: Findings From the Second Australian Study of Health and Relationships. *J. Sex. Res.* **2017**, *54*, 227–240. [CrossRef] [PubMed]
39. Skegg, K.; Nada-Raja, S.; Dickson, N.; Paul, C. Perceived "Out of Control" Sexual Behavior in a Cohort of Young Adults from the Dunedin Multidisciplinary Health and Development Study. *Arch. Sex. Behav.* **2010**, *39*, 968–978. [CrossRef] [PubMed]
40. Štulhofer, A.; Jurin, T.; Briken, P. Is High Sexual Desire a Facet of Male Hypersexuality? Results from an Online Study. *J. Sex. Marital Ther.* **2016**, *42*, 665–680. [CrossRef]
41. Frangos, C.C.; Frangos, C.C.; Sotiropoulos, I. Problematic Internet Use among Greek university students: An ordinal logistic regression with risk factors of negative psychological beliefs, pornographic sites, and online games. *Cyberpsychol. Behav. Soc. Netw.* **2011**, *14*, 51–58. [CrossRef]
42. Farré, J.M.; Fernández-Aranda, F.; Granero, R.; Aragay, N.; Mallorquí-Bague, N.; Ferrer, V.; More, A.; Bouman, W.P.; Arcelus, J.; Savvidou, L.G.; et al. Sex addiction and gambling disorder: Similarities and differences. *Compr. Psychiatry* **2015**, *56*, 59–68. [CrossRef]
43. Kafka, M.P. Hypersexual disorder: A proposed diagnosis for DSM-V. *Arch. Sex. Behav.* **2010**, *39*, 377–400. [CrossRef]
44. Kaplan, M.S.; Krueger, R.B. Diagnosis, assessment, and treatment of hypersexuality. *J. Sex. Res.* **2010**, *47*, 181–198. [CrossRef] [PubMed]
45. Reid, R.C. Additional challenges and issues in classifying compulsive sexual behavior as an addiction. *Addiction* **2016**, *111*, 2111–2113. [CrossRef] [PubMed]
46. Gola, M.; Lewczuk, K.; Skorko, M. What Matters: Quantity or Quality of Pornography Use? Psychological and Behavioral Factors of Seeking Treatment for Problematic Pornography Use. *J. Sex. Med.* **2016**, *13*, 815–824. [CrossRef] [PubMed]
47. Reid, R.C.; Carpenter, B.N.; Hook, J.N.; Garos, S.; Manning, J.C.; Gilliland, R.; Cooper, E.B.; McKittrick, H.; Davtian, M.; Fong, T. Report of findings in a DSM-5 field trial for hypersexual disorder. *J. Sex. Med.* **2012**, *9*, 2868–2877. [CrossRef] [PubMed]
48. Bancroft, J.; Vukadinovic, Z. Sexual addiction, sexual compulsivity, sexual impulsivity, or what? Toward a theoretical model. *J. Sex. Res.* **2004**, *41*, 225–234. [CrossRef]
49. Bancroft, J. Sexual behavior that is "out of control": A theoretical conceptual approach. *Psychiatr. Clin. N. Am.* **2008**, *31*, 593–601. [CrossRef]
50. Stein, D.J.; Black, D.W.; Pienaar, W. Sexual disorders not otherwise specified: Compulsive, addictive, or impulsive? *CNS Spectr.* **2000**, *5*, 60–64. [CrossRef]
51. Kafka, M.P.; Prentky, R.A. Compulsive sexual behavior characteristics. *Am. J. Psychiatry* **1997**, *154*, 1632. [CrossRef]
52. Kafka, M.P. What happened to hypersexual disorder? *Arch. Sex. Behav.* **2014**, *43*, 1259–1261. [CrossRef]
53. Krueger, R.B. Diagnosis of hypersexual or compulsive sexual behavior can be made using ICD-10 and DSM-5 despite rejection of this diagnosis by the American Psychiatric Association. *Addiction* **2016**, *111*, 2110–2111. [CrossRef]
54. Reid, R.; Kafka, M. Controversies about Hypersexual Disorder and the DSM-5. *Curr. Sex. Health Rep.* **2014**, *6*, 259–264. [CrossRef]
55. Kor, A.; Fogel, Y.; Reid, R.C.; Potenza, M.N. Should Hypersexual Disorder be Classified as an Addiction? *Sex. Addict. Compuls.* **2013**, *20*, 27–47. [CrossRef]

56. Coleman, E. Is Your Patient Suffering from Compulsive Sexual Behavior? *Psychiatr. Ann.* **1992**, *22*, 320–325. [CrossRef]
57. Coleman, E.; Raymond, N.; McBean, A. Assessment and treatment of compulsive sexual behavior. *Minn. Med.* **2003**, *86*, 42–47. [PubMed]
58. Kafka, M.P.; Prentky, R. A comparative study of nonparaphilic sexual addictions and paraphilias in men. *J. Clin. Psychiatry* **1992**, *53*, 345–350. [PubMed]
59. Derbyshire, K.L.; Grant, J.E. Compulsive sexual behavior: A review of the literature. *J. Behav. Addict.* **2015**, *4*, 37–43. [CrossRef] [PubMed]
60. Kafka, M.P.; Hennen, J. The paraphilia-related disorders: An empirical investigation of nonparaphilic hypersexuality disorders in outpatient males. *J. Sex. Marital Ther.* **1999**, *25*, 305–319. [CrossRef]
61. Stein, D.J. Classifying hypersexual disorders: Compulsive, impulsive, and addictive models. *Psychiatr. Clin. N. Am.* **2008**, *31*, 587–591. [CrossRef]
62. Lochner, C.; Stein, D.J. Does work on obsessive-compulsive spectrum disorders contribute to understanding the heterogeneity of obsessive-compulsive disorder? *Prog. Neuropsychopharmacol. Biol. Psychiatry* **2006**, *30*, 353–361. [CrossRef]
63. Barth, R.J.; Kinder, B.N. The mislabeling of sexual impulsivity. *J. Sex. Marital Ther.* **1987**, *13*, 15–23. [CrossRef]
64. Stein, D.J.; Chamberlain, S.R.; Fineberg, N. An A-B-C model of habit disorders: Hair-pulling, skin-picking, and other stereotypic conditions. *CNS Spectr.* **2006**, *11*, 824–827. [CrossRef] [PubMed]
65. Goodman, A. Addictive Disorders: An Integrated Approach: Part One-An Integrated Understanding. *J. Minist. Addict. Recover.* **1995**, *2*, 33–76. [CrossRef]
66. Carnes, P.J. Sexual addiction and compulsion: Recognition, treatment, and recovery. *CNS Spectr.* **2000**, *5*, 63–72. [CrossRef] [PubMed]
67. Potenza, M.N. The neurobiology of pathological gambling and drug addiction: An overview and new findings. *Philos. Trans. R. Soc. Lond. B Biol. Sci.* **2008**, *363*, 3181–3189. [CrossRef] [PubMed]
68. Orzack, M.H.; Ross, C.J. Should Virtual Sex Be Treated Like Other Sex Addictions? *Sex. Addict. Compuls.* **2000**, *7*, 113–125. [CrossRef]
69. Zitzman, S.T.; Butler, M.H. Wives' Experience of Husbands' Pornography Use and Concomitant Deception as an Attachment Threat in the Adult Pair-Bond Relationship. *Sex. Addict. Compuls.* **2009**, *16*, 210–240. [CrossRef]
70. Rosenberg, K.P.; O'Connor, S.; Carnes, P. Chapter 9—Sex Addiction: An Overview*. In *Behavioral Addictions*; Rosenberg, K.P., Feder, L.C., Eds.; Academic Press: San Diego, CA, USA, 2014; pp. 215–236, ISBN 978-0-12-407724-9.
71. Kraus, S.W.; Voon, V.; Kor, A.; Potenza, M.N. Searching for clarity in muddy water: Future considerations for classifying compulsive sexual behavior as an addiction. *Addiction* **2016**, *111*, 2113–2114. [CrossRef]
72. Grant, J.E.; Chamberlain, S.R. Expanding the definition of addiction: DSM-5 vs. ICD-11. *CNS Spectr.* **2016**, *21*, 300–303. [CrossRef]
73. Wéry, A.; Karila, L.; De Sutter, P.; Billieux, J. Conceptualisation, évaluation et traitement de la dépendance cybersexuelle: Une revue de la littérature. *Can. Psychol.* **2014**, *55*, 266–281. [CrossRef]
74. Chaney, M.P.; Dew, B.J. Online Experiences of Sexually Compulsive Men Who Have Sex with Men. *Sex. Addict. Compuls.* **2003**, *10*, 259–274. [CrossRef]
75. Schimmenti, A.; Caretti, V. Psychic retreats or psychic pits? Unbearable states of mind and technological addiction. *Psychoanal. Psychol.* **2010**, *27*, 115–132. [CrossRef]
76. Griffiths, M.D. Internet sex addiction: A review of empirical research. *Addict. Res. Theory* **2012**, *20*, 111–124. [CrossRef]
77. Navarro-Cremades, F.; Simonelli, C.; Montejo, A.L. Sexual disorders beyond DSM-5: The unfinished affaire. *Curr. Opin. Psychiatry* **2017**, *30*, 417–422. [CrossRef]
78. Kraus, S.W.; Krueger, R.B.; Briken, P.; First, M.B.; Stein, D.J.; Kaplan, M.S.; Voon, V.; Abdo, C.H.N.; Grant, J.E.; Atalla, E.; et al. Compulsive sexual behaviour disorder in the ICD-11. *World Psychiatry* **2018**, *17*, 109–110. [CrossRef]
79. Hyman, S.E.; Andrews, G.; Ayuso-Mateos, J.L.; Gaebel, W.; Goldberg, D.; Gureje, O.; Jablensky, A.; Khoury, B.; Lovell, A.; Medina Mora, M.E.; et al. A conceptual framework for the revision of the ICD-10 classification of mental and behavioural disorders. *World Psychiatry* **2011**, *10*, 86–92.

80. Park, B.Y.; Wilson, G.; Berger, J.; Christman, M.; Reina, B.; Bishop, F.; Klam, W.P.; Doan, A.P. Is Internet Pornography Causing Sexual Dysfunctions? A Review with Clinical Reports. *Behav. Sci. (Basel)* **2016**, *6*, 17. [CrossRef] [PubMed]
81. Wilson, G. Eliminate Chronic Internet Pornography Use to Reveal Its Effects. *Addicta Turkish J. Addict.* **2016**, *3*, 209–221. [CrossRef]
82. Blais-Lecours, S.; Vaillancourt-Morel, M.-P.; Sabourin, S.; Godbout, N. Cyberpornography: Time Use, Perceived Addiction, Sexual Functioning, and Sexual Satisfaction. *Cyberpsychol. Behav. Soc. Netw.* **2016**, *19*, 649–655. [CrossRef] [PubMed]
83. Albright, J.M. Sex in America online: An exploration of sex, marital status, and sexual identity in internet sex seeking and its impacts. *J. Sex. Res.* **2008**, *45*, 175–186. [CrossRef] [PubMed]
84. Minarcik, J.; Wetterneck, C.T.; Short, M.B. The effects of sexually explicit material use on romantic relationship dynamics. *J. Behav. Addict.* **2016**, *5*, 700–707. [CrossRef]
85. Pyle, T.M.; Bridges, A.J. Perceptions of relationship satisfaction and addictive behavior: Comparing pornography and marijuana use. *J. Behav. Addict.* **2012**, *1*, 171–179. [CrossRef] [PubMed]
86. French, I.M.; Hamilton, L.D. Male-Centric and Female-Centric Pornography Consumption: Relationship With Sex Life and Attitudes in Young Adults. *J. Sex. Marital Ther.* **2018**, *44*, 73–86. [CrossRef] [PubMed]
87. Starcevic, V.; Khazaal, Y. Relationships between Behavioural Addictions and Psychiatric Disorders: What Is Known and What Is Yet to Be Learned? *Front. Psychiatry* **2017**, *8*, 53. [CrossRef] [PubMed]
88. Mitra, M.; Rath, P. Effect of internet on the psychosomatic health of adolescent school children in Rourkela—A cross-sectional study. *Indian J. Child Health* **2017**, *4*, 289–293.
89. Voss, A.; Cash, H.; Hurdiss, S.; Bishop, F.; Klam, W.P.; Doan, A.P. Case Report: Internet Gaming Disorder Associated With Pornography Use. *Yale J. Biol. Med.* **2015**, *88*, 319–324.
90. Stockdale, L.; Coyne, S.M. Video game addiction in emerging adulthood: Cross-sectional evidence of pathology in video game addicts as compared to matched healthy controls. *J. Affect. Disord.* **2018**, *225*, 265–272. [CrossRef]
91. Grubbs, J.B.; Wilt, J.A.; Exline, J.J.; Pargament, K.I. Predicting pornography use over time: Does self-reported "addiction" matter? *Addict. Behav.* **2018**, *82*, 57–64. [CrossRef]
92. Vilas, D.; Pont-Sunyer, C.; Tolosa, E. Impulse control disorders in Parkinson's disease. *Parkinsonism Relat. Disord.* **2012**, *18*, S80–S84. [CrossRef]
93. Poletti, M.; Bonuccelli, U. Impulse control disorders in Parkinson's disease: The role of personality and cognitive status. *J. Neurol.* **2012**, *259*, 2269–2277. [CrossRef]
94. Hilton, D.L. Pornography addiction—A supranormal stimulus considered in the context of neuroplasticity. *Socioaffect. Neurosci. Psychol.* **2013**, *3*, 20767. [CrossRef]
95. Volkow, N.D.; Koob, G.F.; McLellan, A.T. Neurobiologic Advances from the Brain Disease Model of Addiction. *N. Engl. J. Med.* **2016**, *374*, 363–371. [CrossRef] [PubMed]
96. Vanderschuren, L.J.M.J.; Pierce, R.C. Sensitization processes in drug addiction. *Curr. Top. Behav. Neurosci.* **2010**, *3*, 179–195. [CrossRef] [PubMed]
97. Volkow, N.D.; Wang, G.-J.; Fowler, J.S.; Tomasi, D.; Telang, F.; Baler, R. Addiction: Decreased reward sensitivity and increased expectation sensitivity conspire to overwhelm the brain's control circuit. *Bioessays* **2010**, *32*, 748–755. [CrossRef]
98. Goldstein, R.Z.; Volkow, N.D. Dysfunction of the prefrontal cortex in addiction: Neuroimaging findings and clinical implications. *Nat. Rev. Neurosci.* **2011**, *12*, 652–669. [CrossRef]
99. Koob, G.F. Addiction is a Reward Deficit and Stress Surfeit Disorder. *Front. Psychiatry* **2013**, *4*, 72. [CrossRef] [PubMed]
100. Mechelmans, D.J.; Irvine, M.; Banca, P.; Porter, L.; Mitchell, S.; Mole, T.B.; Lapa, T.R.; Harrison, N.A.; Potenza, M.N.; Voon, V. Enhanced attentional bias towards sexually explicit cues in individuals with and without compulsive sexual behaviours. *PLoS ONE* **2014**, *9*, e105476. [CrossRef] [PubMed]
101. Seok, J.-W.; Sohn, J.-H. Neural Substrates of Sexual Desire in Individuals with Problematic Hypersexual Behavior. *Front. Behav. Neurosci.* **2015**, *9*, 321. [CrossRef] [PubMed]
102. Hamann, S. Sex differences in the responses of the human amygdala. *Neuroscientist* **2005**, *11*, 288–293. [CrossRef]

103. Klucken, T.; Wehrum-Osinsky, S.; Schweckendiek, J.; Kruse, O.; Stark, R. Altered Appetitive Conditioning and Neural Connectivity in Subjects with Compulsive Sexual Behavior. *J. Sex. Med.* **2016**, *13*, 627–636. [CrossRef]
104. Sescousse, G.; Caldú, X.; Segura, B.; Dreher, J.-C. Processing of primary and secondary rewards: A quantitative meta-analysis and review of human functional neuroimaging studies. *Neurosci. Biobehav. Rev.* **2013**, *37*, 681–696. [CrossRef]
105. Steele, V.R.; Staley, C.; Fong, T.; Prause, N. Sexual desire, not hypersexuality, is related to neurophysiological responses elicited by sexual images. *Socioaffect. Neurosci. Psychol.* **2013**, *3*, 20770. [CrossRef] [PubMed]
106. Hilton, D.L. 'High desire', or 'merely' an addiction? A response to Steele et al. *Socioaffect. Neurosci. Psychol.* **2014**, *4*. [CrossRef] [PubMed]
107. Prause, N.; Steele, V.R.; Staley, C.; Sabatinelli, D.; Hajcak, G. Modulation of late positive potentials by sexual images in problem users and controls inconsistent with "porn addiction". *Biol. Psychol.* **2015**, *109*, 192–199. [CrossRef] [PubMed]
108. Laier, C.; Pekal, J.; Brand, M. Cybersex addiction in heterosexual female users of internet pornography can be explained by gratification hypothesis. *Cyberpsychol. Behav. Soc. Netw.* **2014**, *17*, 505–511. [CrossRef] [PubMed]
109. Laier, C.; Pekal, J.; Brand, M. Sexual Excitability and Dysfunctional Coping Determine Cybersex Addiction in Homosexual Males. *Cyberpsychol. Behav. Soc. Netw.* **2015**, *18*, 575–580. [CrossRef] [PubMed]
110. Stark, R.; Klucken, T. Neuroscientific Approaches to (Online) Pornography Addiction. In *Internet Addiction*; Studies in Neuroscience, Psychology and Behavioral Economics; Springer: Cham, Switzerland, 2017; pp. 109–124, ISBN 978-3-319-46275-2.
111. Albery, I.P.; Lowry, J.; Frings, D.; Johnson, H.L.; Hogan, C.; Moss, A.C. Exploring the Relationship between Sexual Compulsivity and Attentional Bias to Sex-Related Words in a Cohort of Sexually Active Individuals. *Eur. Addict. Res.* **2017**, *23*, 1–6. [CrossRef] [PubMed]
112. Kunaharan, S.; Halpin, S.; Sitharthan, T.; Bosshard, S.; Walla, P. Conscious and Non-Conscious Measures of Emotion: Do They Vary with Frequency of Pornography Use? *Appl. Sci.* **2017**, *7*, 493. [CrossRef]
113. Kühn, S.; Gallinat, J. Brain Structure and Functional Connectivity Associated with Pornography Consumption: The Brain on Porn. *JAMA Psychiatry* **2014**, *71*, 827–834. [CrossRef]
114. Banca, P.; Morris, L.S.; Mitchell, S.; Harrison, N.A.; Potenza, M.N.; Voon, V. Novelty, conditioning and attentional bias to sexual rewards. *J. Psychiatr. Res.* **2016**, *72*, 91–101. [CrossRef]
115. Banca, P.; Harrison, N.A.; Voon, V. Compulsivity Across the Pathological Misuse of Drug and Non-Drug Rewards. *Front. Behav. Neurosci.* **2016**, *10*, 154. [CrossRef]
116. Gola, M.; Wordecha, M.; Sescousse, G.; Lew-Starowicz, M.; Kossowski, B.; Wypych, M.; Makeig, S.; Potenza, M.N.; Marchewka, A. Can Pornography be Addictive? An fMRI Study of Men Seeking Treatment for Problematic Pornography Use. *Neuropsychopharmacology* **2017**, *42*, 2021–2031. [CrossRef] [PubMed]
117. Schmidt, C.; Morris, L.S.; Kvamme, T.L.; Hall, P.; Birchard, T.; Voon, V. Compulsive sexual behavior: Prefrontal and limbic volume and interactions. *Hum. Brain Mapp.* **2017**, *38*, 1182–1190. [CrossRef] [PubMed]
118. Brand, M.; Snagowski, J.; Laier, C.; Maderwald, S. Ventral striatum activity when watching preferred pornographic pictures is correlated with symptoms of Internet pornography addiction. *Neuroimage* **2016**, *129*, 224–232. [CrossRef] [PubMed]
119. Balodis, I.M.; Potenza, M.N. Anticipatory reward processing in addicted populations: A focus on the monetary incentive delay task. *Biol. Psychiatry* **2015**, *77*, 434–444. [CrossRef] [PubMed]
120. Seok, J.-W.; Sohn, J.-H. Gray matter deficits and altered resting-state connectivity in the superior temporal gyrus among individuals with problematic hypersexual behavior. *Brain Res.* **2018**, *1684*, 30–39. [CrossRef] [PubMed]
121. Taki, Y.; Kinomura, S.; Sato, K.; Goto, R.; Inoue, K.; Okada, K.; Ono, S.; Kawashima, R.; Fukuda, H. Both global gray matter volume and regional gray matter volume negatively correlate with lifetime alcohol intake in non-alcohol-dependent Japanese men: A volumetric analysis and a voxel-based morphometry. *Alcohol. Clin. Exp. Res.* **2006**, *30*, 1045–1050. [CrossRef] [PubMed]
122. Chatzittofis, A.; Arver, S.; Öberg, K.; Hallberg, J.; Nordström, P.; Jokinen, J. HPA axis dysregulation in men with hypersexual disorder. *Psychoneuroendocrinology* **2016**, *63*, 247–253. [CrossRef]

123. Jokinen, J.; Boström, A.E.; Chatzittofis, A.; Ciuculete, D.M.; Öberg, K.G.; Flanagan, J.N.; Arver, S.; Schiöth, H.B. Methylation of HPA axis related genes in men with hypersexual disorder. *Psychoneuroendocrinology* **2017**, *80*, 67–73. [CrossRef]
124. Blum, K.; Werner, T.; Carnes, S.; Carnes, P.; Bowirrat, A.; Giordano, J.; Oscar-Berman, M.; Gold, M. Sex, drugs, and rock "n" roll: Hypothesizing common mesolimbic activation as a function of reward gene polymorphisms. *J. Psychoact. Drugs* **2012**, *44*, 38–55. [CrossRef]
125. Jokinen, J.; Chatzittofis, A.; Nordstrom, P.; Arver, S. The role of neuroinflammation in the pathophysiology of hypersexual disorder. *Psychoneuroendocrinology* **2016**, *71*, 55. [CrossRef]
126. Reid, R.C.; Karim, R.; McCrory, E.; Carpenter, B.N. Self-reported differences on measures of executive function and hypersexual behavior in a patient and community sample of men. *Int. J. Neurosci.* **2010**, *120*, 120–127. [CrossRef] [PubMed]
127. Leppink, E.; Chamberlain, S.; Redden, S.; Grant, J. Problematic sexual behavior in young adults: Associations across clinical, behavioral, and neurocognitive variables. *Psychiatry Res.* **2016**, *246*, 230–235. [CrossRef] [PubMed]
128. Kamaruddin, N.; Rahman, A.W.A.; Handiyani, D. Pornography Addiction Detection based on Neurophysiological Computational Approach. *Indones. J. Electr. Eng. Comput. Sci.* **2018**, *10*, 138–145. [CrossRef]
129. Brand, M.; Laier, C.; Pawlikowski, M.; Schächtle, U.; Schöler, T.; Altstötter-Gleich, C. Watching pornographic pictures on the Internet: Role of sexual arousal ratings and psychological-psychiatric symptoms for using Internet sex sites excessively. *Cyberpsychol. Behav. Soc. Netw.* **2011**, *14*, 371–377. [CrossRef] [PubMed]
130. Laier, C.; Schulte, F.P.; Brand, M. Pornographic picture processing interferes with working memory performance. *J. Sex. Res.* **2013**, *50*, 642–652. [CrossRef] [PubMed]
131. Miner, M.H.; Raymond, N.; Mueller, B.A.; Lloyd, M.; Lim, K.O. Preliminary investigation of the impulsive and neuroanatomical characteristics of compulsive sexual behavior. *Psychiatry Res.* **2009**, *174*, 146–151. [CrossRef] [PubMed]
132. Cheng, W.; Chiou, W.-B. Exposure to Sexual Stimuli Induces Greater Discounting Leading to Increased Involvement in Cyber Delinquency Among Men. *Cyberpsychol. Behav. Soc. Netw.* **2017**, *21*, 99–104. [CrossRef] [PubMed]
133. Messina, B.; Fuentes, D.; Tavares, H.; Abdo, C.H.N.; Scanavino, M.d.T. Executive Functioning of Sexually Compulsive and Non-Sexually Compulsive Men Before and After Watching an Erotic Video. *J. Sex. Med.* **2017**, *14*, 347–354. [CrossRef]
134. Negash, S.; Sheppard, N.V.N.; Lambert, N.M.; Fincham, F.D. Trading Later Rewards for Current Pleasure: Pornography Consumption and Delay Discounting. *J. Sex. Res.* **2016**, *53*, 689–700. [CrossRef]
135. Sirianni, J.M.; Vishwanath, A. Problematic Online Pornography Use: A Media Attendance Perspective. *J. Sex. Res.* **2016**, *53*, 21–34. [CrossRef]
136. Laier, C.; Pawlikowski, M.; Pekal, J.; Schulte, F.P.; Brand, M. Cybersex addiction: Experienced sexual arousal when watching pornography and not real-life sexual contacts makes the difference. *J. Behav. Addict.* **2013**, *2*, 100–107. [CrossRef] [PubMed]
137. Brand, M.; Young, K.S.; Laier, C. Prefrontal control and internet addiction: A theoretical model and review of neuropsychological and neuroimaging findings. *Front. Hum. Neurosci.* **2014**, *8*, 375. [CrossRef]
138. Snagowski, J.; Wegmann, E.; Pekal, J.; Laier, C.; Brand, M. Implicit associations in cybersex addiction: Adaption of an Implicit Association Test with pornographic pictures. *Addict. Behav.* **2015**, *49*, 7–12. [CrossRef]
139. Snagowski, J.; Laier, C.; Duka, T.; Brand, M. Subjective Craving for Pornography and Associative Learning Predict Tendencies Towards Cybersex Addiction in a Sample of Regular Cybersex Users. *Sex. Addict. Compuls.* **2016**, *23*, 342–360. [CrossRef]
140. Walton, M.T.; Cantor, J.M.; Lykins, A.D. An Online Assessment of Personality, Psychological, and Sexuality Trait Variables Associated with Self-Reported Hypersexual Behavior. *Arch. Sex. Behav.* **2017**, *46*, 721–733. [CrossRef]
141. Parsons, J.T.; Kelly, B.C.; Bimbi, D.S.; Muench, F.; Morgenstern, J. Accounting for the social triggers of sexual compulsivity. *J. Addict. Dis.* **2007**, *26*, 5–16. [CrossRef] [PubMed]
142. Laier, C.; Brand, M. Mood changes after watching pornography on the Internet are linked to tendencies towards Internet-pornography-viewing disorder. *Addict. Behav. Rep.* **2017**, *5*, 9–13. [CrossRef]

143. Laier, C.; Brand, M. Empirical Evidence and Theoretical Considerations on Factors Contributing to Cybersex Addiction from a Cognitive-Behavioral View. *Sex. Addict. Compuls.* **2014**, *21*, 305–321. [CrossRef]
144. Antons, S.; Brand, M. Trait and state impulsivity in males with tendency towards Internet-pornography-use disorder. *Addict. Behav.* **2018**, *79*, 171–177. [CrossRef] [PubMed]
145. Egan, V.; Parmar, R. Dirty habits? Online pornography use, personality, obsessionality, and compulsivity. *J. Sex. Marital Ther.* **2013**, *39*, 394–409. [CrossRef] [PubMed]
146. Werner, M.; Štulhofer, A.; Waldorp, L.; Jurin, T. A Network Approach to Hypersexuality: Insights and Clinical Implications. *J. Sex. Med.* **2018**, *15*, 373–386. [CrossRef]
147. Snagowski, J.; Brand, M. Symptoms of cybersex addiction can be linked to both approaching and avoiding pornographic stimuli: Results from an analog sample of regular cybersex users. *Front. Psychol.* **2015**, *6*, 653. [CrossRef]
148. Schiebener, J.; Laier, C.; Brand, M. Getting stuck with pornography? Overuse or neglect of cybersex cues in a multitasking situation is related to symptoms of cybersex addiction. *J. Behav. Addict.* **2015**, *4*, 14–21. [CrossRef] [PubMed]
149. Brem, M.J.; Shorey, R.C.; Anderson, S.; Stuart, G.L. Depression, anxiety, and compulsive sexual behaviour among men in residential treatment for substance use disorders: The role of experiential avoidance. *Clin. Psychol. Psychother.* **2017**, *24*, 1246–1253. [CrossRef] [PubMed]
150. Carnes, P. Sexual addiction screening test. *Tenn. Nurse* **1991**, *54*, 29.
151. Montgomery-Graham, S. Conceptualization and Assessment of Hypersexual Disorder: A Systematic Review of the Literature. *Sex. Med. Rev.* **2017**, *5*, 146–162. [CrossRef] [PubMed]
152. Miner, M.H.; Coleman, E.; Center, B.A.; Ross, M.; Rosser, B.R.S. The compulsive sexual behavior inventory: Psychometric properties. *Arch. Sex. Behav.* **2007**, *36*, 579–587. [CrossRef] [PubMed]
153. Miner, M.H.; Raymond, N.; Coleman, E.; Swinburne Romine, R. Investigating Clinically and Scientifically Useful Cut Points on the Compulsive Sexual Behavior Inventory. *J. Sex. Med.* **2017**, *14*, 715–720. [CrossRef]
154. Öberg, K.G.; Hallberg, J.; Kaldo, V.; Dhejne, C.; Arver, S. Hypersexual Disorder According to the Hypersexual Disorder Screening Inventory in Help-Seeking Swedish Men and Women With Self-Identified Hypersexual Behavior. *Sex. Med.* **2017**, *5*, e229–e236. [CrossRef]
155. Delmonico, D.; Miller, J. The Internet Sex Screening Test: A comparison of sexual compulsives versus non-sexual compulsives. *Sex. Relatsh. Ther.* **2003**, *18*, 261–276. [CrossRef]
156. Ballester Arnal, R.; Gil Llario, M.D.; Gómez Martínez, S.; Gil Juliá, B. Psychometric properties of an instrument for assessing cyber-sex addiction. *Psicothema* **2010**, *22*, 1048–1053.
157. Beutel, M.E.; Giralt, S.; Wölfling, K.; Stöbel-Richter, Y.; Subic-Wrana, C.; Reiner, I.; Tibubos, A.N.; Brähler, E. Prevalence and determinants of online-sex use in the German population. *PLoS ONE* **2017**, *12*, e0176449. [CrossRef] [PubMed]
158. Kor, A.; Zilcha-Mano, S.; Fogel, Y.A.; Mikulincer, M.; Reid, R.C.; Potenza, M.N. Psychometric development of the Problematic Pornography Use Scale. *Addict. Behav.* **2014**, *39*, 861–868. [CrossRef] [PubMed]
159. Wéry, A.; Burnay, J.; Karila, L.; Billieux, J. The Short French Internet Addiction Test Adapted to Online Sexual Activities: Validation and Links With Online Sexual Preferences and Addiction Symptoms. *J. Sex. Res.* **2016**, *53*, 701–710. [CrossRef] [PubMed]
160. Grubbs, J.B.; Volk, F.; Exline, J.J.; Pargament, K.I. Internet pornography use: Perceived addiction, psychological distress, and the validation of a brief measure. *J. Sex. Marital Ther.* **2015**, *41*, 83–106. [CrossRef] [PubMed]
161. Fernandez, D.P.; Tee, E.Y.J.; Fernandez, E.F. Do Cyber Pornography Use Inventory-9 Scores Reflect Actual Compulsivity in Internet Pornography Use? Exploring the Role of Abstinence Effort. *Sex. Addict. Compuls.* **2017**, *24*, 156–179. [CrossRef]
162. Bőthe, B.; Tóth-Király, I.; Zsila, Á.; Griffiths, M.D.; Demetrovics, Z.; Orosz, G. The Development of the Problematic Pornography Consumption Scale (PPCS). *J. Sex. Res.* **2018**, *55*, 395–406. [CrossRef] [PubMed]
163. Griffiths, M. A "Components" Model of Addiction within a Biopsychosocial Framework. *J. Subst. Use* **2009**, *10*, 191–197. [CrossRef]
164. Reid, R.C.; Li, D.S.; Gilliland, R.; Stein, J.A.; Fong, T. Reliability, validity, and psychometric development of the pornography consumption inventory in a sample of hypersexual men. *J. Sex. Marital Ther.* **2011**, *37*, 359–385. [CrossRef]

165. Baltieri, D.A.; Aguiar, A.S.J.; de Oliveira, V.H.; de Souza Gatti, A.L.; de Souza Aranha E Silva, R.A. Validation of the Pornography Consumption Inventory in a Sample of Male Brazilian University Students. *J. Sex. Marital Ther.* **2015**, *41*, 649–660. [CrossRef]
166. Noor, S.W.; Simon Rosser, B.R.; Erickson, D.J. A Brief Scale to Measure Problematic Sexually Explicit Media Consumption: Psychometric Properties of the Compulsive Pornography Consumption (CPC) Scale among Men who have Sex with Men. *Sex. Addict. Compuls.* **2014**, *21*, 240–261. [CrossRef] [PubMed]
167. Kraus, S.; Rosenberg, H. The pornography craving questionnaire: Psychometric properties. *Arch. Sex. Behav.* **2014**, *43*, 451–462. [CrossRef] [PubMed]
168. Kraus, S.W.; Rosenberg, H.; Tompsett, C.J. Assessment of self-efficacy to employ self-initiated pornography use-reduction strategies. *Addict. Behav.* **2015**, *40*, 115–118. [CrossRef] [PubMed]
169. Kraus, S.W.; Rosenberg, H.; Martino, S.; Nich, C.; Potenza, M.N. The development and initial evaluation of the Pornography-Use Avoidance Self-Efficacy Scale. *J. Behav. Addict.* **2017**, *6*, 354–363. [CrossRef] [PubMed]
170. Sniewski, L.; Farvid, P.; Carter, P. The assessment and treatment of adult heterosexual men with self-perceived problematic pornography use: A review. *Addict. Behav.* **2018**, *77*, 217–224. [CrossRef] [PubMed]
171. Gola, M.; Potenza, M.N. Paroxetine Treatment of Problematic Pornography Use: A Case Series. *J. Behav. Addict.* **2016**, *5*, 529–532. [CrossRef] [PubMed]
172. Fong, T.W. Understanding and managing compulsive sexual behaviors. *Psychiatry (Edgmont)* **2006**, *3*, 51–58.
173. Aboujaoude, E.; Salame, W.O. Naltrexone: A Pan-Addiction Treatment? *CNS Drugs* **2016**, *30*, 719–733. [CrossRef]
174. Raymond, N.C.; Grant, J.E.; Coleman, E. Augmentation with naltrexone to treat compulsive sexual behavior: A case series. *Ann. Clin. Psychiatry* **2010**, *22*, 56–62.
175. Kraus, S.W.; Meshberg-Cohen, S.; Martino, S.; Quinones, L.J.; Potenza, M.N. Treatment of Compulsive Pornography Use with Naltrexone: A Case Report. *Am. J. Psychiatry* **2015**, *172*, 1260–1261. [CrossRef]
176. Bostwick, J.M.; Bucci, J.A. Internet sex addiction treated with naltrexone. *Mayo Clin. Proc.* **2008**, *83*, 226–230. [CrossRef]
177. Camacho, M.; Moura, A.R.; Oliveira-Maia, A.J. Compulsive Sexual Behaviors Treated With Naltrexone Monotherapy. *Prim. Care Companion CNS Disord.* **2018**, *20*. [CrossRef] [PubMed]
178. Capurso, N.A. Naltrexone for the treatment of comorbid tobacco and pornography addiction. *Am. J. Addict.* **2017**, *26*, 115–117. [CrossRef] [PubMed]
179. Short, M.B.; Wetterneck, C.T.; Bistricky, S.L.; Shutter, T.; Chase, T.E. Clinicians' Beliefs, Observations, and Treatment Effectiveness Regarding Clients' Sexual Addiction and Internet Pornography Use. *Commun. Ment. Health J.* **2016**, *52*, 1070–1081. [CrossRef] [PubMed]
180. Orzack, M.H.; Voluse, A.C.; Wolf, D.; Hennen, J. An ongoing study of group treatment for men involved in problematic Internet-enabled sexual behavior. *Cyberpsychol. Behav.* **2006**, *9*, 348–360. [CrossRef] [PubMed]
181. Young, K.S. Cognitive behavior therapy with Internet addicts: Treatment outcomes and implications. *Cyberpsychol. Behav.* **2007**, *10*, 671–679. [CrossRef] [PubMed]
182. Hardy, S.A.; Ruchty, J.; Hull, T.; Hyde, R. A Preliminary Study of an Online Psychoeducational Program for Hypersexuality. *Sex. Addict. Compuls.* **2010**, *17*, 247–269. [CrossRef]
183. Crosby, J.M.; Twohig, M.P. Acceptance and Commitment Therapy for Problematic Internet Pornography Use: A Randomized Trial. *Behav. Ther.* **2016**, *47*, 355–366. [CrossRef]
184. Twohig, M.P.; Crosby, J.M. Acceptance and commitment therapy as a treatment for problematic internet pornography viewing. *Behav. Ther.* **2010**, *41*, 285–295. [CrossRef]

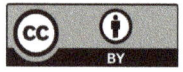

© 2019 by the authors. Licensee MDPI, Basel, Switzerland. This article is an open access article distributed under the terms and conditions of the Creative Commons Attribution (CC BY) license (http://creativecommons.org/licenses/by/4.0/).

MDPI
St. Alban-Anlage 66
4052 Basel
Switzerland
Tel. +41 61 683 77 34
Fax +41 61 302 89 18
www.mdpi.com

Journal of Clinical Medicine Editorial Office
E-mail: jcm@mdpi.com
www.mdpi.com/journal/jcm

www.ingramcontent.com/pod-product-compliance
Lightning Source LLC
LaVergne TN
LVHW070146100526
838202LV00015B/1901